DIABETES
A Guide to Living Well
Updated and Revised 3rd Edition

Ernest Lowe & Gary Arsham, MD, PhD

Foreword by Peter Forsham, MD

CHRONIMED PUBLISHING

Diabetes: A Guide for Living Well © 1997 by
Ernest Lowe and Gary Arsham, MD, PhD

Library of Congress Cataloging-in-Publication Data

Arsham, Gary M.
Diabetes: a guide to living well, third edition

       p.   cm.

Includes bibliographic references and index

ISBN 1-56561-112-8 $14.95

1. Diabetes—Popular works. I. Lowe, Ernest. II.
Title.

RC660.4.A777   1997   616.4'62 88-31040
        CIP

Edited by Brian Jacobson
Editorial Manager: Jeff Braun
Cover Design: Terry Dugan Design
Text Design & Production: David Enyeart
Art/Production Manager: Claire Lewis

Printed in the United States

Published by
Chronimed Publishing
P.O. Box 59032
Minneapolis, MN 55459-0032

10   9   8   7   6   5   4   3   2   1

Notice: Consult a Health Care Professional
Readers are advised to seek the guidance of a
licensed physician or health care professional before
making changes in health care regimens, since each
individual case or need may vary. This book is
intended for informational purposes only and is not
for use as an alternative to appropriate medical care.
While every effort has been made to ensure that the
information is the most current available, new
research findings, being released with increasing frequency, may invalidate some data.

To Diana Silver Arsham and Grace O'Rielly Lowe who could easily write a sequel to this book called *Diabetics: A Guide to Living Well With Them.*

To my parents, Florence and Sanford Arsham and my physician while growing up, Max Miller, who gave me the guidance and freedom to live well.—Gary

To John Menscher and Michael Barricks, whose skilled laser treatment enabled me to keep 20/20 vision.—Ernest

Table of Contents

SECTION VI: WOMEN AND CHILDREN LIVING WELL

Acknowledgments

Many people have made valuable contributions to *Diabetes: A Guide to Living Well*—fellow people with diabetes (patients and friends) and professional colleagues.

We wish to thank Everett Ai, Carol Alston, Robert Barnes, Peter Barrett, Patrick Bean, Ken Burke, Philip R. Calanchini, Larry Catus, Cathy Corum, Leona Dang, Wayne Davis, Joan Enns, Fran Fernandez, Betty Fukuyama, Diana Guthrie, Dwight Holing, Peggy Huang, Larry Hulbert, Chris Kilduff, Barry S. Levin, Maureen McGrath, Nancy Key Nelson, Fran Nereu, Jan Norman, Linda Parker, Sheila Perez, Donna Radcliffe, Vicky Sears, Nanci Stern, Wendy Ullman-Duarte, Helen Wall, Ben and Bonnie Weyhing, Seena Wolf, patients of the Early Treatment Diabetic Retinopathy Study, and the many others who supported our work with their knowledge and experience.

Special thanks go to George Cleveland, formerly of Diabetes Center, Inc., and Caroline Danielson, our editor for the first edition, for helping to bring this book to completion. We are grateful to Donna Hoel and David Wexler of Chronimed Publishing for their assistance and guidance with the second edition, and to Jeff Braun for this third edition.

We are also appreciative of the writing and editorial work for this edition done by Grace Lowe, Ernie's wife. Additionally, she made major contributions to the chapter on Type 2 diabetes, which she has had for 12 years.

Foreword

by Peter Forsham, M.D., Professor of Medicine and
Pediatrics, Emeritus, and former Director, Metabolic
Research Unit, University of California, San Francisco.

Dr. Forsham wrote this for the original edition of
this book, but his insights are just as relevant today
as when he wrote it. Sadly, Dr. Forsham died in
December, 1995, at the age of 80 after 71 years of
diabetes. We miss him, but his legacy, warmth, and
humor live on.

Diabetes: A Guide to Living Well is one of the few books to acknowledge
a difficult fact of life. There are three kinds of people with diabetes: those
who cooperate completely in maintaining a normal blood glucose range;
those who do this part time; and those who never do it. The authors, all
Type 1 diabetics for many years, provide guidance appropriate to all three
groups.

This book covers all the modern ways of maintaining a normal blood
sugar level (not usually exceeding 130 mg/dl or 7.2 mmol/L*) and intro-
duces in a philosophical way the persuasive reasons for doing this. At the
same time, the authors support the individual's right to choose his or her
level of self-care, and they recognize that many choose a level far below
the standard now attainable. Their unique contribution is to offer alternative strategies for increasing the reader's willingness to follow regimens
valuable in diabetes management. Throughout, the hope is expressed that
through lifelong learning and adequate teaching by his or her medical
team, the reader will become increasingly wise.

The authors write from a powerful combination of personal and professional experience. Not only have they lived with diabetes for many
years, but they've also surveyed advanced research in diabetes and medical education to uncover the most effective techniques for improving self-
care and adherence to reasonable regimens. They dismiss ignorant old

---

*Outside the U.S., blood glucose is often measured in millimols per liter
  (mmol/L).

beliefs, some harking back to the days before insulin, when people with diabetes were absolutely forbidden sugar and were told to stay in a mild state of ketoacidosis to survive. Unfortunately, such misinformation from the past still fills some diabetes texts. This book makes little of the old prejudices, introducing instead the latest concepts in treatment of diabetes.

Beginning with tips on mastering the challenge of learning a complex regimen, the book is an operating manual for the individual who wishes to maintain the best possible level of diabetic control. It wisely charts alternative paths for those prepared to quickly gain this goal and those who prefer to move more gradually.

The authors accept the concept that hyperglycemia (or high blood sugar levels) is what I once called toxic. Today we know that the prevention of general vascular disease in people with diabetes is a function of the control of blood glucose, cholesterol, and fat levels in the blood. This is an essential component in the reduction of the risk of diabetic complications involving the eyes, kidneys, nerves, and circulatory system. This *Guide to Living Well* imparts knowledge enabling the reader to manage fat intake on the one hand and to prevent hyperglycemia on the other.

The crowning achievement of this book, however, is its full synthesis of all factors affecting blood sugar level. On the deficit side, mental instability, stress, lack of exercise or rest, and dietary excess, each through different mechanisms, raise the blood sugar level and accelerate the degenerative processes of diabetes. But when a person with diabetes assumes a regimen integrating mental balance, stress management, dietary moderation, and exercise, he or she is reducing long-term risks and ensuring more immediate well-being.

The authors realistically offer routes to this ideal of self-management suited to a broad range of personalities, not just those immediately capable of strong discipline.

In the 1860s, Claude Bernard observed that the condition for a free existence is the constancy of the internal environment. Now people with diabetes can hope to approach this metabolic constancy by controlling the multiple factors that are abnormal in the average patient. This aim is deeply supported by this very practical yet highly philosophical newcomer to the diabetes information scene.

Preface

We wrote *Diabetes: A Guide to Living Well* to give you (1) a command of one of medicine's most demanding regimens; (2) mastery over the threats diabetes presents; and (3) strength to meet its emotional challenges. Throughout the book, we encourage you to choose a regimen individualized to your personal needs and preferences. Most important, we present strategies empowering you to follow the regimen you choose. We wrote this book so you can learn to live well with diabetes.

This third edition not only incorporates the good news from the Diabetes Control and Complications Trial—that blood sugar control reduces complications—but also adds much more about the management of Type 2 (noninsulin-dependent) diabetes. New and improved, user-friendly blood sugar meters and insulin delivery devices have appeared, and there are many new oral medications for Type 2 diabetes. These drugs work differently than sulfonylurea medications, and provide new tools to help manage diabetes. They help make it easier (not easy) for those with Type 2 diabetes to achieve an excellent level of control, often without the need for insulin. Furthermore, the new American Diabetes Association nutrition guidelines are also incorporated in this edition. (Actually, this book foreshadowed these recommendations, even in its first edition.)

The Living Well approach is based on the dual experience each of us brings to the book. We know diabetes professionally and personally. (Your writing team has logged over 120 years of living with diabetes!) We temper medical experts' views with first-hand knowledge of the challenges, threats, and gifts of diabetes.

The basic diabetes lifestyle is a thorough program with strong unity. Control of blood sugar levels is important in avoiding short-term problems, in maintaining a feeling of well-being, and in reducing your risk of long-term diabetic complications. Blood sugar control, along with an active life, balanced diet, and effective stress management, work together to reduce your risk of complications. Emotional balance and self-esteem contribute to stress management and aid you in following your self-care program. Remembering this unity is central to the Living Well approach.

While we devote many pages to the question of blood glucose control, we emphasize throughout the book that you live well by balancing metabolic control with all other aspects of your lifestyle. When you do this, you integrate diabetes into your life and keep it from dominating you.

Individual choice is central to the Living Well approach and can easily be applied while using this book. It is not necessarily a book to be read from front to back. You know better than anyone else what you need to learn first. We encourage you to follow your own sense of priorities.

You may have much to learn, many skills to gain, and behaviors to change as you adopt the Living Well approach, especially if you are new to diabetes. Throughout this book, you will find ideas for making this process of learning and changing easier to handle. You will also find many techniques for increasing your willingness to follow this life-enhancing and demanding self-care regimen.

Ingredients of the Living Well With Diabetes Lifestyle

▷ Find a balance between meeting your needs as someone with diabetes and the other needs in your life. Chapters 1 and 4 offer guidance on striking this balance.

▷ Know how to avoid the acute, life-threatening crises of diabetes. We have highlighted basic life-saving guidelines at the back of this book. Chapter 9 contains a thorough discussion of low blood sugar and insulin reactions.

▷ Know the measures you can take to reduce the risk of developing diabetic complications. Preventive measures are discussed in Chapters 16 and 18.

▷ Maintain the best control of blood glucose levels you can achieve without damaging the quality of your life. Chapters 4 through 8 offer a choice of regimens and instructions for each.

▷ Meet your emotional needs, not just your physical needs. Chapter 15 presents a variety of techniques for maintaining emotional well-being. Chapter 3 describes techniques for dealing with crisis.

▷ Manage stress effectively. Chapter 12 describes the impact of stress on diabetes and techniques for coping with it.

▷ Maintain an active lifestyle, adjusted to your physical condition. Chapter 11 explores the role of physical activity in diabetes management.

▷ Follow a balanced and moderate meal plan. Chapter 10 gives tips on making your food choices delicious as well as healthy.

▷ Work to increase your willingness to follow this lifestyle, and continue learning about it. Chapter 1 surveys actions and beliefs that support continuing adherence to the self-care program you choose. Chapter 3 includes techniques to help you handle the times when you want to rebel.

A Fundamental Guideline to Using This Book

Diabetes is a condition requiring a balance between your own day-to-day decision making in self-care and your doctor's guidance on basic regimen decisions. We include detailed information on three regimens so you can work with your physician and diabetes educator in making decisions about insulin dosage; overall balance between medications, food choices, and physical activity; or treatment of acute problems like ketoacidosis or serious infections. In no way do we encourage you to make these fundamental medical decisions on your own.

In writing this book, we have deepened our own capacity for living well with diabetes. We hope reading it helps you do the same.

Gary Arsham

Ernest Lowe

To The Physician and Other Health Care Team Members

Diabetes: A Guide to Living Well is intended to help your patient to not only live well with diabetes, but also to be a better, more informed, more responsible patient. As you know, with a chronic illness like diabetes, what patients do outside your office is critical to their medical care. You can recommend, monitor, guide, encourage, and exhort, but it is your patient who does or does not follow what you and your patient agree is an appropriate regimen.

This book provides considerable information that should make your patient much more informed and motivated to work with you and other members of the health care team. It encourages the patient to examine the options available, consider the risks and benefits as we understand them today, and, in collaboration with you, choose a level of diabetes management and control that fits the individual situation. We hope this book will help your patient and also make your tasks more satisfying and rewarding.

To Increase Your Chances for a Longer, More Healthful Life

Living well with diabetes means preserving your health and vitality and reducing your risk of developing future diabetic complications. Improving blood sugar control is just one of the things you can do to achieve these goals. The complete Living Well lifestyle asks you to

▷ Improve your control of blood glucose and continue improving it to the best level you are comfortable with (Chapters 4-8).

▷ Learn to handle stress well (Chapter 12).

▷ Follow a meal plan that features overall moderation and low animal fat and high fiber (Chapter 10).

▷ Engage in physical activity regularly (Chapter 11).

▷ Lose weight if you are overweight.

▷ Act to prevent high blood pressure by controlling stress, weight, and salt consumption. Seek treatment for hypertension if your blood pressure is high (above 130/85) (Chapter 18, hypertension section).

▷ Get the amount of sleep and rest you need.

▷ Know the warning signs for each complication. Begin treatment early if symptoms appear (Chapter 18).

▷ Consider taking a multivitamin pill daily. Consider taking one aspirin (enteric coated or plain) every day or every other day to help avoid heart attacks, stroke, and blood clots.

These preventive measures are discussed in detail in Chapter 18. You should also skim through that chapter to find the sections describing what you can do to prevent individual complications.

Introduction

"Nobody asked me if I wanted to have diabetes. I just started feeling lousy, losing weight, and getting thirsty. And there I was—diabetic. I thought my life was ruined. But then I said, 'No, dammit! This may not go away, but I'm going to call the shots. My life is more than a defective pancreas.'" —John, 45 years old, twenty-five years diabetic

"The anger, the frustration, and all of these feelings aren't going to take the diabetes away. You have to find a level ground and decide, 'Okay, this is the way I am now and I'd better learn what I'm supposed to do and what I'm not supposed to do and live with it, because that's the way it's going to be.'" —Norma, 58 years old (In *Focus on Feelings,* from Pyramid Films)

This book is about options and personal choices. We can choose how to live with diabetes. We can't decide not to have it, but we can decide to live a full and satisfying life, rejecting all images of ourselves as ill or disabled. No matter what our physical condition, we can choose to live well. The act of choosing becomes the foundation of our ability to manage diabetes effectively.

Living well depends less on how we care for our diabetes than on how we care for ourselves. Each of us has a pattern of living that includes our individual needs, style, abilities, and physical characteristics. The diabetic regimen we choose will work only if it fits this pattern. We cannot make decisions about diabetes care as if diabetes is the only thing we have to consider in life.

For this reason, the authors of *Diabetes: A Guide to Living Well*—both with insulin-dependent diabetes—emphasize the need to select a self-care program, in conjunction with your physician and health care team, that will work for you as an individual. We encourage you to read this book in whatever order feels right to you. Work on the subjects that interest you the most. Find the level of regimen you can follow comfortably. Work to find a healthy balance between quality of life and care of diabetes. When you exercise this freedom of choice, you are likely to arrive at a program you can live with.

Throughout this book is advice on how you can build willingness to follow the regimen you choose with information on the physical and emotional care of diabetes. In the last decade, dramatic improvements have been made in diabetes care, changes that have made the state-of-the-art regimen more complex. Taking full advantage of these breakthroughs may require you to pay attention to the feelings, beliefs, and patterns of behavior that sometimes divide your will.

Living well with diabetes is easier if you are willing to continually learn about the rapid changes in diabetes management. There are many new skills to be learned and behaviors often need changing as information is updated. We have included hints and strategies in the book to make the learning process easier.

Which Regimen?

If you select anything less than the strictest regimen, you may feel guilt, anxiety, or conflict for making a "bad" choice. These feelings are important to consider in your decision-making process. You must accept your level of care, or the quality of your life will suffer from the conflict you feel. Once you understand the risks and benefits of the different options you can make an informed decision. You need to accept your decision, and realize that it is the best one for you.

Of course, we want to be certain that what we do to take care of ourselves will actually work. However, we have very little certainty at this point. What we do know is that excellent diabetic control reduces the risk of complications. A large percentage of us who maintain good control will escape blindness, kidney disease, and nerve damage. But any one of us can do everything possible to control our diabetes and still experience some degree of disability because of the disease.

Living well with diabetes requires accepting uncertainty, and staying motivated despite this uncertainty. This is such a central issue that we ask you to explore your reactions to it in this questionnaire.

Questionnaire: A Certain Uncertainty

1. As you read the last three paragraphs, how did you feel?
2. How do you handle uncertainties in areas of your life outside diabetes?
3. What attitudes or beliefs could you adopt that would help you deal with the uncertainties that diabetes imposes on your future?
4. What do you think would help motivate you to follow your diabetes management program, even though you have no guarantee that the program will prevent complications?

There are no simple formulas for handling these questions. However, it is dangerous to avoid them. Negative reactions to uncertainty range from abandoning all efforts to manage diabetes to caring for it so compulsively that life holds little joy. Clearly, managing diabetes is a matter of balance—doing your best to live a rewarding life, without dwelling on possible future misfortunes.

One way of neutralizing uncertainty about the future is to make the present rewarding. Learn to accept each moment as a source of benefit, no matter what happens. This way, you are prepared for whatever the future may bring. How do you learn such a profound lesson? Perhaps diabetes itself is the teacher.

Because we believe that diabetes is a teacher about living, we have chosen to make this book more than a manual on testing blood, taking shots, and balancing rutabagas against radishes. Having diabetes is a challenge, a burden, a transformation, and a blessing. So let's accept it as a gracious gift and let it teach us to live our years well.

Section One
Learning To Live Well

Chapter One

Willing To Live Well

Although a cure for diabetes is probably many years away, fundamental breakthroughs in diabetes care have been made in recent years. These breakthroughs include

▷ Home blood glucose tests that give immediate and accurate feed-back on your blood sugar levels whenever you need it.

▷ New insulins and oral drugs (primarily for Type 2 diabetes) that enable you to maintain better control of blood sugar.

▷ Better information about the steps you can take to reduce the risk of developing diabetic complications, including promising new drugs.

▷ Improved treatments for complications, which have allowed thousands of people to save their vision, avoid impotence, survive kidney disease, and reduce the effects of heart disease.

▷ Greater awareness of the emotional and behavioral implications of diabetes.

▷ New knowledge about nutrition and diet.

▷ Recognition of diabetes education as a lifelong learning experience.

These are significant improvements that may enable you to normalize levels of blood sugar, blood fats, cholesterol, and hormones. Also, there is now proof that controlling blood sugar levels and other aspects of body chemistry greatly reduces the risk of developing diabetic complications. The Diabetes Control and Complications Trial (DCCT) showed that people with Type 1 diabetes (insulin-dependent) can reduce the risk of complications up to 70% by maintaining good blood sugar control. It is believed, though not yet proven, that the same is true for those with Type 2 (non-insulin-dependent) diabetes. Preliminary studies support this, and larger studies are underway to test this hypothesis further.

The highest available level of diabetic self-care may enable you to keep blood sugar levels close to normal. Achieving this requires that you learn and follow the most demanding regimen medicine can offer (what we and others call the Intensive Regimen). The DCCT also showed that there is a direct relationship between the level of blood sugar control and the risk of complications. In other words, every bit of improvement makes a difference, so don't be discouraged if your efforts are not always as successful as you would like. More modest levels of control still call for education and the willingness to use what you learn.

Learning To Do What You Choose To Do

It is likely that you will have to change some of your behaviors. Research has shown that individuals usually progress through five stages when they make major changes in behavior: precontemplation, contemplation, preparation, action, and maintenance. Determining where you are in the process can help you make realistic plans for change, so we'll briefly outline these stages. (For further information, see the book *Changing for Good* by James O. Prochaska [William Morrow, 1994]. The book focuses on addictive behaviors related to smoking, eating, and alcohol because most research concerns them, but the stages apply to any type of difficult-to-change behaviors.)

Precontemplation is the stage during which there is no intention to change behavior in the foreseeable future (e.g., six months). At this stage, we do not even acknowledge a problem or a need to change.

Contemplation is the stage where we are aware of a behavior we want to change and are seriously considering it, but have not yet made a commitment to act. This stage can last a long time (knowing where we want to go but not quite ready to get started).

The preparation stage combines intention to act with some initial steps (e.g., preparing a daily log sheet, buying a home blood glucose meter).

The action stage is where the change occurs. It takes a considerable commitment of time, energy, and effort.

Finally, maintenance is the stage where the individual works to prevent returning to old behaviors and incorporate the changes into their everyday life.

Most of us don't move in a straight line through these stages, rather, we spiral back into a preceding stage or stages, each spiral getting us further along until we are successful in the maintenance stage.

It's important to recognize where you are in these stages so you can be realistic about your expectations and not berate yourself if progress is slower or less direct than you would like. The items on the list below will help you focus on the change processes needed to move through the stages.

If you have had diabetes for some time, some items on this list are probably a part of your life already. Adding others can make living with diabetes much easier for you. Check off the ones you already practice and note those you would like to add. Later, if you encounter difficulties, it might help to see if something from this list offers a solution.

1. Believe that treatment for diabetes is effective. If you doubt this, try to understand the basis for your doubt.
2. Recognize that diabetes is a serious condition worth your attention, even if you have few symptoms at present.
3. Balance seriousness with lightheartedness, humor, and detachment.
4. Believe that you are capable of learning and following any regimen you choose.
5. Recognize that you are the one who chooses how you will care for yourself. Make your decisions thoughtfully.
6. Make decisions about diabetes self-care with your other life needs in mind. Don't neglect other important aspects of your life or the overall quality of your life.
7. When choosing how you will care for yourself, find a balance between your preferences and needs.
8. Monitor your stress levels as you work on diabetes care. Use stress-management tools to prevent your regimen from becoming an additional source of stress.

9. Offer yourself healthful rewards for both your efforts and achievements. Recognize that feeling better is itself a reward for improved self-care.
10. Define the tasks required by the regimen you choose. Divide the tasks and the behavioral changes into small, concrete steps. Set goals so you understand clearly what will demonstrate your success. Create a realistic schedule for the learning or change.
11. Explore possible difficulties you may encounter in the process of change. Plan ways of dealing with them in advance.
12. Make a commitment to changing your behavior and learning the skills and information you need.
13. When you feel reluctant to make a particular change, try it for a short time and see how it affects your life.
14. Give yourself positive feedback as you learn, and support yourself when you have difficulty learning. Don't cling to feelings of guilt or failure.
15. When obstacles arise, deal with them and learn from your experience.
16. Evaluate your efforts and achievements, without self-condemnation.

We will briefly discuss each of these 16 factors affecting your self-care program. Why are they important? What is it that makes them relevant?

1. Believe that treatment for diabetes is effective. If you doubt this, try to understand the basis for your doubt.

If you don't believe treatment will improve your health, you will have difficulty managing any regimen. This issue becomes complex with diabetes. As we have said, there is no guarantee that even the best self-care will prevent long-term complications. Effective treatment improves your odds, but you cannot eliminate the risk of developing complications.

However, when you increase your level of blood sugar control, you get a short-term demonstration of effectiveness: You feel better, both mentally and physically. Every measure of control helps, as the DCCT proved.

Gary's Experience
"As my control improves, I feel leaner and healthier. I'm less sluggish, as though my blood has become less viscous with the reduction of excess sugar. I sleep better because I don't have to get up two or three times a night to go to the bathroom. Now, I can recognize much sooner when my blood sugar may be too high, I test to confirm, and can quickly correct it.

I was concerned that I might become preoccupied with diabetes as I tightened up my control. Actually, I find I can be less aware of it because there are fewer symptoms of high blood sugar to remind me."

If you choose loose control, you might still experience the short-term disadvantages of high blood sugar, depending on how high your tests are. But there is a level of effectiveness even here. By maintaining a limited regimen and remaining committed to learning more from it, you keep a positive attitude. You will be in a better position to improve physical control, if and when you choose to do so.

2. Recognize that diabetes is a serious condition worth your attention, even if you have few symptoms at present.

When you exercise a moderate degree of control, you might experience few symptoms of diabetes. Even when blood sugar levels are high, it is possible to become accustomed to short-term symptoms such as thirst, frequent urination, sluggishness, and susceptibility to infection and illness.

Unless complications develop, you might not understand the seriousness of diabetes through your experience with it. Unlike people with arthritis, for instance, you have few immediate and painful reminders. You have to create your own way of remembering that diabetes is an important part of your life.

Respecting Diabetes

Writing down your thoughts can help you define the significance of diabetes in your life. Answer the questions spontaneously, even if the ideas that first come to mind seem inappropriate.

1. What aspects of diabetes make it a serious condition that could have a major impact on your life?
2. Do you ever feel you have no future because of diabetes?
3. Do you avoid looking at problems and difficulties that arise because of your diabetes?
4. Do you sometimes take diabetes too seriously? If so, how?
5. Do you have any doubts about the seriousness of diabetes? If so, see Chapter 18, where complications are described.

3. Balance seriousness with lightheartedness, humor, and detachment.

Diabetes is a lifelong companion, so you might as well make it an agreeable one, threats and all.

You can invoke lightheartedness and humor when dealing with your situation. Speak as though you are referring to another person, someone you are fond of and find gently amusing. You might even try telling your story to the person in the mirror. Or visualize yourself and your dilemmas from a time when you have long since resolved them. Note the clever ways you avoided seeing the obvious solutions back then.

Detachment is not indifference, but rather a viewing of yourself and the problems you face from a larger perspective. From this point of view, you are not attached to the feelings and beliefs that often trap you. You experience and acknowledge them, but you realize that you are more than these limitations, utilizing your resources to break them.

Humor is a powerful way of breaking attachments. When you can laugh at habitual behavior, you feel less controlled by it.

4. Believe that you are capable of learning and following any regimen you choose.

Feeling competent comes naturally to some; however, many people learn to doubt that they can do what they set out to do. Whether your doubts stem from feeling you are dumb, weak, or stuck for life, they are aspects of self-image that you can unlearn. Diabetes can make us feel dumb, despite our ability to learn about or change other areas of our lives. This was especially true before the recent breakthroughs in self-care.

Ernest's Experience

"Out of 48 years of living with diabetes, I spent 30 of them trying to get it under control. I thought I knew what I needed to do, but actually doing it seemed harder than climbing Mount Everest. For one thing, I didn't feel I could ask my doctor for help. That meant I'd have to tell him how out of control I was! I always tried to look like a good patient.

So, I'd study my 1954 *Joslin's Diabetes Manual*. I'd measure the food I ate, pee in the test tube, get more and more uptight. Nothing made any sense to me. I couldn't predict when I would or would not spill sugar. An incredible sense of frustration and failure came with that stinking orange color foaming up at me in the test tube!

Of course, I always felt that I'd done something wrong, no matter how hard tried. No one had ever mentioned that stress affects blood sugar levels strongly, or that urine tests are very imprecise, or that one shot a day of intermediate insulin couldn't possibly prevent large ups and downs in blood sugar levels.

In short, I didn't know that I was in a double bind, being expected to do something but not having the tools necessary to do it. It was like being asked to build a house with bent nails and a hammer without a handle and feeling incompetent because the task seemed impossible."

Today the diabetes tool kit is full of new tools for both physical and psychological self-care, however, diabetes is still not easy to control. If you choose to work toward the highest level of control, your ability to learn and change behavior will be challenged. And even with the best effort, a moderate level of control is the best that can be achieved in some cases due to hormonal factors or high stress levels.

Whenever you achieve less than your goal, don't label yourself a failure. Give yourself credit for what you have achieved, and look to see what you still have to learn or change to reach your goal. (This may be something other than what you set out to learn.) With this point of view, you learn from experience, and you continue to believe in your capacity to learn. (Chapter 15 contains ideas on freeing yourself from the limits described here.)

5. Recognize that you are the one who chooses how you will care for yourself. Make your decisions thoughtfully.

Your doctor, nurse, dietitian, social worker, or diabetes educator cannot make the actual choices for you. Only you can make them. You are the only one who can manage the prescriptions, recommendations, and external pressures in your life.

It can be difficult to accept the responsibility of making choices, especially when the choices conflict with professional recommendations. You may find yourself saying, "I don't have time to do all this testing," or "The cafeteria doesn't have the right kind of food for my diet," or "It's too much hassle to test my blood when I'm at work," or "I carry enough stuff around with me already."

If you make your choices consciously and accept them, you gain power. ("I prefer to sleep an extra few minutes rather than get up to test," or "I don't want to bother fixing a bag lunch.") You also make clear to yourself what the alternatives are, and you may find it easier to make more healthful decisions.

As we said in the beginning of this book, the realization of your power to choose all aspects of your regimen is fundamental to your following it. Your life is under your control; you make the important decisions. If you rebel against your own authority, learning to stop becomes one more item on your learning agenda.

Your medical team can do more than recommend a self-care program. They can help you understand the alternatives available to you, and work with you to identify and overcome barriers you encounter. Don't be afraid to say, "That's going to be hard for me to do because..." In fact, they'll appreciate it.

6. Make decisions about diabetes self-care with your other life needs in mind. Don't neglect other important aspects of your life or the overall quality of your life.

Health professionals often place top priority on your diabetes care and may forget that you have other concerns. Diabetes sometimes demands that you deal with it before all else. However, most of the time you need to balance your diabetes with a host of other issues. If you don't, you

	Specific Need	Actions Called For
Diabetes Care		
Family		
Leisure		
Other Issues		
Education and Intellectual Growth		
Spiritual Concerns		

might run into difficulties concerning other areas of your life. Use the table below to catalog your needs and priorities.

In the table, list important needs in the areas on the left, then use the other categories to help you rank them according to the amount of attention they demand from you.

If this exercise suggests that you have enough concerns to keep an army busy, don't despair. See what can possibly be postponed or dealt with gradually. Dedicate at least a few minutes each day to improving your diabetes care, even if it's a couple of minutes spent planning your next steps. In a month or two, set a date to review your priorities.

Several needs can often be satisfied by a single activity. Dancing or sports, for instance, can help you improve metabolic control while providing enjoyment and social interaction. Better relations with your spouse and mutual support concerning diabetes issues could both be served by participation in a support group or communications workshop. When you find connections between your different needs, you won't have to spend as much time dealing with them individually.

Difficulty	Urgency	Rank

7. When choosing how you will care for yourself,
find a balance between your preferences and needs.

You can't ignore your feelings, but you can't let them dictate your decisions about self-care. The best choices come out of an inner dialogue between your emotional and rational sides, with help from intuition. This dialogue may happen spontaneously, or you may need something to guide your decision making.

One way of opening this inner dialogue is to write it out, taking into account both emotion and logic.

8. Monitor your stress levels as you work on diabetes
care. Use stress-management tools to prevent your
regimen from becoming an additional source of stress.

Learning diabetes care can cause blood sugar levels to increase due to the stress involved. It is important for you to work on diabetes management with an awareness of stress. Let your body remind you when it's time to slow down and relax. (Chapter 12 contains many techniques for dealing with stress.)

9. Offer yourself healthful rewards for both your efforts and achievements.
Recognize that feeling better is itself a reward for improved self-care.

Rewards are an important part of diabetes care because our condition can deprive us of certain pleasures. People often reward themselves with sweets or extra food, but for people with diabetes, this can be a penalty, rather than a prize. You may benefit from creating a positive reward system to offset possible feelings of deprivation.

As you work on learning and changing behavior, rewards help reinforce the effort you make and the changes you achieve. The most substantial rewards come from feeling better physically, and feeling more powerful mentally. There is also evidence that additional bonuses help keep motivation high.

Take a few minutes to write down a variety of rewards you would appreciate, such as gifts, good times, experiences, or even things it would be nice not to do. At the start of a diabetes learning project, promise yourself one reward for effort after a certain period, and another reward when you have successfully completed the learning project.

You May Have Already Won...

1. Gifts I can give myself:

_____

_____

2. Celebrations and other good times I'd enjoy:

_____

_____

3. New experiences I would value:

_____

_____

4. Some things I'd like not to have to do:

_____

_____

---

10. Define the tasks required by the regimen you choose.

Divide the tasks and the behavior changes into small, concrete steps. Set goals so you understand clearly what will demonstrate your success. Create a realistic schedule for the learning or change.

It may seem that learning to manage diabetes is a full-time job. That's why this item is so important. When you divide a large project into small steps and schedule progress over a realistic period, the project becomes more manageable. Make the first step an easy one. No matter how much urgency you may feel, you simply cannot learn it all in one day. Once you have mastered the basic survival skills such as detecting and treating reactions, administering your shot or other medications, and dealing with infections and illness, you can proceed with learning and making changes at a gradual pace.

By setting reasonable and specific goals, you give yourself a much better chance of experiencing success. If you have had very poor control, saying "I'll get my diabetes under control sometime" is too vague. Aiming to achieve an average blood test of 180 mg/dl or 10 mmol/L in one month's time will give you a manageable target, and you will clearly know whether you have attained it. Be sure to set intermediate goals as well, so you can measure progress toward your ultimate goals.

11. Explore possible difficulties you may encounter in the process of change. Plan ways of dealing with them in advance.

You may be one of the blessed who never have trouble doing anything. However, most of us experience some difficulty when making changes. You probably know what troubles you've had in the past, and you have dealt with them. By making some notes at the beginning, you will be able to draw on more creativity than you usually have available when you encounter problems.

Trouble Spots

In the past, I have had trouble learning or following a diabetes regimen because

_____

_____

I have run into trouble in areas other than diabetes because

_____

_____

I have moved (or could move) through the difficulty by

_____

_____

12. Make a commitment to changing your behavior and learning the skills and information you need.

For some people, commitment falls into place easily, without being formalized. But others like to state their intentions in a way that helps them strengthen their will to change, in some cases by making a contract with themselves. If this appeals to you, you can use the following form.

A Contract with Myself

I commit myself to changing this behavior or learning this aspect of diabetes care (be as specific as possible):

_____

_____

I believe this will improve my diabetes self-care by

_____

_____

I believe I am capable of doing this, although I may need assistance in the form of

_____

_____

If I experience difficulties in completing this task, I will use the help processes in Chapter 3 to help me overcome them.

I will learn from the whole experience—setbacks as well as achievements.

(Optional)

I will receive the following reward for effort by (specific date) _____

I will receive the following reward for achievement upon completion

_____

_____

If I do not fulfill this contract I will (specify penalty)

_____

_____

I can reasonably expect to complete this by _____

Signature

_____

Date

_____

13. When you feel reluctant to make a particular change, try it for a short time and see how it affects your life.

Some alterations in lifestyle suggested by diabetes may arouse resistance in you. When this happens, it helps to remember that we often exaggerate the consequences of changes we don't want to make. In our minds, we see only the negative, and blow it up to monumental proportions.

If you do this, you can suspend negative expectations and do a trial run. For instance, test your blood sugar four times a day for a few days, if that's what you're resisting. Make no commitment beyond this period. Then contrast what you actually experience with your prior expectations. Whatever the specific change is, you are likely to find that it's not as bad as you thought it would be.

If you still have trouble beginning, break the task down into smaller steps and try just the first step for a while, then try the second, and so forth.

14. Give yourself positive feedback as you learn, and support yourself when you have difficulty learning. Don't cling to feelings of guilt or failure.

Having diabetes is an emotional strain. Don't make it a greater burden by telling yourself you are a "bad" diabetic. Improve your willingness to manage diabetes well by accepting yourself when you have trouble learning about or following a regimen.

As you learn, acknowledge the improvements, changes, and efforts you make. Don't ignore your mistakes; observe them without blame. They are simply areas requiring further attention. (Chapter 15 includes ideas for supporting yourself and dealing with guilt.)

15. When obstacles arise, deal with them and learn from your experience.

Treat obstacles that you can't seem to overcome as new learning assignments. For example, if you have started to learn home blood testing but are afraid to prick your finger, then your new assignment is to learn to deal with fear, physical discomfort, and negative expectations.

Perhaps the obstacle is total resistance to learning about diabetic complications. Maybe you break into a cold sweat every time you think of the subject. In this case, recognize the opportunity to learn about your feelings of vulnerability or mortality. Before—and probably while—studying complications, you need to work with these emotions. Perhaps you could enlist a friend or relative to help. Other people with diabetes who have dealt with these issues can also give valuable support.

16. Evaluate your efforts and achievements without self-condemnation.

Each time you complete an aspect of your diabetes learning program, take a moment to evaluate your work in a nonjudgmental manner. Look at both how you worked on it and what you accomplished. Give yourself credit for what you have achieved, even when you have not yet reached your final goal. Be honest about the shortcomings of your work, but don't view the shortcomings as a sign of weakness.

The process of evaluation is important in learning to manage diabetes well. Our condition demands a great deal from us. There are many variables affecting diabetic control. Sometimes we can make the best possible effort and still find blood sugar levels outside the limits we try to maintain. It is important not to add negative judgment to the frustration we naturally feel. If we are to continue learning, we must congratulate ourselves for our accomplishments and determine how to improve our diabetes management even further.

Chapter Two

Living Well
At The Beginning
of Diabetes

> "I really felt sorry for myself [when I found out I had diabetes]. I still want to know 'Why me?' I never did anything to deserve this. Why all of a sudden do I have to stick to a diet and take shots for the rest of my life?" —Carol, 17 years old (In *Focus on Feelings*, Pyramid Films)

If you have recently discovered that you have diabetes, take a deep breath, sigh, and relax for a moment. You are going through a crisis. You may be handling the challenges of this time well, or you may feel overwhelmed by them. In either case, it is a demanding situation, and you need all the breaks you can get.

When you first learn you have diabetes, there are three basic demands to handle:

1. Practical tasks. You must learn new skills, absorb new information, make decisions you previously did not have to make, and change aspects of the way you live.

2. Emotional tasks. You need to deal with the emotional impact of being told that you have a lifelong chronic disease that as yet has no cure.

3. Support tasks. You need to mobilize internal and external sources of support.

You may find yourself trying to meet all three needs at the same time, as well as dealing with the other needs in your life. It is very easy to feel overwhelmed in this initial period, so remember that you can't do everything at once. Set priorities with the help of your doctor and medical team.

Practical Tasks

The practical demands of diabetes begin long before you feel ready for them. If you have been in the hospital to get your system under control, you know that you cannot be a passive patient. Your life depends on learning a great amount of information very quickly, especially if you have Type 1 (insulin-dependent) diabetes. Your learning may create anxiety, since it is difficult to understand initially which information is of life-or-death importance. You are still dealing with the emotional shock of the diagnosis, as well as the physical stress of uncontrolled diabetes, so your mind may be functioning with less clarity than usual.

This is an excellent time to learn a fundamental lesson of diabetes education: When you don't understand something or when you feel overloaded with information, tell your doctor or diabetes educator. Ask for an explanation or clarification. Don't just nod your head so the doctor won't think you are stupid. Some health professionals are very good communicators, but others don't notice if you are suffering from information overload.

Sometimes your physician will involve other health professionals. In this case, your basic care will be supervised by the doctor, but the specific educational aspects will be handled by a nurse, dietitian or diabetes educator.

Acute Versus Chronic Health Care

In the past, people diagnosed with Type 1 diabetes were usually hospitalized to get their blood sugar under control. Now, however, this process is often accomplished through office visits and phone contact for both Type 1 and Type 2 (non-insulin dependent) diabetes, assuming the initial symptoms are not too extreme. In either case, you will experience a combination of acute and chronic medical care. Acute care occurs when a doctor deals with a short-term illness or some other emergency. A patient in this situation usually has little involvement other than following a few instructions. When you are diagnosed with diabetes your physician has to quickly restore order to an uncontrolled condition.

However, your doctor and other health professionals also initiate you to a different type of treatment: chronic medical self-care. This involves extensive training that teaches you to take care of yourself for the rest of your life. Within a few years, you might know as much about diabetes as your health professionals. They are there to assist you in this process and take charge when an acute crisis (such as diabetic coma) occurs, however, you are the one who is responsible for your day-to-day care.

Your Treatment Program

Being in charge of your diabetes care may seem to be an enormous responsibility at first, but millions of people with diabetes deal with it and live well every year. Your medical team will provide a lot of support, so you can always get help when you can't figure out what to do. If you consult others with diabetes about the simple questions that arise, you can avoid feeling that you are bothering your medical team with too many questions.

If you feel able to meet the challenge, there are strong arguments for adopting an intensive treatment program from the beginning. The DCCT (a near 10-year NIH multicenter clinical trial) proved that maintaining normal blood sugar levels decreases the risk of developing complications. (Although the trial included only Type 1 patients, many experts, as well as the American Diabetes Association, believe the findings apply to Type 2 patients as well. A British study dealing with Type 2 patients should give us more answers.) This will be the most intense period of diabetes learning you will go through: What you learn will remain with you for years. If you begin with a loose level of management, you might have a hard time tightening your regimen later. Maintaining excellent patterns of self-care from the beginning also increases your chances of benefiting from any future advances in research, such as islet cell transplants.

Some people are able to begin diabetes self-care at this level very easily. Others feel too overwhelmed by the shock of diagnosis to begin with such a detailed program. If you feel it is more than you can handle at this time, start with a more moderate regimen, but think of it as a temporary decision. When you have adjusted to the demands of diabetes, reconsider the intensive regimen. For those with Type 2 diabetes, the regimen for tight control is not as complex, but it can be just as challenging to get medications, eating, and activity habits to an optimal level.

Another factor affecting the level of care you adopt is the experience and attitude of your physician. As a whole, the profession is moving toward tighter control, but there are still varying opinions on this matter. In the past, Type 2 diabetes was inappropriately not considered a serious disease. If you want to maintain strict control and your doctor doesn't support this choice, you will need to find one who does. On the other hand, if your physician urges strict control and you do not feel ready for it, you can probably negotiate for looser control. Create a plan for moving in the direction your doctor recommends over the next few months. If a difference of opinion remains, you might need to find a new doctor.

Diabetes: A Lifelong Learning Experience

Living well with diabetes requires learning for the rest of your life. You probably already know what a powerful teacher diabetes is, with its many challenges and surprises. You are in the midst of learning the details of care, some of which have life-or-death significance. At this stage, you need to determine which aspects of care have such vital importance. (See "Diabetes Survival Kit" at the back of the book.) You may also be changing aspects of your lifestyle and dealing with the emotions that occur when diabetes is diagnosed.

Diabetes treatment is continuously evolving, so you can expect to continue learning about it for many years. As you grow older you may learn some of life's important lessons sooner than your friends without diabetes. Our physical condition requires us to accept vulnerability and mortality and to value the preciousness of life. The experience that accompanies such learning can be seen as a benefit of our condition.

Learning About Diabetes

To avoid feeling overwhelmed by the amount you have to learn following your diagnosis with diabetes, divide the learning into manageable lessons. Work out a schedule and identify the resources that can assist you. There may be a series of classes at a local hospital or clinic, a diabetes educator (usually a nurse or dietitian) may be available, or your local chapter of the American Diabetes Association may offer educational programs and support groups. Don't worry if your doctor plays a minor role in the educational process. In many cases, other members of your health care team will have more experience and training in this field.

Emotional Tasks

Ask a dozen people how they reacted to being told they have diabetes and you will probably hear a dozen different stories: "It really scared me. My uncle had diabetes and he died when he was 40." "No big deal. I don't let things like that get to me." "I was angry for months. I thought it would destroy all of my plans." "I just pulled the covers over my head and felt numb."

The only "right" way to feel is the way you are feeling. In the midst of learning about diabetes management, give yourself time to experience your particular emotions. If you deal with feelings on your own, be sure you set aside time to do this. Some people use writing, some take long solitary walks, others pray or meditate. (See Chapter 15 for ways of handling your feelings.)

If you prefer to have assistance, remember that it is available, even if you think you are isolated. There may be people available in your present support network; if not, you have guaranteed membership in the community of people with diabetes. Some people also find value in a few sessions with a counselor, psychologist, or social worker.

Some common reactions to being told you have diabetes are described in the following paragraphs. To some extent, these feelings can be offset by information, but you may find that the feelings persist even when you "know better." It may be simply your way of reacting to situations. The section on emotions in Chapter 15 offers ways to deal with some emotional habits.

You may feel helpless or unable to assume the new responsibilities diabetes assigns to you. If so, it helps to discuss your feelings with other people with diabetes. Their reassurance comes from knowing that feelings of being overwhelmed diminish as you begin taking care of yourself.

You may be depressed, fearful, or angry over the many changes in lifestyle you are expected to make. Some of the changes are specific to diabetes, but many of them are the basis of healthful living. Regular physical activity and a balanced diet are recommended for everyone. The schedule required by people with diabetes can be much more flexible now, with multiple daily insulin injections or the insulin pump.

Perhaps you are depressed about the possibility of developing complications and dying early; stories and statistics of the casualties of diabetes may lead you to believe you are doomed to disability and an early grave. However, recent advances in diabetes care offer the means of preventing or delaying the onset of diabetic complications. (See Chapters 16-18.)

You may feel frustrated about the restrictions you believe diabetes imposes on your life. Actually, diabetes closes very few doors to you. You are not allowed to fly a plane solo or have a job where an insulin reaction would threaten the safety of others. However, most roles you seek are open to you, including the role of mother or father.

Often, people react to diabetes by doing everything right, but at the same time creating so much anxiety that they feel terrible. If you are caught in this pattern, make relaxation and stress management a high priority. You will benefit from sorting out the aspects of diabetes care that are most critical. Until you do this, the slightest mistake in self-care can seem threatening.

Another reaction is to be unconcerned, insisting that diabetes will have no effect on your life. At some level, you may even believe that you don't really have the disease. Once you get your blood sugar under a moderate degree of control, diabetes has few outward signs. What a "nice" disease it seems to be. The temptation to do little to control it may be strong, especially when you are already getting by with managing the disease. In Type 1 diabetes, there is even a "honeymoon period," a few months during which insulin requirements temporarily decrease. However, after this period, they go up again.

Living well with diabetes calls for accepting it as a fact of life, and one of major significance. The more you ignore it through minimal self-care, the greater the impact it can have. If you follow a full regimen, you will lessen the risks and ensure that your body will be able to benefit from future advances in treatment or a cure.

Support Tasks

In the beginning, you can find support for dealing with both practical and emotional issues concerning diabetes. Relatives, friends, other people with diabetes, and professionals may be called upon at this time. You will need comfort, encouragement, and honest feedback on how you are handling things. You may have countless questions that seem too minor to take to your doctor, especially with Type 1 diabetes. Or perhaps you want information on cutting the costs of the supplies you need.

Some people are blessed with abundant support networks. Others feel isolated and don't know where to turn. If you feel there is little support available to you, give yourself a chance to be surprised. You may have more resources than you think. Even if you know few people, you are probably no more than two or three phone calls away from dozens of people who are willing to help you cope.

Wherever you live, there are people nearby who are well informed, positive, and helpful. You can contact others through your physician, pharmacist or other health professionals, the American Diabetes Association, the American Association of Diabetes Educators or the Juvenile Diabetes Foundation, or through people you already know. Let them know you are looking for people who have a positive outlook and who don't mind talking with others about diabetes. If you encounter people who only complain or tell horror stories, stay away from them. You need support, not discouragement. (See Chapter 14 for more on networking.)

Beginning Well

This questionnaire is designed to help you bring order to the process of adjusting to diabetes. Use your answers to help you sort out your new priorities. Determine what requests you need to make of your health care team and support network. What changes do you need to make in your life to handle this crisis well? If the challenge of diabetes feels overwhelming, begin with small steps you can easily handle. The most important thing is getting started.

1. Your Support Network

The people I can count on for emotional support include

_____

_____

The people who will help me with practical problems such as getting to an appointment with the doctor or bringing food when I'm ill include

_____

_____

(If you have trouble asking for help) I wouldn't want to ask for help because

_____

_____

How would you answer a friend who gave you this reason?

_____

_____

(If you feel you need more support) I can increase my support network by:
_____ Contacting the American Diabetes Association, the American Association of Diabetes Educators, or the Juvenile Diabetes Foundation.
_____ Joining a support group (either general or diabetic).

_____ Asking my minister for help.

_____ Asking my doctor or pharmacist to help me get in touch with other people who have diabetes.

_____ Going to a social worker or psychologist.

_____ Other

(If there are people in your life who are discouraging or otherwise negative) I can neutralize this "antisupport" by

_____ Asking the person involved to change.

_____ Changing how I respond.

_____ Avoiding the person.

_____ Having more contact with people who show a positive attitude.

_____ Other

The personal strengths I can call on within myself at this time include

_____

_____

A past crisis I handled well was

_____

_____

2. Your Physical Care

_____ I know which aspects of diabetes management have life-or-death significance. (See Diabetes Survival Kit at back of book.)

_____ I feel satisfied with my physician.

_____ I feel my physician is adequate, but I would like him/her to

_____ I feel I need a different doctor because

I feel most certain about the aspects of diabetes care I've checked below:

_____ Insulin or medication dosage

_____ Insulin reactions (low blood sugar)

_____ Blood testing

_____ Urine testing

_____ Diet and meal planning

_____ Exercise or other physical activities

_____ The effect of stress on diabetes control

_____ The interactions among all of these

(If your budget is limited) Have you located the least expensive source of diabetes supplies? A local ADA chapter might be able to refer you to medical discount shopping services. Also refer to the Appendix.

3. Your Emotional Care

My emotional reactions to the diagnosis of diabetes include the items I've checked below:

_____ Anger

_____ Fear

_____ Anxiety

_____ Depression

_____ Guilt

_____ Lack of feeling

_____ Calm

_____ Other

I am dealing with these reactions by

_____

_____

My overall response to the diagnosis of diabetes includes the items I've checked below:

_____ I feel overwhelmed by diabetes and find it difficult to handle.

_____ I am upset because I have to make too many changes in my life.

_____ I feel anxious about the things I have heard about complications.

_____ I am concerned that diabetes will make it impossible to achieve my life goals.

_____ I am worried about doing all the diabetes procedures correctly.

_____ I have withdrawn into myself.

_____ I don't believe that diabetes is any big deal or that I have to change much.

_____ I am dealing well with my feelings and with the practical challenges that diabetes has presented.

_____ Other

I can reduce my negative response to diabetes by

_____

_____

4. Your Diabetes Learning Program

_____ I have a good sense of what I know and what I still have to learn.

_____ I feel confused and need help figuring out what is important to learn.

_____ I have enrolled in a diabetes instruction class.

I have subscribed to

_____ *Diabetes Forecast*

_____ *Diabetes Self-Management*

_____ *Diabetes Interview*

(See Appendix for addresses.)

Review your answers and put 1, 2, or 3 stars by them to indicate their importance to you. Use this ranking to guide your use of this book.

Chapter Three

Help!

There are times when life gets difficult; diabetes has a way of adding to those difficulties we already face. Our self-care regimen is demanding, both to learn and to practice. We meet a variety of immediate and long term health crises. We are threatened by low blood sugar, delayed meals, lost insulin, missed injections or pills, coma, infections, depression, anxiety, denial, difficulties in relationships, and countless other diabetic complications.

You may have come to this chapter because you are in one of those situations. You may be in the midst of a diabetes crisis and need help handling your feelings and actions. Or you may feel unable (or unwilling) to continue learning what you need to know to care for yourself. Here you will find a number of tools to help you understand what is happening. You will also find what you need to do to move on.

While you can do much to help yourself, you might need help from your medical team or personal support network. Don't be afraid to ask for help. If the specific crisis you are handling is an aspect of your physical care, call your doctor, nurse practitioner, or diabetes educator for help.

We offer a variety of methods to suit individual styles and situations. You may want to work through the whole sequence laid out here, or you may need to use only one or two of the methods. Choose the course that is right for you.

We recommend beginning with relaxation and detachment. This will help you gain perspective and work more effectively.

Tools For Rescuing Yourself From A Crisis

Relaxation

When you have trouble—especially when your health is at stake—a natural response is to become tense and frustrated. When you become tense, it is difficult to find solutions to problems. It is a good idea to begin the process of rescuing yourself by relaxing as deeply as possible, before doing anything else.

If you have healthful techniques for relaxing that work for you, use them. Eating, drinking, watching television, and other common distractions don't count as healthful techniques. You may already be using stress management practices described at the end of Chapter 12 or others that you learned elsewhere.

If you need to relax right now, try this:

▷ Begin by saying something like: "My only job right now is to relax." For the moment, put all other concerns aside.

▷ Then, focus on your breathing, especially the feeling of it as you exhale. You can even sigh as you breathe out, if you like.

▷ Your body will respond now, if you talk with it. Say, "My right arm is becoming heavy." Repeat this phrase as many times as necessary.

▷ Now, repeat the phrase for your left arm: "My left arm is becoming heavy." Continue the exercise with your legs.

Within five to ten minutes, your body will translate the feeling of heaviness into relaxation. You can help the process by focusing on the heaviness that develops as you go along, rather than the tensions that remain.

Prayer and meditation can be the most effective means of relaxation you can use. These practices help you gain insight into the problems you are dealing with. Learn to pay attention to the supportive voice inside you guiding you toward better health decisions. Other techniques of relaxation are described at the end of Chapter 12.

Detachment

When difficulties arise, we often feel closed in. We lose perception and creativity because we focus on what is wrong. Finding solutions is much easier if we can gain some distance from the difficult situation. This is especially true with serious circumstances, such as pregnancy, or someone who is developing complications. No matter how urgent the need to achieve a particular goal, it is more likely to be attained if anxiousness can be calmed.

Following are a number of ways you can gain detachment from your reactions in a difficult situation. Once you have the basic idea, you will be able to find a method suited to your needs.

▷ Adopt an attitude of curiosity. Look at your situation as an artist or scientist who says, "Hmmm, very interesting. Let me explore what is happening."

▷ Remember a time when things were going well for you, or when you felt very calm and peaceful. See or feel the places, happenings, and people that were part of this special time. Let the remembrance of positive feelings come into the present, reminding you that you are more than someone having a problem.

▷ Think of an area of your life in which you are successful. Appreciate the strengths and skills you demonstrate here. Imagine your success if you were to act with these qualities on the problem you are now facing.

▷ Speak in the past tense when describing the difficulties you are working on now. Look back on them from a time in the future when they have all been overcome and you have made great progress. See this as one of the many steps needed to reach your goal.

▷ Describe your problems as those of someone you care for and understand and whom you see very clearly. Give this person credit for the effort he or she has made and assure them the challenge will be met.

▷ Find a humorous point of view for perceiving the situation you are in. Laughter is a healing agent and is good for the imagination.

Central to the idea of detachment is letting go of any judgments about yourself and your ability to handle problems. Even if you are dealing with total rebellion against the diabetes regimen, suspend the self-condemnation that often goes along with it. You are acting with great power. You just haven't learned to use that power to promote living well.

Finding Out What Is Going On Now

You may understand what is causing your present crisis and your difficulty in dealing with it. However, if you have only a vague sense of what is happening and why, you need to develop more awareness of your problem and its source. The following exercise may help you.

Write a brief statement summarizing what you know about the problem you are facing. This summary will help you clarify the problem and identify the solution. Draw on your answers to any of the following questions in the analysis.

▷ What are the facts of your situation? Which aspects appear to be outside your control? Which ones are within your control?

▷ When you examine how you are feeling about the problem, what are your strongest emotions? Where in your body do you feel them?

▷ Consider your thoughts. Are there beliefs or attitudes that make you feel unwilling or unable to deal with this situation, such as "I can't cope with crisis," "It's too late for me to change," "It's not fair," "I shouldn't have to," "I don't want to"?

▷ In your behavior, what is it that you find difficult to do (or to stop doing)? Break down the behavior into small parts. Figure out which are the most difficult.

▷ What pictures come to mind when you consider the problem? Do they help you understand what is happening?

▷ Is there something you are holding onto by having this problem—some positive benefit, such as increased attention from someone you care about?

▷ Is there something you are avoiding? What undesirable result might come if you were free of the crisis?

▷ Is something else happening in your life that needs attention or is distracting you from what you are trying to accomplish with diabetes?

Some people are most comfortable doing this sort of work on their own, perhaps by writing notes in a journal. Others appreciate talking through a crisis with a friend or relative who is a good listener. A diabetes support group is another good setting for exploring such issues. If no progress is made in any of these ways, a few sessions with a counselor might help you sort things out.

Creating Your Solutions

Sometimes, a clear understanding of what is happening is all we need to get past an obstacle. "Oh, I was hung up on that old belief 'I'll die by the time I'm 50,' just like Mom. No wonder I was stuck. It's time to get on with learning to live!" When this happens, tension is released and we can move forward.

This may be a time when you need action, not just understanding. If so, take the role of creator, designing the solutions to your problem. View the situation without blame or judgment. In the work you have just done, identify the specific beliefs, feelings, and behaviors that cause you stress and generate options for dealing with them.

Some guidelines for this process include the following:

▷ Affirm your ability to handle the situation. Recognize that you choose your responses to what is happening and can make new choices.

▷ Pay attention to your feelings throughout the process, but do not be trapped by them. Use the techniques for detachment described above when negative feelings seem to dominate. Remember, your feelings are created within you and you have the power to change them. Ask yourself, "Is this how I want to feel?" If it isn't, create new feelings or attitudes.

▷ Work with the information generated in the previous sections to help define your next steps concerning your situation.

▷ Identify the specific goals you want to reach. What changes will let you know you are out of the crisis?

▷ Brainstorm a list of specific actions that will help you move forward. Write down any ideas that come to mind, then search the list for those you feel prepared to take. Choose the one that will enable you to take a first step.

▷ Imagine yourself taking the actions you need to overcome your problem. Let scenes unfold in your mind in which you discover new answers. (Also use this visualization to reinforce actions you chose in the previous step.)

▷ Take a first step, no matter how small. Action restores your confidence to take further action and is also an antidote to anxiety.

▷ Give yourself space for breaks, relaxation, exercise, and entertainment. In most crises, time off increases your ability to find solutions.

If you do everything possible and still feel that you are getting nowhere, look for further help from your health care team and personal support network. You don't have to do this by yourself. Some challenges in living well with diabetes can be met only with outside support.

(See Chapter 15 for more on working with feelings and beliefs. Chapter 14 can also be of aid in a crisis. If you are dealing with the threat or diagnosis of complications, see Section Five.)

Section Two
Living Well
With Diabetic Control

Chapter Four

Diabetes—
Defining The Choices

Before we developed diabetes, our bodies performed a number of vital functions spontaneously, without our ever having to give a thought to them. The pancreas released insulin whenever it sensed that our blood sugar level was above a certain point. Hormones from other glands kept insulin from lowering blood sugar to dangerous levels. (These counter-regulatory hormones inhibit insulin action or stimulate the release of sugar into the bloodstream.) We maintained a delicate balance, with blood glucose usually ranging between 60 and 120 mg/dl (3.3 and 6.6 mmol/L). We enjoyed a natural control of our sugar metabolism and, as a result, other factors such as blood fats (including cholesterol and triglycerides) remained at normal levels.

When we develop Type 1 diabetes, insulin production from our pancreas is reduced or eliminated. (See Chapter 6 for Type 2 diabetes.) Blood sugar soars to readings two to five times the normal level, sometimes higher. Blood fats increase. Counter-regulatory hormones such as adrenaline increase because of physical stress and drive our blood sugar levels even higher. Our whole system is out of control.

When we begin taking insulin, we regain a sense of control, but with an enormous difference. We need to be consciously involved in the metabolic control process. We have to make decisions about many things that we never had to worry about before, such as the timing of meals and insulin injections, and the effects of exercise and stress on our blood sugar level.

Making decisions that result in normal blood glucose levels requires information and skill, whether we have Type 1 or Type 2 diabetes. We need to be able to measure our blood sugar level at any moment; we need to be aware of the factors determining that level such as diet, activity, medication, and stress; and we need to know how to vary those factors to regain balance when test levels are too high or too low. Finally, we need support to maintain the regulated lifestyle that makes real control of diabetes possible.

Until the last few years, most of us were unable to achieve a good level of control. Only in mild cases of diabetes was it possible to avoid swings in blood sugar levels far outside the normal range. Urine tests gave imprecise information about the actual blood glucose level at the time of testing. Once-a-day injections of intermediate or long-acting insulin could not provide the insulin activity needed to handle blood sugar increases after each meal. The oral medications for Type 2 worked for some, but not all. We knew little about the way emotional stress raises and lowers blood sugar. And the need for emotional support was scarcely recognized.

All of this has now changed. Home blood glucose testing gives fairly precise readings of blood sugar levels any time we need them. An insulin pump or two to four insulin injections each day can provide a supply that more closely matches our varying need for insulin. We have several new oral medications that provide more options for those with Type 2 diabetes. Physicians are encouraging us to make necessary alterations in insulin dose, diet, and exercise to keep blood glucose levels close to normal. Recognition of the effect of emotional stress on diabetic control has brought a new emphasis on learning to deal with stress more effectively, and we are finally admitting the need for emotional support— something required by anyone living with a chronic medical condition.

It is now possible to bring diabetes under control rather quickly (as required during pregnancy, for instance). Many of us have learned to achieve an average blood sugar level that was impossible five to ten years ago. And without an urgent short-term need, many of us have gained this level of control simply because we want to live well with diabetes.

The level of regimen needed to maintain optimal control of diabetes is both demanding and liberating. This book outlines a step-by-step process for learning this regimen in an organized and safe fashion. This process is for people who want intensive diabetes management, which takes commitment, effort, time, a modest amount of money, and close teamwork with health professionals.

For those with Type 2 diabetes, it is just as important to achieve optimal control. Diabetes of either type is a serious disease, and complications develop with both types. For those with Type 2, the steps may be less complex, but not necessarily easier. They may involve lifestyle changes in diet and exercise, as well as an adjustment in medication by a physician or nurse practitioner.

Not everyone is prepared to follow this path. Some people like to move gradually or are less motivated than others. Some have major concerns other than diabetes competing for their energies. Others may be held back by certain beliefs and emotional reactions that make them feel unable to change. For one reason or another, many people choose to remain at a level of moderate or even loose management.

There are also medical reasons that argue against following this path. The pros and cons should be weighed by you and your physician. Because of the increased likelihood of hypoglycemia, patients with significant cardiovascular or cerebrovascular disease might be adding undue risk to an already compromised circulation of nutrients (oxygen and glucose). Patients with hypoglycemic unawareness—decreased symptoms due to a variety of reasons that are not fully understood—may be advised not to follow the intensive regimen. Patients with advanced kidney disease have less predictable insulin action and may find the intensive regimen very difficult to manage.

Although many reasons favor the path of intensive management, it is important not to bias this choice. If those with diabetes who do not adopt this regimen feel that a less rigorous program is ineffective and futile, they may abandon all efforts to control their metabolism.

You may feel that you have no control; your blood sugar levels may soar and plummet crazily. Even so, it is vitally important that you do not condemn yourself as weak or incompetent. By accepting yourself and your past choices, you gain the power to make new, more healthful decisions about self-regulation. If your present choice is a moderate or loose regimen, give yourself credit for what you are doing and continue doing it. You will feel better, and this alone may help you decide to tighten your level of management.

If the Word Control Sounds Like Fingernails on a Blackboard...

Most of us believe that living well is living with freedom. Yet when we have diabetes, we are told that we must control our metabolism, our blood sugar, and our eating. Sometimes it seems as though every aspect of our lives requires some kind of control.

One problem is with the word control itself. *Roget's Thesaurus* lists the synonyms for control as whip hand, subjugation, domination, suppression, oppression and tyranny. Verbs associated with control include browbeat, bully, restrict, and corner. It doesn't sound like a very pleasant place to visit, much less live. No wonder controlling our diabetes often feels like a burden. Yet control is one of the most frequently used words in articles on diabetic management, and we have not been able to come up with many adequate substitutes.

We can purge control of its negative connotations by evoking the image of metabolic order it truly represents. When we work to gain control of diabetes, we are seeking to take over a task our bodies previously handled. If anything, this opportunity of exercising control is a challenge. We are cooperating with and helping direct our life processes. We are not simply managing diabetes; we are managing our lives.

Discovering Your Present Levels Of Control

We are considering two aspects of control here: the actual level of control you achieve and the level of regimen you follow to control your metabolism. The actual level of control you achieve is measured by home and lab tests and the way you feel. The level of regimen is defined by what you do. Before telling you about the different possible levels, we are going to suggest that you find out about them by determining what your own level is at present. The following questionnaire helps you do this.

Finding Your Level

Circle the number following the statement that is most true for you. Your doctor's office can supply results of your lab tests if you have had tests done.

A. Level of Control

1. My last fasting blood glucose test in the lab or doctor's office was
   less than 120 mg/dl (6.6 mmol/L) 3
   between 120 and 180 (6.6 and 10) 6
   between 181 and 240 (10 and 13.3) 9

higher than 240 (13.3) 12

Don't know or NA (not applicable) 7.5

2. My last hemoglobin A1c test was

less than 8% 3

between 8 and 9.9% 6

between 10 and 12% 9

higher than 12% 12

Don't know or NA 7.5

3. My last test for total cholesterol was

less than 201 2

between 201 and 225 4

between 226 and 240 6

higher than 240 8

Don't know or NA 5

4. The average of my home blood glucose tests for the last seven days is

less than 120 mg/dl (6.6 mmol/L) 2

between 120 and 180 (6.6 and 10) 6

between 181 and 240 (10 and 13.3) 9

higher than 240 (13.3) 12

Don't know or NA 7.5

5. The approximate percentage of my home blood glucose tests for the
last seven days that were between 60 and 140 mg/dl (3.3 and 7.7
mmol/L) is

more than 75% 3

between 50 and 75% 6

between 25 and 50% 9

less than 25% 12

Don't know or NA 7.5

6. If you do not test blood or urine, or if you do so less than twice a
week, circle 12 here and skip to question 8. 12

7. I test urine for sugar regularly, and I almost never have a positive
urine test (one or more +). 2

My tests are negative (-) at least half the time and usually not higher
than 1/4%. 4

My tests vary greatly, sometimes negative, sometimes 1 or 2%. .6

My tests are usually over 1%. 8

Not applicable, because I test only blood sugar. 5

8. When you test for ketones in your urine, the test is

always negative 2

always negative unless I am ill or under stress (or I have Type 2 and rarely test) 4

occasionally positive (1-3 times a month) 6

frequently positive (1+ times a week) 8

NA 5

9. I have had severe low blood sugar in the last month (severe = strong symptoms such as confusion, shakiness, sweating, pounding heart, etc.)

Never 2

1-4 times 4

5-10 times 6

More than 10 times 8

10. I have been unconscious from a reaction or failed to awaken to a reaction occurring during sleep in the last year. If yes, circle 16. If no, skip to question 11. 16

11. I have had symptoms of high blood sugar (frequent urination, nighttime urination, thirst, and lethargy) in the last month.

Never 2

1-3 times 4

4-10 times 6

More than 10 times 8

12. I have normal weight. 3

I am slightly overweight (up to 10% above normal) 6

I am moderately overweight (10-20% above normal) 9

I am very overweight 12

13. I seldom have illness or infections, and I recover or heal easily when I do. 1

I have occasional illness or infection, and I recover somewhat slowly. 3

I am frequently ill or have infections, and I heal slowly. 4

14. My energy level is good and I recover from exertion easily. 1

I occasionally feel lethargic. 2

I tire very easily and need to rest frequently during the day. 4

15. In the last year I have been hospitalized because my diabetes was out of control.

Never 4

Once 9
More than once 16

B. Level of Regimen

These questions cover only the aspects of diabetes regimen that relate to metabolic control.

1. I am on an intensive insulin regimen (2 or more injections per day, using both regular and intermediate or long-acting insulin or the insulin pump) and vary dosage according to blood sugar tests. . .3
I take two injections per day but rarely vary dosage from day to day. 6
I have only one injection of insulin each day. 9
NA 6

2. In the last two months I have forgotten or deliberately not taken insulin or oral meds.
Never 4
1-2 times 12
More than twice 16
NA 10.5

3. I test blood glucose levels two or more times a day. 3
I test blood glucose levels at least twice a week, or urine at least
once a day 6
I test blood or urine at least twice a week. 9
I seldom (or never) do any home urine or blood tests. 12

4. When my control is off (high or low blood sugar) or
when there are changes in my routine (schedule, activity,
food, or stress), I know how to alter insulin, diet, or activity
to compensate for the changes. I can return to normal quickly. .2
I make some general adjustments
but sometimes don't get back to normal for a few days. 4
I know when my control is off,
but I rarely do anything to compensate. 6
I don't know anything about adjusting insulin,
food, or activity to maintain control. .8

5. I measure or accurately estimate the amount of food I eat and
keep the prescribed balance of carbohydrate, protein, and fat. .3
I usually eat in moderation and have a general awareness
of the balance of carbohydrate, protein, and fat. 6

I eat pretty much what I want to, but not to excess. 9

I frequently eat excessively or irregularly. 12

6. I seldom eat sweets, and I minimize intake of other simple carbohydrates (such as dried fruits and fruit juices). 3

I eat small portions of sweets and other simple carbohydrates. . . .6

I usually eat small portions, but I binge at least once a week. 9

I eat all the sweets and fruit I want. 12

7. I eat as little animal fat as possible (butter, fatty meat,
luncheon meat, high fat cheese). 3

I eat small amounts of animal fat and
rarely eat excessive amounts. 6

I usually eat only small amounts of animal fat,
but at least once a week I binge. 9

I eat all the animal fat I want. 12

8. I eat complex carbohydrates and high fiber foods (whole grains,
vegetables, etc.)

at most meals 2

about half the time 4

rarely 6

never 8

9. When I have overeaten or know that a large meal is coming, I use
extra insulin or exercise to compensate for the extra calories

nearly always 2

usually 4

rarely 6

never 8

10. I have moderate to strenuous physical activity regularly
(the equivalent of 20 minutes of exercise with heart rate 120+). .2

I have moderate physical activity, but it usually
varies quite a bit from day to day. 4

I am relatively inactive or irregular in my level of activity. 6

I am very inactive or very irregular in my level of activity. 8

11. When I am under emotional stress, I feel able to cope well,
and the stress does not seriously affect my blood sugar level. . . .2

I try to cope, but my control may be off for the next few tests. . .4

I don't cope too well, and my blood sugar level
may be high for a day or more. 6

I forget everything I know about coping,
ignore my diabetes, and my blood sugar stays high. 8

Add up the numbers you circled for parts A and B and enter your totals here:

Part A: Level of Control _____
Part B: Level of Regimen _____

Now see what your level of control and level of regimen are.

Level of Control	Score	Level of Regimen	Score
Optimal	34-42	Intensive	28-42
Moderate	43-65	Moderate	43-63
Loose	66-90	Loose	64-84
Minimal	91+	Minimal	85+

Although general ranges are derived from the authors' experience and have been tested, they have not been fully validated. However, your score should give you a sense of where you are and what you need to work on.

Completing this exercise can be challenging, perhaps even unpleasant. If your results were not as positive as you thought they would be, don't blame yourself. Acknowledge the choices you have been making and the reasons you have been making them. Give yourself room to begin making new choices. You might go through the regimen part of the questionnaire and check the places where you marked the higher numbers. These will indicate areas for needed improvement in management that you may feel willing to begin at this time. A little later in this chapter, there is another exercise that will help you choose the overall level of management you wish to exercise.

In your answers to this questionnaire, you have a general profile of your current metabolic control regimen and your level of control. You may feel comfortable with this level of management, or other concerns may take priority. On the other hand, you may wish to improve control as your next step in living well with diabetes. You may wish to assume the intensive regimen, or you may prefer to make the change in stages, working first to gain loose or moderate control.

Benefits Of Achieving Optimal Control

The first thing you need to consider in choosing your level of diabetic regimen is what you can gain from the best level of control. You know achieving it will take effort, how will it benefit you?

Since the second edition of this book, the findings of a landmark study have proven that blood sugar control matters! That is very good news.

The better your control, the less likely you are to develop long term complications of diabetes. The NIH-sponsored Diabetes Control and Complications Trial (DCCT) demonstrated that good blood sugar control can delay or prevent the development of diabetic retinopathy, nephropathy, and neuropathy in those with Type 1 diabetes. Although the participants were only Type 1, the American Diabetes Association and most diabetes specialists believe that the findings apply to Type 2 as well, since it appears that abnormal blood sugar is the main cause. The Kumamoto Study from Japan has also provided early support for the same benefits as in Type 1. The United Kingdom Prospective Diabetes Study, with results due in 1998, may provide more definitive answers specifically for those with Type 2 diabetes.

The DCCT firmly established the importance of measuring the average level of blood sugar over a 2- to 3-month period using the HbA1c (hemoglobin A1c) lab test. The study showed that the lower your average blood sugar levels, the less likely you were to develop complications. Even though the study participants on the intensive regimen did not reach normal levels, their risk of complications was reduced by up to 70%, and every step toward normal helped!

The HbA1c has become the most important measure of overall control. It is recommended that desirable level for adults is below 7%, and for children is below 8%. Because labs differ in testing procedures, normal values may be different from those on which the above targets are based. In this case, adult targets should be less than 1 percentage point above the lab's top range of normal, and children less than 2 percentage points. This is the target for the intensive regimen. The consequences of the moderate and loose regimens would be higher HbA1c levels, and greater risk of complications. (See Chapter 5 for more on HbA1c.)

Beginning the learning process necessary to achieve optimal control often brings an immediate emotional benefit to those with diabetes. Many report a sense of greater power, less depression, and less anxiety. This emotional high helps us through the initial period of greater regulation required until we have learned the regimen. Once we have done so, we will experience greater freedom. We can deal with irregularities of diet, mealtimes, activity, and stress, and still obtain greatly improved blood sugar levels.

The first physical benefits start soon after control is improved. When blood sugar levels are closer to normal, we simply feel better. We have more energy; we need less sleep; we are less likely to grow fatigued. Also, our immune systems work more effectively, so we are less likely to become ill or have infections that get out of control. When we do become seriously ill, we are better able to compensate for the effect of the physical stress on blood sugar, and we are less likely to develop ketoacidosis, a condition that can lead to diabetic coma. In formal studies, those with diabetes who maintained good control had many fewer hospitalizations—a considerable economic benefit.

Women who improve metabolic control develop fewer vaginal and urinary tract infections and consequently find greater enjoyment in sex. In addition, their menstrual periods become more regular. Adolescents are less likely to experience a delay in beginning menstruation. With strict control leading up to and continuing during pregnancy, the risks for both mother and child are greatly reduced. (During pregnancy, careful management of diabetes is necessary. See Chapter 19, Living Well As A Diabetic Woman.)

For children, optimal control encourages normal patterns of growth and development. (Growth is sometimes stunted when blood sugar is poorly controlled in childhood.) Fluctuations in insulin requirements caused by growth spurts and the hormonal changes during puberty are more easily handled with the intensive regimen. Also, parental awareness of the emotional side of diabetes can help children live well with the more demanding regimen.

These are the short-term benefits we can experience directly, but that's only half the story. Laboratory tests of people with diabetes in good control show that several important measures of physiological balance also reach normal levels. These include elements in the blood that are responsible for clotting, the levels of cholesterol and triglycerides which contribute to heart and circulatory disorders, the release of hormones; and the thickness and fragility of capillaries (the thinnest blood vessels). All of these levels tend to be abnormal when blood sugar is high.

Although we don't experience immediate symptoms from these abnormalities, their presence is not healthful. They are the building blocks from which diabetic complications are constructed over time. In the long run, high blood sugar levels increase the chance of developing heart disease, circulatory problems, blindness and other vision problems, kidney disorders, and neuropathy (nerve malfunctions).

These future possibilities encourage us to follow a demanding regimen in the present. This works most effectively when it takes the form of healthy concern, rather than chronic anxiety.

Studies are now accumulating that document the effect of improved short-term control. Capillary thickness, growth hormone levels, excessive fats in the blood, and factors affecting clotting become normal when blood sugar levels are brought under control. In this way, a major, but subtle, aspect of the illness of diabetes can be erased. We can live well with diabetes now and provide a basis for a future without major complications.

But what if complications have already set in? Is it too late to bother with control? No, but talk to your doctor about the cautions mentioned earlier in the chapter concerning cardiovascular disease, neuropathy, and kidney disease. Even at this stage, one may benefit from improved control. The DCCT clearly showed that good control will slow or stop the progression of complications. In some cases, complications may be reversed or their impact lessened by careful management. Whether or not existing complications can be reversed, one's chances of avoiding or slowing the development of other complications are also improved. The immediate physical benefits and the emotional lift gained by taking control help one deal more effectively with the fears that usually accompany the diagnosis of a complication. (One additional caution: Control must be improved gradually if retinopathy or kidney disease at any stage has already started. See Chapter 18, Complications Simplified, for details.)

Optimal control of diabetes offers immediate and long-term benefits. However, there is no guarantee that it will prevent future complications or reverse them once they have started. But it does improve our odds, reducing the risk of developing complications. The decision to gain optimal control must be made in terms of the present benefits, which include having a body that functions more healthfully now and has less risk of developing complications later.

The Costs Of Gaining Optimal Control

What are the costs of better control? Economically, there is a moderate cost—one that many insurance companies are now covering. Blood test strips are much more expensive than urine test materials, but there are ways of cutting corners (and the strips) to save money. During the most intensive testing (four to six times a day for the first weeks), the cost ranges from $15 to $25 a month by the economy route, and up to $100 a month without cutting costs. Those with Type 2 diabetes will not need to test as often (once or twice a day at varying times), so the costs are much lower. Many people use a meter to read the strips, at a cost of $50 to $200. Often there are discounts and rebates that will lessen the cost. With most meters, it is also necessary to use an entire strip. The only other piece of equipment is an automatic fingersticking device that lessens the chance of pain. It costs around $15.

During the first months of intensive management, there is a significant cost in time and energy. Collecting information, testing, keeping records, and figuring out what the records mean can become a major project. But it is probably no more complex than learning to drive. Depending on how much new information you have to acquire, the task could take anywhere from three to ten hours a week.

Another cost at the beginning: You need to regularize all aspects of life that affect blood sugar, making changes that may or may not be simple. The more you do this, the more quickly you will reach the point where you do not have to be so regular. It is much easier to learn how to keep your blood sugar within limits if you follow set routines during the training period. Without this regularity, it is difficult to know what is causing tests to be too high or too low. Once you establish a routine, you'll enjoy much more freedom.

One potential liability when maintaining strict control is that you are likely to have more low blood sugar or insulin reactions (this is not as likely for Type 2 diabetes). This is especially true if you have usually had high blood sugar levels or are irregular in activity or diet. (Often, fear of reactions is one of the reasons a person with diabetes will keep blood sugar high.) Meanwhile, you will need to sharpen your awareness of the cues indicating that a reaction is on its way, and be sure to always have some form of sugar with you. With home blood testing, you can easily check whether those funny feelings are the result of low blood sugar or some other cause, such as anxiety. Also, hypoglycemic unawareness is becoming more recognized, and researchers are studying the causes.

Testing is especially important if you find that your reaction symptoms have become more subtle. Some people experience a decrease in the output of stress hormones that signal the appearance of an insulin reaction. They also exhaust the glycogen (sugar reserves) stored in the liver. When this develops, blood sugar can drop quite low without triggering the usual alarms—shakiness, sweating, increased pulse, and so forth. If you feel it has become difficult to tell when an insulin reaction is occurring, talk with your doctor; it is an important consideration when determining the level of control you will try to maintain. Although hypoglycemic unawareness used to be considered a form of diabetic nerve disease that developed in people with diabetes for many years, it is now realized that this can also happen early in diabetes.

We have included in the following pages many safeguards against low blood sugar. In Chapter 9, we give comprehensive information on reactions, including tips on recognizing and treating them.

Weighing the Costs and Benefits

Take a moment to consider how these benefits and costs of optimal control balance out for you.

What value do you place on the benefits we have described?

Which are the most important to you?

Do any of the costs seem particularly heavy to you?

If so, what could you do to lighten them?

A Choice Of Regimen

Given the benefits of optimal control, one might conclude that the it should be the only regimen offered to people with diabetes. Options and choices are among the main principles underlying this book. We cannot ignore the obvious fact that diabetes care is just one of the many items we must manage in our lives. Until the next set of technical breakthroughs, optimal control will depend on a set of lifestyle changes and an educational process requiring time and intense effort. Many who are not prepared to make these changes or have extraordinary demands on time and energy might choose to ignore their diabetes if they feel they cannot follow the optimal path.

This is why we offer a choice of regimens along a continuum of self-care. The choices we make are reflected in our day-to-day actions, whether our regimen for diabetes management is intensive or loose. These actions are performed with or without the knowledge and support of our physician or health care team. It makes sense to recognize this and support each person in the choices they make. With this approach, you can begin at a level you feel comfortable with and proceed at a pace that is right for you.

The Intensive Regimen

The first choice we will consider is the regimen that allows you to gain nearly normal blood sugar values in a few months. This optimal control of diabetes depends upon a number of innovations in self-care, knit together into a state-of-the-art management program. This is usually called the intensive regimen.

The Intensive Regimen

1. Home blood sugar testing (blood glucose monitoring) two to four times a day (as many as six times a day at the beginning). For those with Type 2 diabetes, testing will be one to two times a day (more frequently in the beginning), and performed at different times each day to determine blood sugar levels overnight, and before and after meals. For both types, HbA1c's less than 7% (or less than 1 percentage point above the lab's norm).

2. Insulin injections two to four times a day, often using both rapid-acting and intermediate or long-acting insulins, or continuous insulin delivery by insulin pump. For Type 2 diabetes, it will include working with your health professional to determine the optimum combination of pills and/or insulin, if good nutrition and physical activity are not sufficient.

3. Knowledge of food values and ability to follow a meal plan that ensures normal body weight, diabetic control, and reduced risk of complications.

4. An active lifestyle, an exercise program, or both, followed regularly.

5. Ability to alter medications, food intake, and activity level to compensate for irregularities and the effects of stress.

6. Knowledge of the role of physical and emotional stress in diabetes and the ability to manage both.

7. Commitment to continue diabetes learning, maintain motivation, and meet one's emotional needs.

The staples of diabetes care are all here—insulin, pills, meal plans, physical activity—but we've added several new ingredients. In this approach, home blood glucose monitoring allows precise feedback about blood sugar levels, which enables you to make more precise decisions about medications, activity, and diet. For Type 1, where blood is tested several times a day, multiple injections or the pump can provide a level of insulin appropriate to blood sugar levels. For Type 2, optimum adjustment of medications, food, and activity allow relatively stable and near normal blood sugar levels over a 24-hour period. For both, a HbA1c less than 1 percentage point above normal.

Awareness of the effect of stress on diabetic control helps you understand puzzling swings in blood sugar levels. More effective stress management helps to reduce the metabolic effect of these swings. Furthermore, the intensive regimen recognizes that the demands of the regimen itself may become a source of stress. Therefore, it includes ways to make these demands less burdensome and to help you stay motivated. For the regimen to work in the long run, it must serve as a foundation for the rest of your life.

Who Needs the Intensive Regimen?

Some people will choose this path simply because they want to do their best in everything they do or because they have strong motivation to live as healthfully as possible. However, others will make this choice because of a specific and immediate health need.

The intensive regimen is especially recommended for:

▷ Women who are pregnant or are planning to become pregnant.

▷ Patients beginning to develop diabetic complications such as nerve and kidney disorders, circulatory problems, heart disease, retinopathy, and other eye disorders. (If retinopathy or kidney disease has started, you may need to proceed gradually. See Chapter 18, Complications Simplified.)

▷ Children whose growth is significantly behind schedule.

▷ Patients with other chronic illnesses or conditions, where the consequences of high blood sugar make the other chronic conditions worse.

People in these categories often choose to make optimal control a high priority despite other aspects of their lives that might interfere. If personal obstacles are making it hard for you to make this level of commitment, you may wish to seek assistance such as individual counseling or a support group. If you decide to continue with a moderate or loose regimen because other problems are more pressing, you can review your decision periodically to see if a new choice is possible.

You may need to adopt a somewhat less strict version of the intensive regimen if you have difficulty recognizing the symptoms of an insulin reaction. After living with diabetes for many years, the usual signs of low blood sugar can diminish or disappear because of hormonal changes. Your doctor can order tests to determine whether this has happened to you. If your hormonal output is normal, then you need to sharpen your awareness of the physical signs of low blood sugar. Medicines for some other conditions (typically beta blockers for high blood pressure) can also lower your ability to recognize symptoms.

The Moderate Regimen

If we discussed only the intensive regimen, some of you, unable or unwilling to devote yourself to diabetes care in such a concentrated fashion, would be left out in the cold. If you are facing extraordinary personal demands, a lack of motivation, or emotional obstacles, you may need a regimen particular to your needs. A slower pace with less structure will allow you to deal with your concerns and periodically review your choice of regimen. It is possible to include in the moderate regimen many aspects of the intensive regimen so that you can significantly improve your control. We are talking about various levels of self-care, not an all-or-none situation.

The Moderate Regimen

1. Regular home blood glucose testing (at least two or four times a week, preferably daily, and as needed) combined with daily urine tests.

2. One or two insulin injections daily, usually with a combination of rapid-acting and intermediate or long-acting insulins. (The insulin pump is not recommended with this regimen.) For those with Type 2, the moderate regimen would probably use fewer medications, and perhaps one insulin injection. The HbA1c would probably be in the 8-9% range (less than 2-3 percentage points above normal). Bringing the HbA1c lower would require a more complex and intense medication and eating program.

3. Knowledge of food values and ability to follow a meal plan that ensures close to normal body weight and moderate diabetic control.

4. An active lifestyle, a regular exercise program, or both.

5. Ability to make cautious adjustments in medications, food intake, and activity level to compensate for changes and the effects of stress.

6. Knowledge of the role of physical and emotional stress in diabetes and the ability to manage both.

7. Commitment to continue diabetes learning, maintain motivation, and meet your emotional needs.

The moderate regimen differs from the intensive regimen in the level of feedback and control it provides. Testing is less rigorous and, as a result, the insulin and/or pill dosage cannot be so finely tailored. Without frequent blood tests, those with Type 1 have too little information to make precise daily adjustments in insulin dosage, food, or activity. Caution is recommended. For this reason, the insulin pump or more than two insulin injections a day are not usually recommended for anyone on either the moderate or the loose regimen. Those with Type 2 will be eating less carefully, and taking medications that do not result in target HbA1c. When optimal control is very difficult to achieve, this may be the best option.

Home blood sugar testing is an important part of the moderate regimen, even when it is done only a few times a week. The accuracy of the results, compared with urine tests, helps to build motivation to improve control. Having the strips on hand means that you can easily see how stress, a large meal, or an unusual level of exercise affects blood sugar. When you are ill, you can handle blood sugar and ketone problems more accurately. If you have difficulty detecting insulin reactions, you can use the tests to confirm hypoglycemia and become more aware of its symptoms.

Sometimes, success in improving control has the unexpected effect of dramatically increasing your motivation. If you now feel that you could never handle the intensive regimen, you may find that the act of beginning to improve management gives you greater willingness later. Whether or not this occurs, you will feel much better about yourself than if you just continued in your old ways, believing that you could not control your diabetes. You will be dealing with one of the most important issues in your life—living well with diabetes.

The Loose Regimen

For those of you who may feel that even the moderate regimen is too restrictive or too demanding, you have a third choice. In the loose regimen, the focus is on identifying whatever you are willing to do to begin improving control, and then doing it. In this regimen, we emphasize building willingness and a positive attitude, even though you may now be living with a low level of control. One important element for those who maintain a level of loose control is to realize that it is a choice they have made; it is not something that just happens to them. It is useful to define this as a level of regimen rather than as a rebellion against, or a neglect of regimen. Both authors have managed their diabetes at this level in the past. Each of us has the right to choose how we live with our bodies. Learning to accept the choices we make helps us move on to more healthful choices.

The Loose Regimen

1. Knowledge of blood testing techniques, even though tests may be done infrequently. Urine testing occasionally, including testing for ketones, especially when ill.

2. One or two insulin injections daily. (More injections or the insulin pump are not recommended without regular blood sugar testing.) HbA1c is likely more than 3 percentage points above normal. People with Type 2 diabetes will take a pill, a combination of pills, and/or insulin on a schedule prescribed by their physicians. If taking a combination of pills and/or insulin, you are already very close to a regimen that could result in optimal blood sugar and HbA1c levels. Work with your diabetes educator or physician to explore improving your blood sugar levels.

3. Eating a healthful diet, usually in moderation.

4. Caution in adjusting medications , food intake, and activity level. If you have Type 2 diabetes, or have not received adequate instruction in adjusting your own insulin, consult your physician before making any changes in your medication. Once a Type 2 individual achieves a target blood sugar level, changes in the regimen will be relatively infrequent, and usually only if insulin were one of the medications.

5. Commitment to continue diabetes learning, maintain motivation, and review obstacles to improve control.

You may choose the loose regimen because your attention is focused on other areas in your life. If you choose this level, remember that the time you give to improving your diabetes management will probably help you manage the rest of your life better. Recognize that you are increasing the likelihood of developing serious complications associated with diabetes.

Choosing Your Regimen Level

If you have not decided which level of regimen to follow, answering these questions may help you do so.

1. I need to achieve improved control soon because

_____ I have diabetic complications.

_____ I am pregnant.

_____ I am planning to become pregnant.

_____ I am a child whose growth is significantly below normal.

_____ I have another major illness.

2. I should be cautious about initiating an intensive regimen because

_____ I do not experience the usual symptoms of low blood sugar and it is difficult for me to detect low blood sugar.

_____ I have significant kidney, cerebrovascular, or cardiovascular disease.

_____ I have beginning diabetic retinopathy or nephropathy.

3. The reasons I have for wanting to improve my control of diabetes include

4. a. Other major problems that need my attention are

_____

_____

b. I could gain assistance and support in dealing with these issues by

_____

_____

c. Could I postpone working on any of these to gain time for diabetes?

_____

_____

5. The external support I now have for dealing with diabetes is

_____ abundant

_____ adequate

_____ inadequate

6. In making this decision, I also have to consider

_____

_____

Review your answers, discuss them with your physician and those close to you, and then make a decision you are happy with.

7. Given the above, my choice of regimen is

_____ intensive

_____ moderate

_____ loose

Chapter Five

The Intensive Regimen

This chapter and the chapters on moderate and loose regimen are intended primarily for those with Type 1 diabetes. If you have Type 2 diabetes, the next chapter is targeted for you. The terms intensive, moderate, and loose apply to Type 2 regimens, but in different ways. While the steps toward optimal control can be just as challenging, and the commitment just as important, they are less complex than Type 1. Whether you have Type 1 or Type 2 diabetes, this chapter will provide useful information about diabetes management, insulin use, and behavior change.

You learn much more easily when you divide large projects into manageable steps. You can see each task more clearly, and make visible progress toward your goal. This is especially important when learning the intensive regimen and making the necessary lifestyle changes. How you learn the regimen can make the experience safer and more useful. You may already have some of the required skills or knowledge, but we urge you to review all of the information in this book, especially chapters on stress and physical activity. You may learn information you haven't seen elsewhere.

Eleven Steps to Optimal Control

1. Create a positive foundation. Be sure you have a positive setting for learning the intensive regimen, a physician, diabetes health care team, or diabetes educator who agrees with your goals, and support from family, friends, and others with diabetes.

   If you become frustrated or discouraged during this process, review the information in Chapters 3 and 15.

2. Under your doctor's supervision, have a lab test your hemoglobin A1c and blood lipids (triglycerides and cholesterol) to indicate your present level.

   This gives you a benchmark by which you can measure the effect of your new regimen.

3. Learn the skills and information necessary for the intensive regimen.
   a. Learn how to test blood sugar and urine.
      The criteria of diabetic control.
      An effective record-keeping system.
      The meaning of each laboratory test relevant to diabetic control.
   b. Review Chapter 9, "Living Well With Reactions." This is important because you may experience different signs of reaction when your metabolism is under better control. You may also experience more frequent reactions.
   c. Survey the basics of diabetic metabolism (how your system processes food and liquids to produce energy).
   d. Understand the different factors that determine blood sugar level.
4. Regularize meals, activity, and schedules during this period of learning. Later, you will have greater freedom.
5. Begin the period of intensive testing and record keeping without making any changes in regimen (unless your doctor requests changes). Keep detailed records, and observe how you respond to your present regimen.
6. With your doctor's and/or diabetes educator's guidance, select the intensive insulin regimen best suited to you. Begin this regimen and make the adjustments needed to obtain the highest possible level of control. Those with Type 2 diabetes will need to consult their doctors to determine if their oral medications should be changed or insulin added or modified.
7. Observe the variations in blood sugar level caused by changes in food, exercise, stress, illness, and other factors.
   a. People with Type 1 diabetes need to learn to vary insulin dosage. But with either type of diabetes, you need to learn to vary diet and exercise to compensate for high or low tests and changes in routine.
8. Have new lab tests taken after two or three months to determine the effect of your new regimen and to establish your ongoing regimen.
9. Assess your progress and determine what, if anything, is needed to further improve control.
10. Take steps to maintain your motivation for continuing at this level of management.
11. Celebrate!

Step 1: Create a positive foundation

You are starting one of the most positive and challenging things you can do for yourself as a person with diabetes. The rewards at physical and emotional levels are profound. You will have to overcome many obstacles to gain these rewards. Your first step is to make sure that the foundation for this work is also positive. This includes creating realistic expectations, neutralizing past failures, organizing professional and personal support, and becoming familiar with the things you can do if progress stops.

One of the most useful expectations to have about this process is that it will take time. You can't just flip a switch and gain instant control. People who focus on gaining control quickly will find that the process takes one to two months, and sometimes longer. It is possible to become discouraged, even when committing to an intense effort. This is particularly true for people with physiological problems such as partial immunity to insulin, as well as those with a high level of emotional or environmental stress. These people often follow the diabetic regimen perfectly and improve their control, but still experience large fluctuations in blood sugar level.

If at first you don't succeed, find out what else you need to do. Discuss what is happening with your doctor or diabetes educator; be patient with yourself and give yourself credit for what you have achieved. Sometimes improving diabetic control requires a stress management class, couples counseling, or a less stressful job. A more highly purified insulin may be needed to overcome immunity that can develop after years of injections. For those with Type 2 diabetes, one of the newer medications or new combinations of medications can help gain better control.

Occasionally, it is necessary to accept a lesser degree of control because you are unwilling or unable to make the necessary changes. If so, spare yourself the additional stress of feeling guilty. Respect your decision and keep the postponed changes on your agenda.

In the Introduction we discussed ways to safeguard against failure. There is probably no more important place to apply them than when learning the intensive regimen. If you begin down this path and then feel you are failing, it is time to use Chapters 3 and 15, to help overcome the obstacles you are encountering. You are not really failing; you just have something else to learn before you can succeed. Although you may feel a sense of urgency about the learning, it is helpful to not be judgmental. Transform obstacles into a part of the learning process by letting them define the next lessons you need to master.

Those of us who have tried to improve our metabolic control may have to set aside a history of frustration and lack of success. In the past, we did not have the tools needed to achieve our goal. It is important to let go of the feeling, "I'll never get this right." It is time for a new effort.

The fear and sense of urgency that inspire many to learn the intensive regimen need to be balanced with more positive motivation. Fear is a powerful feeling that can move us for a time, but our progress is steadier and more enduring when it comes from a positive sense of self.

Ernest's Experience

I'm afraid I have to confess, I didn't really begin to take control of diabetes until the ophthalmologist told me I had a high risk of going blind. I learned fast then. I enjoy the world's beauty too much to lose my vision of it.

But soon I realized that everything I was doing was for all of me, not just to save my eyes. I was giving myself a degree of love and respect that I'd always withheld before.

After a few months, I had the first hemorrhage in my left eye. And then, after laser treatment, I had another hemorrhage, and yet another. I could see only a blur through that eye. I had to face the strong possibility of losing vision in both eyes. When the difficulties started, I half expected to give up on my intensive regimen with the childish feeling, "It didn't do any good, anyway." So why didn't I? It's simple: I feel better loving and respecting myself, no matter what the outcome of my actions may be. I am living well, despite the possibility of losing my sight.

As I'm writing, I'm watching cows swishing their tails in the shade of a large oak, against golden hills. Above my keyboard there's a lovely bronze statue of Krishna, a flute-playing god who herds cows in Indian mythology. Once, when I asked my eye doctor what he thought would happen with my eyes, he answered with an unconscious pun, "We'll just have to wait and see." I replied, "I certainly hope so." I waited, and I'm seeing. The laser treatment was successful.

Fifteen years after laser treatment I am pleased to tell you that I have not had a hemorrhage for eight years. There are very small leaks of blood that give me more floaters than most people my age. But I see this beautiful world—the trees I plant, the flowers I grow, and that statue of Krishna—with 20/20 vision.

Another part of this first step is reviewing and strengthening your support system. A key element is, of course, your physician. You need one who is well informed about the newer approaches to diabetes care and who endorses your increased role in diabetes management. Your doctor should also have access to a diabetes educator and additional team members as needed. Discuss what you are doing with your doctor and determine guidelines for the management decisions you are to make at each step. Most physicians are pleased to see their patients taking greater responsibility, and support their independence fully. Doctors often make it possible to discuss test results and special problems by phone and provide twenty-four hour access in case of emergencies. Ask about this if your doctor doesn't suggest it.

The encouragement of your family will help during this time. Let the people close to you know what you are working on and what it means to you; share your concerns and expectations. Ask for the help you need or for changes in family patterns that interfere with your efforts to improve management. If you are in a negative family situation, you will need to take action to neutralize your family's influence, and look for support from others.

You should also let your friends know about your project and ask them for assistance. This is very helpful when you are attempting to make basic lifestyle changes. Friendships often revolve around habitual behavior and may be threatened when you begin changing habits. You can reduce the threat and gain valuable aid if you communicate the importance of the changes you are making. Realize that some friends may be too attached to their old image of you; if they offer little support, let that be their problem, not yours.

Support from others with diabetes, especially those who are also learning the intensive regimen, is second only to the guidance of your physician and diabetes educator during this period. Individual contacts or a support group can offer encouragement and reinforcement, as well as share practical tips on details of management. Some physicians even organize a buddy system or support group for people working on improving control. Such groups can be organized by a few individuals working on their own, or through their local American Diabetes Association chapter.

The final task in this initial phase is remembering the support and guidance you can give yourself when you feel stuck, frustrated, confused, or discouraged. It is likely that you will reach this point one or two times in the coming months; it is a natural part of the process. While you are still full of enthusiasm, plant the seeds for the times when you may forget how creative you are. Glance through Chapters 3 and 15, and review your strengths and skills. You might even write a note to yourself to be opened when you feel that you can't go on. Remind yourself of your accomplishments when you feel there is nothing you can do.

Summary of Step 1

Begin by creating a positive foundation for the work of learning the intensive regimen. Review your support system and strengthen it where it is weak. This includes support from yourself as well as from your doctor, diabetes educator, family, friends, and others with diabetes. Remember that this is a fail-safe process designed to help you overcome any obstacles that may arise.

Step 2: Have laboratory tests taken to provide a benchmark of control

Discuss with your physician the tests that will provide an accurate indication of your present level of control. These usually include hemoglobin A1c, fasting or random glucose, and blood lipids (fats, triglycerides, and cholesterol). (These are described in Step 3.) The results of these tests, along with your other records, tell you how far you have to go to obtain optimal control. More importantly, they tell you how far you have come after a few weeks of learning. The feedback you receive when you compare the next set of lab tests with these results may be very encouraging. Or, if there is little improvement, the new tests (together with your records of home tests, diet, stress, and exercise) will help you determine what to do next.

Step 3: Learn the skills and information basic to the intensive regimen

3a. Learn How to Test Blood Sugar and Urine.

Learn to test your blood for glucose (the type of sugar predominant in human blood). Learn the relationship of this test to urine tests, and the meaning of different laboratory tests your physician requests. Also, learn a record-keeping method that makes it easy to monitor your day-to-day control.

Self blood glucose testing is possibly the greatest advance in diabetes care since the discovery of insulin. It provides accurate information about the level of your blood sugar. On the basis of this information, you can make decisions regarding insulin dosage, exercise, food intake, stress, and reactions. It is one of the keys to achieving both optimal metabolic control and greater freedom in your life.

You can understand the importance of this tool if you consider the automatic "testing" process in people who do not have diabetes. There is a continuous monitoring of blood sugar levels, with feedback to the pancreas and other organs that release hormones to maintain normal levels. The information is available within seconds; insulin and other hormones regulating blood sugar levels begin acting immediately. When blood sugar levels rise after a meal, the pancreas releases insulin into the bloodstream. If a person without diabetes feels stressed or if blood sugar falls because of exercise, glucose is released by the liver, and adrenaline and other hormones inhibit the action of insulin. Through these processes, blood glucose levels are kept between 60 and 110 mg/dl (3.3 and 6.1 mmol/L). Throughout the day and night, a person without diabetes secretes a relatively steady level of insulin. Upon eating, extra insulin is released to keep the blood sugar in the normal range.

When you develop Type 1 diabetes, you begin to lose most or all of your ability to produce insulin. You still generate the other hormones that cause blood sugar to rise and fall, but the key hormone that allows cells to utilize blood sugar is missing. Your body signals high blood sugar, but there is little or no response from the pancreas. Those with Type 2 diabetes either have a pancreas that doesn't produce enough insulin to meet the body's needs, or a body that isn't able to use insulin properly usually as a result of malfunctioning insulin-receptor cells. (Insulin receptors absorb glucose in muscles and other body tissue.)

You need to enter into the control process consciously, injecting insulin or taking oral medication and monitoring blood sugar levels by tests and by how you feel. Your feelings indicate when blood sugar levels are too low and you are having an insulin reaction; they also indicate when blood sugar levels are high. But you cannot feel the difference between normal (60–110 mg/dl [3.3–6.1 mmol/L]), moderately high (111–180 mg/dl [6.1–10 mmol/L]), and very high (181–240 mg/dl [10–13.3 mmol/L]) levels. Until the last dozen or so years, the only daily tests were urine glucose sticks or tablets that give only a rough idea of blood sugar level. They do not give precise feedback; they only indicate whether you are a little out of control or very out of control. They do have their use in diabetes care, but it is limited.

Self blood glucose testing gives information on your level of control at the time of the test. You can get an accurate reading (within 10 to 20% of the actual value) in the critical area where urine tests only read "negative" (below 180 mg/dl [10 mmol/L]). With this feedback, you can tell when you need extra insulin (or less food) and how much. You know when you are having an insulin reaction and you do not mistake the symptoms of an anxiety attack for those of low blood sugar. You know the effect on blood sugar level of a particular meal or snack, or a period of exercise. By making conscious decisions about this information, you can guide your body to a level of metabolic control that is near normal.

Precise feedback of blood sugar level has an impact on the behavior of many who do blood testing. It becomes easier to deal with the craving for a hot fudge sundae when you've seen your blood sugar shoot up to 450 mg/dl (25 mmol/L) after eating one. A much-postponed stress management class becomes a high priority when you've seen a distressing day at work produce a record high in blood sugar. With home blood glucose testing, you have a tool for understanding how you live with diabetes. You begin to understand the reasons for the highs and lows, and you gain the ability to do something about them. That's living well!

Self Blood Glucose Testing

Many people now use meters for reading their strips. It's more convenient and accurate than making a visual estimation based on color. For this reason, pregnant women and those using the insulin pump should use meters. People with color blindness or other visual impairment need them as well. Anyone fascinated with gadgetry may find that the little machine boosts their motivation to test.

Since a variety of strips and meters are available we will not give specific testing instructions here. The new meters are more user-friendly, faster, smaller, and much more automatic than the old meters. We encourage you to attend a class in blood glucose testing or have your procedures and interpretation checked by your physician or nurse. Training is often provided by the meter vendor. We will, however, offer some tips and cautions that will help you with your home blood testing.

To ensure the accuracy of your readings, test where it is at least 60° F, or breathe on the strip while the blood is on it to keep it warm. Many of the newer strips are usable over a wider temperature range—check the information that comes with your strips. Use the sides of your fingertips; they are less sensitive. Never use such a small drop of blood that you have to smear it on the strip (the blood should stay liquid during the testing time). Some of the newer strips, however, allow you to add more blood if the initial drop was not sufficient. Never use gauze to remove the blood (it may scrape off the test material). If timing is not automatic, keep your timing within three to five seconds of the required time (don't estimate). Never use test strips after they have expired.

If you visually read the test strips, estimate blood sugar levels when the colors fall between those on the container. A chief source of error is choosing one of the "official" scores when the actual color is midway between those given. Do not match your test strip with a color chart other than the one on the container from which it came. BG Chemstrips can be visually read, and their color is stable for about a month. This means you can bring your most recent test strips to your care provider to be read in a meter. Compare your visual estimates with the meter reading; this feedback will sharpen your reading accuracy.

Here are a few of the objections and concerns about home blood testing that are raised by users.

"I'm afraid it'll hurt." We already stick ourselves at least once a day to take insulin, yet fingertips seem more sensitive than thighs and upper arms. Actually, there is little pain, especially along the sides of the fingertips. Often you hardly feel the prick. With the automatic devices adjusted to the proper depth, you almost never notice when the lancet strikes. The anticipation of the pain is usually far worse than anything you actually experience. It is a good idea to rotate from finger to finger, just as insulin shots are given in a different site each time. This decreases the possibility of your fingertips becoming sore from repeated pricks.

In development are "non-invasive" meters that will read your blood sugar through the skin, without requiring a drop of blood. Rumor is that they may be quite expensive, at least initially. (See Chapter 21.)

"Won't it be terribly expensive if I start testing several times a day?" Costs can be lowered two ways. First, with visually read tests, you can cut the strips lengthwise (in two) with a scissors. If you have sharp eyes you can cut them into three or four strips, once you have learned to interpret the readings accurately. (Be sure to put unused strips back into the container right away. Cut strips have been tested and found to give reliable results, even when stored cut for a month. Some meters allow for using a half strip, but with most you must use a whole one.)

Second, buy strips from a discount mail-order firm (see Appendix). If you have health insurance, check if testing equipment and supplies are covered. Some medical plans are now covering these costs. The American Diabetes Association, the American Association of Diabetes Educators, and the American Dietetic Association are lobbying at state and national levels to require insurance companies to cover these needed expenses.

"Won't I get discouraged if I see too many high tests?" You probably will, but deal with the discouragement by remembering that this is only one of several steps in learning to control your blood sugar. High tests indicate that you have more to learn, not that you are weak or unable to control yourself. Use the tests to increase your motivation to master the regimen.

"Can children handle home blood testing?" Children can do it, with the proper support and guidance of adults. (It helps if the adults stick their own fingers and test their own blood a few times to offer encouragement and a good example.) Four- and five-year-olds have learned the testing procedure, though they are usually a few years older before they begin doing their own tests. In fact, once they are trained in testing, children become excellent instructors of their peers.

"How often do I have to test?" Curiosity may lead you to do frequent testing at first. It is satisfying to be able to determine the exact impact of food, activity, or stress on your blood sugar levels. For the first month or two of the intensive regimen, you may need to test up to six times a day to understand your pattern of response. This includes tests before each meal, at bedtime, and, at least part of the time, one or two hours after a meal. These "postprandial" tests give you informative feedback on the impact certain foods have on your blood sugar.

"I can tell whether I'm high or low by how I feel." This is true only if you are very high or very low. Usually, you cannot sense much without actual symptoms. You can learn to sense blood sugar levels in the midrange (70–200 mg/dl [3.8–11.1 mmol/L]) by using the feedback from your blood tests. For a few weeks, write down your guess before testing. Write down the level you think you are at (given what you know about what you have eaten and done since the last test), and also write down the first number that comes to your mind. See if you come close to your actual test using either method. Most studies have shown that we are not as accurate as we think in estimating our blood sugar; the above exercise can help you determine this. Even if you are correct half the time, that's not good enough. A meter will do much better.

With optimal control of diabetes, the test values you attain can be close to the blood sugar levels of a person who does not have diabetes. The following table gives the target glucose levels recommended by the American Diabetes Association, as well as levels of hemoglobin A1c (see page 69, "Lab Tests Your Physician May Order"). It also shows values that indicate where action should be taken to improve them. Note that action is not automatically indicated if the value is above the goal—there is a midzone that is close enough to the goal that significant action is probably not required.

Glycemic Control for People with Diabetes

Biochemical index	Nondiabetic	Goal	Action suggested
Preprandial glucose (mg/dl) [mmol/L]	<115 [6.3]	80–120 [4.4–6.6]	<80 [4.4] >140 [7.7]
Bedtime glucose (mg/dl) [mmol/L]	<120 [6.6]	100–140 [5.5–7.7]	<100 [5.5] >160 [8.8]
Hemoglobin A1c (%)	<6	<7	<8

For the Physician: These values are for nonpregnant individuals. "Action suggested" depends on individual patient circumstances. Such actions may include enhanced diabetes self-management education, comanagement with a diabetes team, referral to an endocrinologist, change in pharmacological therapy; initiation or increased SMBG, or more frequent contact with the patient. HbA1c is referenced to a nondiabetic range of 4.0–6.0% (mean 5.0%, SD 0.5%).

These are demanding standards, requiring full practice of the intensive regimen. If you can achieve them, great. If not, keep working to improve your control. Remember that you are acceptable even when your test results are not. You and your doctor may agree on a higher set of target levels to begin with if these seem too difficult to attain. You may also have to shift your targets up if you have too many insulin reactions.

By checking your blood sugar one to two hours after a meal, you will begin to learn how the food you have just eaten is affecting your sugar level. Your goal should be less than 180 mg/dl (10 mmol/L) 1 1/2 to 2 hours after your meal (postprandial). This information will refine your skill in using your intuition, symptoms, feelings, and blood tests to predict how different foods will affect your control. Knowing this, you will be in a better position to choose the target blood sugar levels appropriate for you.

The Intensive Regimen

Urine Testing

In the intensive regimen, urine testing is still very useful to check for ketones in the urine. You should keep ketone test supplies on hand, especially when you are ill or stressed. Both tablets and strips are available.

The traditional test for sugar in the urine is useful in the moderate and loose regimens. However, for those on the intensive regimen, the test does not offer the precise feedback needed to maintain optimal control. For this reason, it is covered in Chapter 7, "The Moderate Regimen."

Metabolic Record Keeping

Keeping precise records that you and your doctor can learn from is as important as doing the testing itself. At the beginning, we recommend that you log your tests, diet, activity level, and stress. (Once control is established, less detailed records will be sufficient.) During this period, you are a scientist studying your own metabolism. The information you gather will help you learn about your individual patterns of response.

Here are two different forms you can photocopy for a daily log and periodic summary of your records. Other logs provided by the meter and insulin companies are also available. For the daily log, you can choose a simple form that allows you to see the pattern of test results easily but does not allow detailed recording of food and activity, or a more elaborate form that provides space for detailed record keeping. (See pages 106-108 for examples of filled-in logs in Step 7 below.) Many meters now have memories to record test results; they can also be linked to computers for printouts and analyses.

Daily Diabetes Log I

Date Time	Insulin Dose	Breakfast Test	Lunch Test	Dinner Test	Bed Test	Illness, change of pattern, stress

Daily Diabetes Log II

Date Time	Blood Test & Reactions	Insulin Dosage	Activity & Exercise	Food	Comments: stress illness, etc.
———	———	———	———	———	———————
———	———	———	———	———	———————
———	———	———	———	———	———————
———	———	———	———	———	———————
———	———	———	———	———	———————
———	———	———	———	———	———————
———	———	———	———	———	———————
———	———	———	———	———	———————
———	———	———	———	———	———————
———	———	———	———	———	———————
———	———	———	———	———	———————
———	———	———	———	———	———————
———	———	———	———	———	———————
———	———	———	———	———	———————
———	———	———	———	———	———————
———	———	———	———	———	———————
———	———	———	———	———	———————
———	———	———	———	———	———————
———	———	———	———	———	———————
———	———	———	———	———	———————
———	———	———	———	———	———————
———	———	———	———	———	———————
———	———	———	———	———	———————
———	———	———	———	———	———————
———	———	———	———	———	———————
———	———	———	———	———	———————
———	———	———	———	———	———————
———	———	———	———	———	———————
———	———	———	———	———	———————

When you miss a test, indicate your estimate (for example. "low," "high," or "150." Include reactions in the blood sugar test column, with the amount of food used to treat it in the food column. Grade reactions as mild (1), strong (2), or severe (3). Indicate the type of insulin if more than one type is used.

Grade activity for each period of the day relative to what is normal for you at that time: 1 = minimal activity, 2 = less activity than usual, 3 = your normal level, 4 = more activity than usual, 5 = maximum activity. Include the duration of time of activity or exercise.

Under "Food," indicate calories or exchanges and anything out of the ordinary, such as delayed meals. If you calculate only carbohydrates, indicate over- or underconsumption. Also, note the particular foods consumed and your post-meal test, if you performed one.

Under "Comments," include stressful events, whether or not you sensed an emotional response. Note difficulty with sleeping, periods of tension or relaxation, emotional highs, and physical occurrences such as illness, menstruation, or low energy—anything that can help explain the variations in your tests.

Remember, these records are not useful only to your doctor or diabetes educator; they are most valuable to you. Analyze and learn from them, and make changes based on what you learn. By recording this information, you enable yourself to see the patterns of your life with diabetes. (The interpretation of these records is discussed in Step 7.)

Lab Tests Your Physician May Order

When you regularly test your blood sugar at home, traditional fasting blood glucose lab tests become less important. However, it can provide a quality check on your testing technique. Bring your materials and test yourself at the same time your blood is drawn at the lab; if there is a significant difference (more than 10%), ask your doctor or nurse to review your procedure.

The lab is able to do other tests with the same sample of blood. Hemoglobin A1c (HbA1c or glycosylated hemoglobin or glycated hemoglobin), gives an overall evaluation of blood sugar control. This test measures the amount of glucose that has bound to hemoglobin in red blood cells. The average blood cell lasts for two to three months; the test results give an approximate summary or average of your blood sugar levels over that period. Higher readings usually indicate a need for changing regimen or level of adherence. See the table on page 65 for ADA target levels. The DCCT showed that every measure of improvement in blood sugar helps avoid complications. There is also evidence of a threshold effect at HbA1c levels of less than 8.1%. (This means that HbA1c levels of less than 8.1% may further reduce the risk of complications.) Aim for the ADA target values in the intensive regimen.

Test methods vary among labs, so different values may be used to evaluate your test. Ask your doctor, diabetes educator, or the lab technician for those being used in your test. Efforts are being made to standardize the test procedure, which will likely conform to the technique used in the DCCT. As a general rule, less than 1 percentage point above the labs upper limit of normal is a good target for someone with diabetes for example, if the upper limit of normal in the lab is 6%, the target would be less than 7%).

Another lab test, though not yet widely used or available, measures the average blood glucose level for a three-week period. It's called a fructosamine test and is marketed under the name RoTag. It can be useful when you and your care provider are making frequent adjustments in your regimen and want prompt feedback.

Another set of blood tests reflects overall control. These tests measure certain blood fats (or lipids). High levels of cholesterol or triglycerides are often associated with high blood sugar values. Their presence over long periods contributes to the development of diabetic complications. These blood fats are also major contributors to the development of heart and blood vessel disease, conditions which affect diabetics at a rate two to four times greater than those without diabetes. These blood lipids should be tested every year or two to see if they are in the normal range. For children, if values are in the range of acceptable risk, tests can be repeated every five years. If your test levels are high and you are working to reduce them with diet and control, it is helpful to be tested every two or three months. It is also useful to measure high-density lipoprotein (HDL) cholesterol, the "good" cholesterol (the more you have, the better).

Values for Blood Lipids

The following table gives the ADA recommended acceptable, borderline, and high risk levels for adults.

Lipid levels for adults

Risk for adults with diabetes	Cholesterol (mg/dl)	HDL cholesterol (mg/dl)	LDL cholesterol (mg/dl)	Triglycerides (mg/dl)
Acceptable	<200	—	<130	<200
Borderline	200–239	—	130–159	200–399
High	≥240	≤35	≥160	≥400

Total cholesterol below 200 mg/dl is considered acceptable; between 200 and 239, borderline high; and 240 or greater, high.

Those with diabetes should not only have total cholesterol measured, but also their low-density lipoprotein (LDL) and high-density lipoprotein (HDL) cholesterols and triglycerides measured. LDL levels of 130 mg/dl or less are considered acceptable; 130–159, borderline high risk; and 160 or greater, high risk. Although desired HDL levels are somewhat controversial, levels less than 35 mg/dl are considered a risk factor, and those greater than 60 are considered protective. Rather than looking at HDL levels, some consider the ratio of total cholesterol to HDL cholesterol a better measure of risk. A higher HDL level means a lower (and more desirable) ratio; ratios between 3.5 and 4 to 1 considered satisfactory. Triglycerides should be less than 250 mg/dl, and treated with medication if greater than 500.

CAUTION: These numbers are subject to your specific situation; how they apply to you should be discussed with your physician.

Tests and Our Emotions

It is natural to feel discouraged or guilty when tests show that you are not in very good control. If the tests are high enough, you may feel like quitting. At times such as these, remember that you don't have to feel guilty about your errors and limitations. Use them to guide your next steps of learning, and turn the discouragement and guilt into motivation for change.

3b. Learn How to Recognize and Treat Insulin Reactions

This step is so important that we have devoted an entire chapter to it (Chapter 9), which should be read regardless of what you may already know about insulin reactions. The symptoms of reactions change; they become more subtle when our metabolism is well controlled. Because our blood sugar is closer to normal, irregularities in food, activity, or schedule can cause reactions to occur more frequently at first.

In addition, it can be difficult to recognize the symptoms of a reaction. This is sometimes caused by changes in the production of hormones that signal low blood sugar. Again, review Chapter 9 to increase your awareness of early reaction symptoms and ensure that you wake up during nighttime hypoglycemia.

3c. Survey the Basics of Diabetic Metabolism

Diabetes is a disorder of metabolism, the process through which the food we eat becomes energy and replenishes our tissues. When we have diabetes, we play an active role in this process, doing things that occur automatically in nondiabetics. Thus we need to learn about our metabolism, especially as it relates to blood glucose.

Let's begin with some praise for blood glucose. We spend so much time trying to control it that we sometimes forget how vital it is to our lives. Glucose is a major fuel for all of our cells, and is the only source of energy for the brain and nerve tissue. We realize the importance of glucose when we experience the confusion associated with an insulin reaction—a sign that not enough glucose is reaching the brain. We can respect our blood glucose, even as we work to keep it within acceptable limits.

Carbohydrates are our main source of glucose. The different forms of starch and sugar in fruits, vegetables, beans, grains, and dairy foods are all transformed into glucose through the digestive process. (A small amount also comes from protein and fat, but these foods go through slower metabolic cycles and do not contribute as much to the production of glucose.) Once in the bloodstream, glucose is used to provide energy for our life processes and activities, or it is stored. It can be stored as glycogen in the liver or in the muscles, or it may be converted to fat and stored as adipose tissue.

In those without diabetes, glucose levels are maintained by the interaction of a number of hormones. These hormones increase or decrease the blood sugar level to keep it between 60 and 120 mg/dl. The hormones act in response to a variety of factors, primarily food, exercise, illness, and stress. When the pancreas senses an increase in blood sugar, it releases insulin. This enables glucose to enter cells that would remain closed without insulin—closed and without fuel.

When we develop Type 1 diabetes, we lose this automatic release of insulin. Blood sugar reaches very high levels (sometimes up to ten times the normal level) because the pancreas cannot produce enough, if any, insulin. Without adequate insulin, glucose molecules are unable to pass through cell walls, and the cells begin to burn fats instead. This process is not as efficient as sugar metabolism, and the byproducts—ketones—contribute to the ill feelings that are normally present when diabetes is first diagnosed. Once diagnosed, Type 1 diabetes must be treated with injected insulin to supplement or replace the insulin from the pancreas.

But insulin is only one of the hormones affecting blood sugar levels; several others work to raise and lower the amount of circulating glucose. Glucagon, also produced by the pancreas, stimulates the release of glucose from the liver. (This substance is available for treating reactions when a person is unconscious.) Low blood sugar or stress hormones cause the pancreas to release glucagon into the bloodstream. The hormones released when we are under stress include cortisol and epinephrine, both from the adrenal gland. In addition to stimulating glucagon, they inhibit the action of insulin. Another hormone that opposes the action of insulin is growth hormone, released by the pituitary gland.

In those without diabetes, these hormones work together, raising and lowering blood sugar to maintain proper levels. When activity increases, they increase the glucose available to support it. When a person is under stress, they ensure that the muscles and nervous system are supplied with enough glucose to function properly. After eating, the balance shifts to accommodate the influx of glucose.

When diabetes develops, insulin, the hormone most important in lowering blood sugar, is no longer available in adequate supply. However, the others continue to flow freely, and contribute to dramatic increases in blood sugar level. Even when insulin therapy begins, the interaction between insulin and other glucose-increasing hormones is not the same. The insulin is usually administered in fixed doses rather than precisely measured doses the body delivers in response to varying needs. The automatic cycle between blood sugar level and insulin release is broken. The only thing that can begin to replace this process is testing blood and making decisions about insulin dosage, food, and activity based on test results.

Research scientists and medical engineers are attempting to create devices that will artificially restore the automatic process. Though good progress is being made, these devices are probably years from general availability. For now, we have the challenge of playing an active role in one of nature's more complex processes.

3d. Understand the Factors Determining Blood Sugar Level

Metabolism is an internal process that is continuously responding to external factors. Diet, activity, insulin, medication, and emotional and physical stress influence our sugar metabolism and the resulting blood sugar levels. Before we can effectively control these levels, we must understand why they fluctuate. We will review each of the factors influencing blood sugar level and explore how they work together. (Here we discuss only their effect on blood sugar; later we will discuss other ways they are important in diabetes management.)

Knowing how these factors influence blood sugar level allows us to understand why tests are unexpectedly high or low. Here, we will describe the day-to-day aspects of each factor; later we will consider the occasional aspects or those that affect only some of us.

Major Influences on Blood Sugar Level In Type 1 Diabetes

Universal	Particular
(These factors affect all people with Type 1 diabetes.)	(These factors are temporary or affect only certain people.)
Insulin	
Types	Immunity to insulin action
Dosage	Interaction with other drugs (medicine, alcohol, marijuana, etc.)
Site of injection	High blood sugar levels inhibit action of insulin
Schedule	Too high dosage
Rebound from reactions	
Diet	
Total calories	High fat consumption inhibits insulin action
Distribution of calories among fat, carbohydrate, and protein	
Rate of absorption (glycemic index)	
Fiber	

Universal	Particular
(These factors affect all people with Type 1 diabetes.)	(These factors are temporary or affect only certain people.)

Activity

Universal	Particular
Typical level	Exercise increases blood sugar when it is higher than 250 mg/dl (13.8 mmol/L)
Frequency and level of exercise	
(There is a delayed lowering of blood sugar as well as the immediate effect with strenuous exercise.)	

Stress

Universal	Particular
Physical tension/relaxation	Infection, illness, fever and other physical stresses raise blood sugar
Possible increase or decrease caused by emotional stress	Growth spurts
	Over- and undereating when stressed

Other

Universal	Particular
Overall degree of regularity	Effects of marijuana, cigarettes, alcohol and other recreational drugs
Menstruation, menopause and pregnancy all affect control	
Socioeconomic—Not having enough money for insulin, testing supplies, and proper diet	

Insulin The effect of injected insulin on blood sugar level depends upon the type(s) of insulin used, the level and schedule of dosage, the site of injection, the timing of injection in relation to meals, the level of blood sugar, and a number of other factors. Variations in any of these factors can cause changes in blood sugar level.

The type(s) of insulin you use determines the pattern of insulin activity in your body throughout the day. A rapid-acting insulin, such as regular, can begin acting as soon as thirty minutes following injection and reaches its peak two to five hours afterward. Its effect is over in four to eight hours. A new insulin analog, lispro, is even more rapid acting. It is very quick in onset and peaks about an hour following injection, with a duration of only two to four hours (see Chapter 21 for more on insulin

The Intensive Regimen

analogs). Because you can take lispro at the time of eating, you have the advantage of knowing precisely how much you will need; if you eat more, you can take more. You can also avoid reactions from delayed meals, and because of the short duration of action, avoid the delayed hypoglycemia (2-3 hours after meals) that can occur with regular insulin. NPH, on the other hand, begins acting in one to four hours, and peaks in six to twelve hours, with a duration of twelve to twenty-four hours. Each type of insulin has its characteristic profile of action. Often, rapid-acting insulin is combined with an intermediate or long-acting insulin to create a series of insulin peaks. These are matched to mealtimes and a "basal" level to accommodate the body's ongoing needs for energy, and to keep the processes functioning properly.

(Human insulin, now available because of genetic engineering, appears to act sooner, peak earlier, and have a shorter duration than animal insulin. This is particularly true for the duration of human ultralente.)

In addition, each person has an individual pattern of response to insulin. This is why the times in the following table have so great a range. One person may find regular insulin taking effect in thirty minutes, another may wait an hour. The onset, peak, and duration of action all vary from one person to another.

You should know the pattern of insulin action your present regimen provides. When does each insulin peak for you? How long is it active? Do your mealtimes coincide with the times of maximum insulin activity? (Your physician or diabetes educator can help you understand your insulin profile.) Blood testing allows you to adjust insulin dosage and scheduling to match the varying need for insulin. In practically every situation, this requires at least two shots a day.

Timing of Insulin Action (in hours)

Type	Lispro	Regular	Semilente	NPH	Lente	Ultralente
Onset	$\frac{1}{10}$	$\frac{1}{2}$-1	1-3	1-4	1-4	4-6
Peak	$\frac{1}{2}$-1	2-5	2-8	6-12	6-12	8-20
Duration	2-4	4-8	8-16	12-24	18-28	24-30

Note: Table derived from several sources, each of which gives different figures. Insulin activity varies greatly from person to person and between animal insulin and human insulin, so these times should be used only as guidelines. Times for Ultralente are for human Ultralente.

The ability of insulin to lower blood sugar is decreased by high blood sugar levels. At normal levels (70-110 mg/dl [3.8-6.1 mmol/L]), one unit of insulin will usually lower blood glucose around 30 mg/dl (1.6 mmol/L). With a high level (such as 300 mg/dl [16.6 mmol/L]), it might take three units of insulin to lower it by the same amount. This is one reason blood sugar levels can skyrocket and remain high for several days. If stress or a food binge pushes tests to high levels and the usual insulin dose is taken, its effect is inhibited by the excess sugar. Extra insulin at times such as these enables you to regain balance.

High fat levels in the blood also reduce insulin's ability to lower blood sugar. Often, you will experience a high test after a meal unusually high in fat but not necessarily high in carbohydrates. The insulin is not able to do the same amount of work in the presence of excess fat. If your diet is high in fat, lower your fat intake to increase the effectiveness of your insulin and improve your cardiovascular health.

A frustrating aspect of insulin therapy is the high blood sugar levels that often result from having low blood sugar; this is the rebound from an insulin reaction. One of the body's responses to the stress of a reaction is to release glucagon, which releases glucose from the liver. It is possible to have high blood sugar levels within an hour of hypoglycemia. This can happen even if we don't overeat when treating the reaction. (This spontaneous rebound can be a lifesaver if one passes out from very low blood sugar.) Hypoglycemia caught in an early stage usually doesn't produce this increase.

Occasionally, the rebound effect becomes a regular part of a diabetic regimen. This can occur when excessive doses of insulin result in regular periods of low blood sugar that are not sensed as reactions (usually occurring during sleep). The body's natural defenses bring blood sugar to a level above normal by the morning test, and insulin may be mistakenly increased. (This Somogyi reaction is discussed in Chapter 9.) High levels before breakfast can also be caused by a normal physiologic predawn rise in blood sugar called the "dawn phenomenon." If this is the case, predinner or prebedtime insulin should be increased. Near-normal 3:00 a.m. blood sugars paired with high prebreakfast sugars suggest the dawn phenomenon. Near-normal bedtime and low-normal or hypoglycemic 3:00 a.m. levels with high prebreakfast levels suggest the Somogyi reaction. If all three levels are high, more insulin is probably needed.

Two other variables of insulin usage have a more subtle effect: the location of the injection and the timing of the injection relative to when you eat. Being aware of these variables increases your ability to fine-tune control after you have mastered the basics, but they are not nearly as important as the facts described above, especially in the beginning of your effort to improve control.

The site of insulin injection affects the timing of its action. Insulin injected into the abdomen is absorbed most rapidly; in the thigh, most slowly; and in the arm, at a moderate rate. In one experiment, the time of absorption was approximately 60 minutes for the abdomen, 75 minutes for the arm, and 90 minutes for the thigh. However, injection site does not seem to be a factor when using lispro, the very fast acting insulin. The different absorption times can be used strategically: Inject in the abdomen when blood sugar is high or when you want to eat soon, and in the leg when a meal may be delayed or when blood sugar is low. (It is necessary to rotate injection sites; change the location of your shot each day within any area of the body.)

If the site of injection is exercised vigorously, absorption is hastened. An arm swinging a tennis racquet or legs pumping while running will quickly activate the insulin injected into them. If you are about to exercise and have recently taken an injection, eat before such activity unless blood sugar is high. If you want to bring down high blood sugar, giving your shot in the area that is exercised will hasten the process.

The timing of injection in relation to mealtime is another variable of insulin therapy. Unless blood sugar is below 80 mg/dl (4.4 mmol/L), insulin should usually be taken between one-half and one hour before meals (unless it is lispro, which can be taken anytime within 15 minutes of eating, or even just as you begin). This allows the insulin to begin working at the time your blood glucose begins to increase from a meal. If you wait until just before a meal or after it, blood sugar is already high by the time the insulin begins to take effect. Shorten the wait if you have reactions before or during a meal.

Recreational and medicinal drugs can significantly affect blood sugar levels, by increasing or decreasing the effectiveness of insulin and other hormones that regulate metabolism. Alcoholic beverages, especially when taken on an empty stomach, increase the ability of insulin to lower blood sugar. Alcohol also interferes with the liver's production of glucose. Drinking before a meal can lead to reactions especially if insulin has just been taken. After a drink or two, it can become difficult to notice the symptoms of a reaction. Drinking enough to become drunk increases the risks further. Nausea, vomiting, dehydration, and reduced awareness play havoc with diabetic control and can lead to ketoacidosis or severe reactions.

People with diabetes should use alcohol only in moderation and with awareness. Avoid drinking on an empty stomach, when blood sugar is low, or after strenuous exercise. Accompany a predinner drink with some carbohydrates. Know the carbohydrate content of your favorite beverages and take it into account in your diet. In some cases, alcohol must be avoided completely. This is an important issue to discuss with your doctor.

Marijuana affects blood sugar by breaking down glycogen, a form of sugar stored in the liver and other body tissue. The release of glycogen increases blood glucose levels. There is no doubt about marijuana's other effect: inducing the "munchies." This drug-induced hunger combined with weakened inhibitions wreaks havoc on a marijuana user's diet. As with alcohol, marijuana decreases the awareness of an insulin reaction until it is far advanced, because the sensations of being high mask the symptoms. The more powerful forms of marijuana carry the added risk of dependency.

Prescription Drug Interactions with Insulin

Many common prescription drugs can seriously affect blood sugar levels by their interaction with insulin. Some reduce insulin's ability to lower blood sugar, or otherwise increase blood glucose. These include diuretics such as Lasix or Thiazide, often used to rid the body of excess water for weight reduction, or for heart disease and high blood pressure. (There are options available for those with diabetes. Talk with your physician and see Chapter 18.) Others include Isoniazid (an antituberculosis drug) and estrogens or steroids that increase glucose production in the liver.

Other drugs add to the hypoglycemic (blood sugar-lowering) effect of insulin, sometimes causing serious insulin reactions. These include anticoagulants (Coumadin), sulfa (Gantrisin), tranquilizers (Thorazine), MAO inhibitors (Nardil and Parnate), and propranolol (Inderal). Propranolol and other "beta blockers" are potentially dangerous because they minimize the usual signs of an insulin reaction—sweating and rapid heartbeat. They are primarily used to treat high blood pressure.

The over-the-counter drugs most likely to influence blood sugar are decongestants and antihistamines.

Ask whether any drugs prescribed for you affect insulin or blood sugar, especially when you go to a doctor other than the one you see for your diabetes. Use your blood test results to determine whether you should change your insulin dosage while taking the prescribed medication.

Another unique condition of insulin therapy is that some people with Type 1 diabetes develop insulin resistance, resulting in decreased effectiveness. (In extreme—but rare—cases, insulin dosage has been increased to hundreds of units per day.) Resistance is caused by antibodies created by the immune system in response to impurities in insulin or to the insulin from a particular animal. Today, all insulin is extremely pure. However, anyone who has been taking insulin for several years could develop some degree of insulin resistance. It can usually be overcome by using human insulin. When the change to more highly purified insulin is made, insulin requirements can decrease by as much as one-third. In those with Type 2 diabetes, insulin resistance is a basic part of the disease and present in nearly everyone. Its causes are different from Type 1. (See the next chapter on Type 2 diabetes.)

Summary The types of insulin, dosage, schedule of injection, and blood glucose levels themselves are the most important factors influencing blood glucose level. With the intensive regimen, the goal is to have peaks of insulin activity coincide with the times immediately following meals. This is achieved by taking at least two injections of insulin per day, usually mixing rapid-acting and intermediate or long-acting insulins. You should be familiar with the pattern of insulin activity provided by your regimen.

The action of insulin is inhibited by high blood sugar levels (over 240 mg/dl [13.3 mmol/L]) or by high fat consumption. When blood sugar is very high, each unit of insulin is less effective.

Because of the delay before insulin begins to act, injections should usually be taken 30 to 60 minutes before meals (except for lispro insulin). The site of injection has a significant effect on the timing of insulin activity; the abdomen provides the most rapid absorption, the arm moderate, and the thigh the slowest.

When insulin reactions occur, low blood sugar levels trigger a stress response resulting in high blood sugar, even if one has eaten moderately to treat the reaction.

Insulin's ability to lower blood sugar can be inhibited or increased by interaction with recreational and prescription drugs. This can result in reactions or unexpected high blood sugar tests.

Meal Planning

The food you eat is the second major factor affecting blood glucose level.

We can see the impact of the total calories consumed on a given day and how they are distributed between meals and snacks. A small lunch on the run or a missed snack can cause low blood sugar and a reaction. Overindulgence at one meal results in high tests afterwards. Heavy eating throughout a day can cause blood sugar levels to remain high for several days if adjustments are not made.

A regular schedule of eating, and a consistent caloric intake are necessary aspects of learning to manage diabetes. With regular home blood glucose testing, you can determine the effect of variances in regimen, and you can learn to correct them by adjusting day-to-day insulin dose and exercise. (Once you have mastered your regimen, it is possible to vary food intake and schedule and still maintain good control.)

Another aspect of meal planning affecting control is the rate at which foods are converted into blood sugar. Although its utility is still being debated, nutrition researchers have developed a glycemic index to measure the conversion rate for different foods. They have determined, for instance, that potatoes raise blood sugar as fast as a drink of glucose syrup. Pasta and beans, on the other hand, are absorbed much more slowly and result in a smaller increase in blood sugar. (See Chapter 10.)

Carbohydrate, fat, and protein all have different absorption rates. Simple carbohydrates (sugars and highly refined starches) usually reach the blood stream quickly, peaking between 15 and 30 minutes. Complex carbohydrates (most starchy vegetables, whole grains, and beans) take between 30 and 90 minutes to reach their maximum impact on blood sugar. Fats take approximately 90 minutes; proteins take approximately 3 hours. (Absorption rates vary greatly among specific foods. Chapter 10 presents a more detailed discussion of this subject.)

A well-balanced meal allows a gradual, sustained intake of nutrition, avoiding the sudden high peak of blood sugar that a meal of simple carbohydrates causes. The amount of fiber in our diet also affects absorption rate. High-fiber diets tend to slow the rate. High fat content interferes with the action of insulin, causing a need for higher doses. However, fat tends to slow the absorption of other foods eaten at the same time.

Significant variations in caloric consumption or dietary balance can result in unexpectedly high or low blood glucose levels. For instance, high blood sugar caused by eating simple carbohydrates can be followed by a serious reaction. Not enough slowly absorbed food is in the intestine to provide a steady, continuous supply of blood sugar. A large meal of steak and potatoes in the evening can elevate blood sugar levels the next morning because the food is digested slowly and the fat decreases insulin effectiveness. Knowing how these factors apply to you, supplemented by results of your blood glucose testing, will help you maintain control.

Summary The total calories consumed, caloric distribution between meals and snacks, and the types and combinations of foods consumed determine the impact on blood sugar level. Until you have learned the entire regimen, you should eat the same amounts of food (in terms of calories or grams of carbohydrates or exchanges) at the same times each day.

Simple carbohydrates (sugars, fruits, juices, milk) are converted to blood glucose within minutes; complex carbohydrates (starchy vegetables, whole grains, and beans) take from 30 to 90 minutes; fats take approximately 90 minutes; proteins can take up to three hours. In general, fats and proteins have relatively little influence on your blood sugar compared to carbohydrates. High-fiber foods are absorbed more slowly, and tend to slow the absorption rate of other foods as well. High fat consumption inhibits the action of insulin.

A diet that is high in fiber, low in fat, and minimizes the consumption of simple carbohydrates results in more stable blood sugar levels. This is probably the best diabetes meal plan.

Activity

This is the third major influence on blood sugar. Control is affected by our pattern of activity as well as any periods of special exercise or work. Changes in activity can cause increases or decreases in blood sugar levels and may result in insulin reactions. As with other factors determining blood sugar level, the more regular you are in your daily activities, the easier it will be to achieve optimal control.

Physical activity and time of exercise affect blood sugar in several ways. First, there is an immediate lowering due to the energy spent. The more strenuous the exercise, the faster blood glucose goes down. If insulin has not been decreased, or food increased, a reaction is likely to occur (unless blood sugar level is high to begin with). Furthermore, during and following exercise, blood sugar levels decrease as the muscles absorb and store glucose in addition to what they are burning. This process can continue for several hours after vigorous exercise. For this reason, reactions may occur long after you have finished the activity, because glucose levels are depleted by muscles that need to replenish their stores.

Once you have learned to adjust diet and insulin dose, it becomes easier to avoid reactions caused by exercise. In fact, the increased glucose storage means you will enjoy more stable blood sugar levels. When levels begin to fall, more glucose is available to bring them back to normal.

If you lead an active life, especially if you are able to follow a consistent exercise program, there is an added benefit: your sensitivity to insulin is increased. This means that exercise will lower your blood sugar more and insulin will be more effective. Insulin dose can be decreased by a few units, or more if you were previously sedentary. A conditioning program is an exercise regimen in which you function at peak three times a week for a least twenty minutes. Breathing is heavy and pulse is at the level defined for your age.

You don't have to exercise strenuously to gain benefits from physical activity. Moderate movement, such as walking or working in the garden, can have a significant effect on blood sugar levels, compared to sitting and reading or watching television. This is important, as you may need to avoid heavy exercise. If complications have developed, it can be harmful to engage in exercise programs that fail to respect your physical limitations. If you have early signs of complications, you should discuss your exercise program with your doctor.

Ironically, the ability of exercise to reduce blood sugar is diminished when levels are higher than 250 or 300 mg/dl (13.8 or 16.6 mmol/L), especially if ketones are present. When we need it most, the effect of exercise is reversed, and blood sugar might increase. If your blood sugar level is higher than 250 mg/dl (13.8 mmol/L), do not try to bring it down with exercise, especially when acetone tests are positive. At this level, your body doesn't perform well and you won't enjoy it anyway. (See Chapter 11 for more on exercising with high blood sugar levels.)

Summary Physical activity helps lower and stabilize blood sugar levels, with the greatest benefits gained from regular exercise. Changes in activity level must be balanced by corresponding adjustments of diet or insulin dose in order to avoid reactions. When complications are developing, medical guidance in choosing appropriate physical activity is necessary.

Chapter 11 gives more detail on all of these subjects.

Stress

Stress is the fourth major influence on blood sugar level. When we are presented with physical or emotional challenges, we adapt through a complex set of chemical and muscular changes. This physical adaptation is called the stress response, which itself is neither negative nor positive in itself. Hans Selye, the noted student of stress, draws a distinction between distress (negative), and eustress (positive). We need the stress response to function; it mobilizes us for action and organizes our defenses to maintain vital functions when we are ill or injured. However, in people with diabetes one aspect of the stress response becomes a challenge. To protect the brain and ensure energy for action, stress produces a rapid change of blood sugar level, often an increase.

Perhaps you have experienced a severe flu in which your urine or blood sugar tests were high even though you ate little. This is a classic example of the diabetic stress response triggered by a physical disorder. Other physical stressors include injury, burns, infections, severe pain, dehydration, surgery, hypothermia (extreme chill), intense exercise, and insulin reactions. These triggers cause blood sugar to increase drastically, insulin to be less effective, and, if the condition persists, toxic ketones to build up in the bloodstream.

If you experience any of these physical stresses, monitor your response by testing your blood sugar and urine ketones. Continue taking insulin, with extra injections as needed, and contact your physician if you do not return to normal blood sugar levels and absence of ketones within a day. There is danger of experiencing ketoacidosis (diabetic coma) if any serious physical disorder is not treated properly. The risk is decreased if you act immediately to compensate for the effect these disorders have on your control.

You don't have to be seriously ill for a physical stress to affect your blood sugar level; when you have a high test that you can't explain, determine what is causing the increase, for example an infected cut, a sunburn, or fatigue.

Emotions can trigger the stress response as easily as a physical disorder. In fact, the body can't really tell the difference. An argument, a disappointment, or a thrilling discovery can cause a release of hormones that raise or lower blood sugar. Frustration or depression that continues for days can cause elevated blood sugar levels throughout the period. (The effect we are describing here is independent of any food indulgence you may have during stressful times. This habit adds to the hormonal effects of stress to produce even higher blood sugar levels.)

So stress is another variable that helps you understand why your test results change, even when you are following your regimen carefully. Being aware of stress can help you adjust to the effects it has on your metabolism (and even control it).

Unfortunately, there are few studies that explain how emotional stress affects diabetic management. Like many other aspects of our condition, stress appears to be highly individual in its effects. Some experience relatively little change in blood sugar level after a stressful experience; others experience dramatic increases in blood sugar, or find that it decreases when they are under stress. The effect often depends on the type of emotion aroused, the duration and intensity of the experience, one's ability to express the feelings through communication or action, and the level of blood sugar at the time the incident begins.

Use blood glucose testing to do your own research on emotional stress in diabetes. When you have had a difficult day, an argument, a fright, or a disappointment, check your blood sugar level. See if it is significantly higher or lower than what you would expect on the basis of the day's activity and food. Some find that a stressful experience can raise blood sugar to 400 mg/dl (22.2 mmol/L), or even higher. Also, note whether you have reactions from particular types of stress, such as when you have expressed your feelings strongly. A decrease in blood sugar level is also possible. It is also helpful to keep notes on your observations in a section of your diabetes log. After a while, you will understand how your system responds to emotional stress.

People with diabetes who experience high stress levels often find that their blood sugar levels decrease when they take time to relax. A holiday or vacation can cause more insulin reactions, not only because of increased exercise, but also because greater calmness means that fewer stress hormones (which counteract insulin) are at work. Studies are beginning to demonstrate that regular periods of relaxation can lower insulin requirements for many with diabetes.

Summary Severe physical stress, occurring as the result of illness, infection, or injury, increases blood sugar levels and the development of ketones in the blood and urine. Monitoring blood sugar and urine ketone levels and consultation with a physician are recommended when a person with diabetes encounters such stress.

Emotional stress can raise or lower blood sugar levels, depending on a number of factors. (It can also stimulate the development of ketones.) Those with diabetes need to observe how they respond to stress, and learn to adjust insulin, food, and exercise accordingly. Stress management and relaxation training can reduce the impact of stress on diabetic control.

Hormonal Changes in Women

Menstruation, pregnancy, and menopause trigger changes in hormone levels that affect control for diabetic women, especially those with Type 1 diabetes (see Chapter 19 and the personal example from one of Gary's friends below). Variations in control during a woman's menstrual period are well known but little research has been conducted. It appears from individual reports that the impact on blood sugar levels varies from woman to woman and at different phases of a woman's period. This is another area in which women with diabetes become their own researchers. Birth control pills may also affect blood sugar levels. Use your blood sugar tests to determine what changes occur before and during your menstrual period. You may need to make changes in insulin dose or food intake to compensate.

The following anecdote from a friend and fellow ADA volunteer illustrates how hormones affect blood sugar (not just monthly), and the usefulness of individual "research." While Nancy and I were sitting at the airport, she showed me tables that she carries with her and uses daily. I was impressed and thought that the tool she uses and the insights behind it would be useful to our readers, especially those women using or considering using the pump. Nancy uses an insulin pump, which enhances her ability to manage blood sugar levels.—Gary

The Special Challenges to a Woman with Diabetes

Note: I am a woman who has had Type 1 diabetes for 35 years. I became a "pumper" soon after reading a workbook entitled *Pumping Insulin* (by John Walsh, PA, CDE, and Ruth Roberts, MA; Torrey Pines Press). As a result, I was convinced that I need to be responsible for figuring out the details of my condition, with the help of my physician.

I learned that many people with diabetes require more than one basal rate throughout the day. (This was certainly true for me.) The basal rate is the amount of insulin my body needs to keep my blood sugar at a normal level, in a "fasting" state. The pump delivers this automatically, at a rate that I set. I also learned that I could best determine appropriate basal rates using the fasting basal test procedure. I was prepared to perform a series of fasting basal tests in order to determine the appropriate basal setting at various times of the day.

But I was not prepared for the realization that even with the disciplined approach I had taken to establish my basal rates, my blood glucose readings fluctuated throughout the month. Working to eliminate as many variables as possible, a "wildcard" was apparent.

I should mention that I am approaching the age of menopause. Observing my inability to find a consistent set of basal rates at various times of the month, I began to suspect that a fluctuation of my hormone levels might be the culprit. After all, I had long known that insulin needs were greatly affected by my menstrual cycle. However, I didn't know how much until I became more diligent in my own data collection as a pumper, and until I had a tool—the pump—with which to make immediate changes in my basal insulin levels. Furthermore, my physician suggested that the frequent fluctuations might by attributed to the beginning stages of menopause. We decided to try regulating my hormones using birth control pills. The pills have a different color depending on the week of the month they are to be taken.

Indeed the changes in my basal requirements began to take on a pattern of stability for a week, only to change the next week. The change seemed to correspond with the different colors of birth control pills (related to a change in the hormone level dose). I performed a basal test to determine the new settings, and discovered that a difference of 0.1 units per hour in my basal settings produced a significant change.

By this time, I was far enough into my personal research project to need a method of tracking my observations. I developed my own form for recording results of my basal tests, and a four-week chart for my basal settings. At first I faxed the results of each basal test to my physician, and he recommended the appropriate change in my basal settings. While on rapid-acting insulin, I adjusted the basal rate two hours before the desired change. Now using the faster-acting lispro (Humalog), I make a change in basal rates one hour before the adjustment is needed. I discovered that three to four different basal settings during a 24-hour period best covers my needs.

As you can see from the following chart, my basal rates during the green pill week vary from 0.7 to 0.9 units per hour. But in a yellow pill week they vary from 0.9 to 1.2 units per hour.

After working through this process for all four weeks of the month, I developed a routine for adjusting my basal rates according to my hormone levels. After changing pill colors, I waited for two unexplained high blood glucose readings (normally on the second day of the week). At this point, I moved to the next set of basal settings. By recording my basal settings for each of the four weeks (colors) of the month, I had a formula for achieving more stable control of my blood glucose.

I am now committed to taking basal tests whenever my blood sugar levels are consistently too low or too high with no apparent explanation. As suggested in *Pumping Insulin,* I break the test into four types: a nighttime test (which is a fasting test), a morning basal test, an afternoon basal test, and an evening basal test. I start with a blood glucose of 80 to 120 mg/dl (4.4 to 6.7 mmol/L) two hours or more after a meal, then test every hour for a period of five to six hours. For convenience sake, I begin with the nighttime test at 3 a.m. Often, this single nighttime test is sufficient to identify the necessary adjustment, though sometimes more diligent nighttime testing is required. After my nighttime rates are established, I perform the morning test, skipping breakfast and testing each hour. The afternoon test is performed two hours after a midmorning meal, again testing on the hour. The evening test is performed in the same manner. I record my blood glucose readings on my testing form.

Now I can make changes on my own; my physician has taught me how to adjust my basal rates according to my test results. I record my new basal settings on the four-week chart so I can compare it with other weeks in the month, and have it available for the next month. When I see my physician (every three months), I give him a copy of my current four-week basal settings.

The process would be similar for women whose hormone levels are consistent without the use of birth control pills. I suggest that you talk with your physician about this and any other options. This process and the use of Humalog have allowed me to reduce my HbA1c levels to within the "normal" nondiabetic range. As a child I used to "paint by number;" as an adult woman with diabetes, I "control by color." (For more information specifically for women with diabetes, refer to Chapter 21.)

Sample Basal Rates—Four Weeks of the Month

Week 1—Green pill

	12	1	2	3	4	5	6	7	8	9	10	11
AM	0.8								0.7		0.8	
PM	12	1	2	3	4	5	6	7	8	9	10	11
				0.9								

Week 2—Brown pill

	12	1	2	3	4	5	6	7	8	9	10	11
AM	0.9						1.0					
PM	12	1	2	3	4	5	6	7	8	9	10	11
				0.9								

Week 3—White pill

	12	1	2	3	4	5	6	7	8	9	10	11
AM	0.9						1.0			1.2		
PM	12	1	2	3	4	5	6	7	8	9	10	11
				1.0								

Week 4—Yellow pill

AM	12	1	2	3	4	5	6	7	8	9	10	11
	1.0				0.9						1.2	
PM	12	1	2	3	4	5	6	7	8	9	10	11
				1.2								

Sample Basal Test—Week 4 (Yellow pill)

	12AM	1	2	3	4	5	6	7	8	9	10	11	12PM
Starting Basal	1.0				0.9						1.2		
BG Reading							105	137	155	157	125	80	73
Adjustment							+.1	+.1	+.1	+.1	-.1	-.1	-.1
New Basal	1.0				0.9		1.0				1.1		

Pregnancy The physical changes that occur in pregnant women with diabetes include an initial reduction in insulin requirement, and after the first two or three months, an increase. Pregnant women with Type 2 diabetes who haven't previously needed insulin may now be required to use it. Every stage of pregnancy should be supervised by a physician who has worked with women with diabetes and is committed to optimal control.

During menopause, profound hormonal changes occur that can affect blood sugar levels. Unfortunately, little research has been conducted, and the influences seem to vary from woman to woman. There is also the risk of mistaking hot flashes for low blood sugar, and vice versa. This is a time when home blood testing can help a woman avoid confusion.

Puberty During puberty, physical and emotional changes greatly affect blood sugar levels. In some cases, insulin dosage may have to be doubled to compensate for the shifts in hormone levels. When teen rebellion becomes a factor, going through puberty requires special strategies for teens with diabetes and their families.

Summary of Step 3d

All of these factors work together and the interaction between them is what determines your blood sugar level. Sometimes these factors balance each other, and sometimes they add to each other's effect, causing a substantial increase or decrease. Even after a period of intense jogging, you can still find a high blood sugar level if you are stressed because you were almost hit by a car. On the other hand, if you consume only quickly absorbed carbohydrates before jogging, you can have a reaction an hour or two later because the blood sugar was expended during exercise and no reserves remain. If you get depressed because blood sugar tests have been high, the emotional reaction can push them even higher. If you don't adjust insulin dosage to compensate for high levels, each unit becomes less effective and blood sugar can go up even more.

This all sounds very complex, but if you stabilize as many factors as possible during this period of learning the intensive regimen, you will be able to determine which factors are affecting your blood sugar at any given time. This is the reason for the next task.

Step 4: Regularize meals, activity, and schedules during the learning period

Regularizing your life will afford you much more long-term freedom in diabetes management. While learning the intensive regimen, you should eat the same number of calories (or food exchanges) in each meal and snack; and maintain a similar activity and exercise level from day to day. Also, maintain the same insulin dosage until instructed to alter it according to your tests and don't vary the timing of injections or meals by more than one hour.

Without this step, it will be difficult to understand how your system responds to the variables affecting metabolic control. If your diet, activity, schedule, and stress levels change each day, you lack the stability needed to establish the best insulin dosage. It will be difficult to learn how to vary insulin, diet, and activity to compensate for blood sugar levels that are too high or too low.

After a month or two of following this routine, you can live with much less regularity and still maintain good blood sugar levels. You will have learned how your system functions, how the different aspects of your regimen affect you, and how to vary them to obtain good control. You will also have learned some internal signs that alert you to your level of control. You will understand what has caused a high test or insulin reaction, and you will have the ability to make changes to balance the highs and lows. Thus, a relatively brief period of increased regularity will give you greater long-term freedom.

This does not mean you should become compulsive and create a new source of stress in your life. Keep things as regular as possible from day to day, and observe how diet and activity create opportunities to study variances in regimen. (Remember, this is guilt-free learning.) Allow yourself to take a day or two off from the routine now and then; you will return to it with renewed discipline. The changes you make will last if you achieve them through willingness rather than force.

Some people find it difficult to achieve greater regularity, either because of outside demands or their own emotional reactions. Work schedules and levels of activity change frequently; daily exercise may not fit into busy lives; or you may want to retain your idea of freedom.

Even if you find it difficult to make your life more systematic for a few months, you can still improve control. Test as often as possible and record the results with your notes on diet, activity, and stress. Review these records with your doctor or diabetes educator to get a better idea of what makes your blood sugar rise and fall. By doing so, you will be more willing to attain greater control because the effects of your lack of routine will be apparent. (If you would like to understand the reasons for your reluctance, use the exercises in Chapters 3 and 15.)

One way to make this period of increased regularity more acceptable is to offer yourself a reward. For some, the benefits of improved control are reward enough. However, others need to reinforce their motivation by giving themselves a special experience or gift. After so many weeks of following strict regimen, you become eligible for that trip or event or object you have been wanting. And you can plan for smaller rewards as you reach milestones along the way. (See Chapters 1 and 2.)

Step 5: Begin a Period of Intensive Testing and Record Keeping

Many of us experience a sense of excitement as we begin testing blood sugar at home. For the first time, we are able to observe how our system is affected by food, exercise or inactivity, and stress. We can determine if a queasy feeling is an insulin reaction, stress response, or merely an unexplained queasy feeling. We can measure the effect of a few cookies or extra slices of bread and butter. We have the feedback essential to living well and maintaining diabetic control.

In the beginning, your doctor or diabetes educator will probably ask you to observe your blood sugar readings without making any changes in regimen. You will need to keep records for several days, along with detailed notes on food, exercise, stress, and any changes that might affect your tests. (Use one of the logs in Step 3.) During this initial period, you will learn most quickly if you test before every insulin injection, before each meal, one to two hours after each meal, and at bedtime. Also, test your blood sugar when you suspect that you are having an insulin reaction. If there are any signs of having reactions while sleeping, set the alarm and test around 2:00 or 3:00 in the morning (see Chapter 9 for signs of Somogyi reactions).

This may sound like a lot of finger pricks (up to seven or eight a day), but testing this often is necessary for only a few weeks, and the information you gain is invaluable. With it, you and your diabetes team will be able to tailor your insulin, diet, and activity to achieve a high level of metabolic control.

It is useful to assume the role of a scientific observer, rather than a judge of right and wrong, as you maintain your test results. You are likely to find the variances in blood sugar level puzzling at first. It is easy to believe that you have done something wrong. However, you will learn faster if you simply record the results (even if it is the result of a binge) and move forward, without blame. Record all of your tests; don't exclude tests because you know they will be high. This will help you understand how high your tests actually are. You are in the process of learning to control blood sugar; you can't possibly have everything under control already.

Step 6: Selecting the Ongoing Insulin Regimen

By using the information from your blood tests, you and your doctor can decide what (if any) changes are needed in your insulin regimen, such as the type, dosage, and timing of insulin you take. The insulin regimen you choose must meet the following criteria.

Criteria for Insulin Regimen

1. Timing and dosage of insulin provides continuous, low-level availability throughout a twenty-four hour period (basal insulin), as well as peaks of insulin action following meals.
2. The majority of tests are between 70 and 150 mg/dl (3.8 and 8.3 mmol/L).
3. Hemoglobin A1c is below 7%.
4. Insulin reactions are infrequent, and their impact is minimized.
5. Normal body weight is maintained (excess weight is lost).
6. Flexibility in dealing with stress and day-to-day changes is ensured.
7. The convenience of the individual with diabetes is respected.
8. In children, normal growth and development are maintained.

A variety of insulin regimens are available that satisfy these criteria. These regimens include using multiple injections each day, mixtures of different types of insulin, and the continuous infusion of insulin provided by the pump. The DCCT, on the other hand, defined the intensive regimen as three or more injections a day. So, if you have Type 1 diabetes, you are more likely to improve your blood sugar if you take at least three shots a day than if you follow the two-shot regimen. Nonetheless, you may be able to achieve your target levels with two injections if your eating and activity patterns are fairly consistent. For those with Type 2 diabetes who take insulin, two injections per day are more likely to help you achieve your blood sugar targets. With these alternatives, you can tailor the pattern of insulin action to meet your needs.

Determining the Total Insulin Dose

The following are general guidelines, developed from averages for many patients. Your specific dosage will be determined by your physician, taking your needs into account. We are providing this information so you will understand what is happening, not because this is a do-it-yourself step.

Recommended starting levels for intensive insulin regimens are:

1. In newly diagnosed patients: 0.5 units of insulin per kilogram per day (a 132-pound person weighs 60 kg; 0.5 x 60 = 30 units of insulin per day).
2. During the "honeymoon" period, when insulin requirements temporarily decrease for the newly diagnosed: 0.4 units per kg per day.
3. For established patients previously treated with more than 0.9 units per kilogram per day: reduce dose between 20 and 25 percent. (A 132-pound person taking 60 units would reduce dose by 12 to 15 units.)
4. For patients previously treated with 0.7 to 0.9 units per kilogram per day, use 0.7 units per kilogram per day.
5. For patients previously treated with less than 0.7 units per kilogram per day, use previous total dose unless it is inadequate.

Your total daily insulin dosage is the first thing to be determined by your physician. When changing from a single daily injection to a more intensive treatment plan, insulin requirements usually decrease. The total dosage of insulin you take each day is determined by your body weight and level of activity.

For those within 20 percent of their ideal body weight, and without illness or high levels of emotional stress, the daily dose varies between 0.5 and 1.0 unit of insulin for each kilogram of weight (1 kilogram = 2.2 pounds; 150 lb. ÷ 2.2 = 70 kg).

After the daily dosage of insulin is determined, your physician will recommend one or two types of insulin to be distributed by two or more injections a day. Many studies have been conducted attempting to find the best method of treatment. It appears that the specific insulin regimen is not as important as the total program of self-care. However, as noted earlier, the DCCT achieved its results using an intensive regimen of three or more injections (or the pump) per day. One study completed in Florida compared the control of patients using the insulin pump, twice-a-day injections, and four-times-a-day injections. Home and lab tests indicated excellent control in each of the three regimens. The researchers concluded that selecting an insulin regimen could be a matter of patient preference. Patient success was based on the full intensive regimen, not just the insulin regimen.

So it appears that you can choose the intensive insulin regimen that matches your personal preferences, if you are willing to follow all other aspects of the intensive regimen. (In some cases, certain factors can make one regimen more effective than another. Your physician will discuss these if any apply to you. Since the publication of the DCCT findings, more diabetes practitioners are recommending three or more injections per day.) The critical elements are your awareness and willingness to make adjustments each day to maintain optimal control.

Insulin Regimens For Optimal Control

1. Two injections of intermediate (NPH or Lente) and rapid-acting insulin; one before breakfast, and one before dinner.
2. Three injections; intermediate and rapid in the morning, rapid before dinner, and intermediate at bedtime.
3. Three injections; rapid and Ultralente before breakfast and dinner, and rapid before lunch.
4. Four injections; rapid before meals, and intermediate at bedtime.
5. The insulin pump provides both a continuous low-level flow of insulin (basal) and bursts of insulin before meals.

These regimens have been used and studied in research trials. Other programs can be developed that may better suit your individual needs; the variations are nearly endless. The types of insulin now available allow you to work with your doctor to find the regimen that works best for you.

(Convenience is the only advantage of the single-injection regimen; this will be discussed later, in the chapters on moderate and loose regimens.

For anyone seeking optimal control, at least two shots a day combining intermediate and rapid-acting insulin are required.)

Some people dislike injections and resist the idea of taking several a day. Insulin pens, pre-filled disposable ones or loaded with insulin cartridges, can make multiple injections more convenient and user friendly. They are easy to carry, easy to use, and inconspicuous. Most people who try them continue to use them, especially for injections away from home. An alternative to injections using a syringe is jet injection. This is a needle-free method that administers insulin at a high pressure through the skin's surface.

Gary Does Away with the Needle

I used a jet injector (Medijector) for over eighteen years. I began using it initially because of curiosity, with the hope that it would make my life somewhat easier. I didn't have a particular dislike for injections (after twenty years of them); I simply found this method of taking insulin faster and more convenient.

For those who want to avoid the pain of needles, jet injection is generally more comfortable. For me, the occasional discomfort is associated with a larger volume of insulin, the type of insulin, or tougher skin.

Another benefit of the jet injector is the reduction in insulin dose due to improved absorption. When I switched, I could cut my dose in half, though most people don't experience such dramatic changes.

If you are considering switching to jet injection, consult your physician; using it requires a prescription. The relatively high cost is covered by most medical insurance. If it isn't, it will pay for itself over time, compared to the cost of disposable needles. Some new and improved devices use disposable "nozzles" so cleaning and sterilizing is not required.

When two or more injections are taken each day, you can adjust the peaks of insulin activity and the ongoing insulin availability to meet your individual needs. In fact, this individualization is essential. Your physician will use your home blood sugar tests to determine the best schedule for you. With some effort, you can have near-normal blood sugar levels throughout the day. When tests are high, you can take action to bring blood sugar down.

The Regimens

1. The least demanding of the intensive insulin regimens is the two-injection plan, in which rapid-acting (regular) and intermediate (NPH or Lente) insulin is taken thirty to sixty minutes before breakfast and dinner. (In the Florida study, two-thirds of the total dose was taken before break-

fast, with two-thirds of the shot intermediate insulin, and one-third rapid-acting insulin. The predinner shot was equal parts of the two types of insulin. In the DCCT, this regimen was considered a "conventional" insulin regimen, and it did not include all the other components of the intensive regimen, such as frequent blood sugar tests and insulin adjustments.) Your doctor will select your dose according to your test results, and your meal and activity patterns. The peaks of the rapid-acting insulin handle the increase in blood sugar caused by breakfast and dinner. The peaks of the intermediate insulin handle the lunch and overnight needs. Pre-mixed intermediate and rapid-acting insulin is available in 70/30 and 50/50 ratios, and may work for you.

The gradual action of intermediate insulin provides continuous low-level activity. Greater convenience is the major advantage of this regimen. The disadvantage is that one has less flexibility in the timing and size of lunch. If tests are high at midday, an extra shot of rapid-acting insulin might be needed.

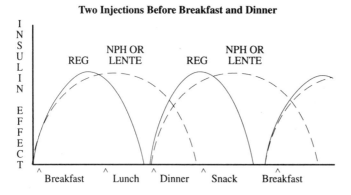

Two Injections Before Breakfast and Dinner

2. The second plan is essentially a variation of the first. The main difference is that the evening shot is divided, with rapid-acting insulin taken before dinner and intermediate at bedtime. This allows better overnight coverage for those who need more low-level insulin action while they sleep enabling them to wake up with normal blood sugar levels. This plan has the same disadvantage as the first.

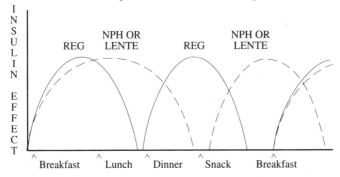

Three Injections Intermediate and Rapid

3. Plan three requires three injections daily, with a mixture of rapid-acting and Ultralente twenty to thirty minutes before breakfast and dinner, and rapid-acting only before lunch. (The long-acting Ultralente makes up 40 to 50 percent of the total dosage. The rapid-acting is divided equally between the three shots.) The rapid-acting insulin covers meals while the Ultralente provides a continuous low-level supply of insulin throughout a twenty-four- hour period.

This regimen affords a great flexibility, allowing one to change mealtime or size and activity plans, and to compensate for high blood sugar levels before each meal. (This is helpful for shift workers or those whose schedules change often.) The disadvantage of this regimen is the action time of each Ultralente injection; it can take up to four days to determine the effect of a change in dosage. Furthermore, the rate of absorption of this insulin varies, which can result in periods of sustained hypoglycemia. This regimen is advisable only when your physician has experience with the characteristics of Ultralente. Also, the only Ultralente presently available in the U.S. is human, which has a shorter duration of action than the animal source. However, Ultralente can also have an unpredictable peak of action, unlike the animal source.

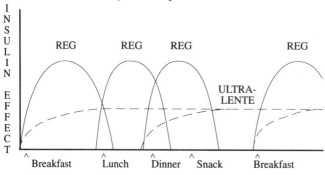

Three Injections Rapid and Ultralente

INSULIN EFFECT

REG   REG   REG   REG

ULTRA-LENTE

Breakfast   Lunch   Dinner Snack   Breakfast

Gary's Ultralente Anecdote

My personal experience using Ultralente is only a case history. There is little support for it in the diabetes literature. I include this updated version from the 1st and 2nd editions as background that demonstrates the utility of the animal Ultralente insulin, with its basal level of activity. Insulin manufacturers are now working to develop genetically engineered insulin analogs that will mimic this insulin (see Chapter 21).

Until 1995, I took one injection of Ultralente each morning. I supplemented the Ultralente with rapid-acting insulin only when I was planning to have a large meal or found my blood sugar too high, and I had reasonably good control over twenty-four-hour periods. I had not been bothered by the reported unpredictable action time of Ultralente, and I found the extended duration of action helpful in preventing early-morning hyperglycemia. I liked the combination of convenience and control that I could obtain with this regimen. It was certainly not for everybody and now, given the unavailability of animal source Ultralente, I would not recommend it as a one injection a day regimen for people with Type 1 diabetes, although it might be useful for those with Type 2 diabetes who require insulin.

I began using Ultralente insulin many years before it became medically fashionable. I found that I could obtain better control with fewer reactions using Ultralente, rather than mixing Lente and Semilente. Since Lente insulin was a fixed-ratio mixture of 30 percent Semilente and 70 percent Ultralente (I believe Lente is now formulated to produce that combination of activity, rather than as a mixture of the two), I began mixing Semi and Ultra to find the ratio that worked for me. As I adjusted the amounts, I found that I was gradually decreasing the Semi and increasing the Ultra. Finally, all I was taking was Ultralente. Thus, before anyone had written about using Ultra for "basal" insulin levels, I was using it as my only insulin. My own experience suggests that it was an underused insulin. Increasing attention is being paid to it, particularly the differences in the peaks and duration of action between human and animal Ultralente. Many physicians and users in the U.S. and England are unhappy that the animal source Ultralente has been discontinued, since they have found the human Ultralente not as effective. Hopefully, new insulin analogs will be useful substitutes.

If you are interested in trying this, I suggest you discuss it with your physician and work out a program that you monitor carefully. Perhaps you will start with one of the more typical regimens, using Ultralente (once or twice a day with rapid-acting before meals, as needed). Home blood glucose testing makes it easier to figure out what is working well for you.

Ernest Becomes an Ultralente Convert

My earlier regimen of NPH, and rapid-acting insulin before breakfast and dinner, began producing unacceptable results when I increased my daily exercise. Various adjustments failed to achieve normal blood sugar levels in the morning. After discussing it with Gary and my regular physician, I shifted to a combination of Ultralente and rapid-acting insulin before breakfast and dinner. The result: fewer reactions and better balance throughout the day.

4. The fourth insulin regimen includes three injections of rapid-acting insulin thirty minutes before meals (if you're using lispro, 5 minutes before eating) and one injection of intermediate-acting insulin (NPH or Lente) at bedtime. This plan allows one to adjust dose according to meal size, however meals must not be delayed because blood sugar can rise. This is because the action of a regular dose is declining by the next meal (or absent if you're using lispro with its very short duration of action). The intermediate insulin before bed provides low-level insulin action needed throughout the night. If you're using lispro, you may need an additional dose of intermediate in the morning. The distribution of total insulin dosage throughout the day is highly individualized, and is best determined by your physician and your blood glucose patterns.

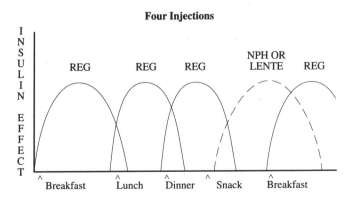

Four Injections

The Intensive Regimen

5. The external insulin pump creates a fifth insulin regimen that comes closest to the natural pattern of insulin availability found in people without diabetes. There are two manufacturers that sell pumps; each pump has different features. Both are effective, and choosing is a matter of individual preference regarding ease of use and desired features. The device pumps a small amount of insulin at regular intervals under the skin (usually in the abdominal area) through a tube and needle (or catheter) that remain implanted day and night. This is the "basal" insulin rate that can be adjusted to match the metabolic rate of an individual. (See the anecdote on page 86 for a discussion on the basal rate.) Before a meal or snack, the user triggers a measured burst or "bolus" of extra insulin to handle the increase in blood sugar from the food. These measured bursts are also used to lower blood sugar when it's too high. The inserted tube and needle is usually changed every two to three days. Some tube sets allow the needle to be removed immediately after insertion, leaving behind a soft, flexible tube. Some pumps also disconnect easily from the inserted part of the tube. This allows short term disconnects without the need for reinserting a needle.

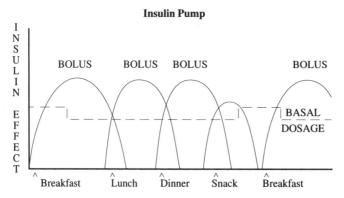

Insulin Pump

Although the insulin-pump user is wearing a tiny computer, using the pump still requires an active role in management. Four to seven blood tests each day are recommended as standard procedure; these allow you to adjust the premeal boluses to balance blood sugar levels. Those using the pump must also be aware of reactions (whose warning signs can become quite subtle) and the danger of sudden increases in blood sugar due to crimping of the tube or a rare pump malfunction. The pumps have many built-in safety devices to alert you of malfunctions.

Many of us have become pump users, experiencing improved control and increased flexibility. (See Gary's anecdote below.) Wearing a device that is connected to one's abdomen can be a constant reminder of diabetes, and it takes some getting used to. However, most users adjust within a few weeks, and its presence passes from consciousness. This reminder can become physically uncomfortable if an infection develops at the insertion site. This is not common, but it does happen. The pumps are also relatively expensive, costing around $4000-$5000. Often, most or all of the expense is covered by insurance if it is medically necessary and justified. Thousands of people are now using the insulin pump. Substantial progress has been made to overcome the pump's infrequent technical failings, and excellent models are on the market.

The pump is a viable option for anyone who wants to maintain optimal control and gain increased flexibility and freedom. If you are interested in using the pump, talk with your physician and people who use it. (There are "pump support groups" that meet to share tips and experiences. It is likely that your local ADA chapter, diabetes educator, or pump supplier can put you in touch with one.) Remember, the pump is not a replacement for active participation in managing your diabetes. An excellent book is available that should be read by all pump users titled *Pumping Insulin,* by John Walsh and Ruth Roberts, San Diego, Torrey Pines Press, 2nd edition, 1994. It is full of detailed information, procedures, and tips, as well as support and guidance for the everyday issues of living with a pump. Also useful is *The Insulin Pump Therapy Book: Insights from the Experts,* edited by Linda Frederickson, published by Minimed Technologies, 1995. Minimed is one of the two current pump manufacturers.

Nearing the end of the research and development phase are implantable pumps, which are about the size of a hockey puck, and are inserted under the skin. Concentrated insulin is injected monthly through the skin into a reservoir in the pump; the pump is programmed and controlled using a hand-held remote. The tubing goes from the pump into the abdominal cavity, where it delivers the insulin in a more physiologically normal way. (See Chapter 21.) The implantable pump will likely be deemed non-experimental by the FDA relatively soon.

Gary Goes On The Pump

For 41 years, the first thing I did every morning when I awoke was take an insulin injection. With the pump, I can wake up like everybody else, and just brush my teeth.

In some ways, this is the most dramatic change in my life since going on the pump. I no longer need extra time in the morning to take my insulin, and the day doesn't have to begin with a somewhat unpleasant task.

What convinced me to change a regimen that enabled me to avoid significant complications for over 40 years? There was no question in my mind that my blood sugar control would be improved. However, I was somewhat skeptical of the glowing reports and testimonials I heard regarding increased freedom and flexibility of lifestyle. It wasn't until I began speaking at national meetings with diabetes educators who had diabetes and were using pumps! Since they were practicing what they were preaching, I figured there must be something to this. With my own physician's support and recommendation, I gave it a try. While it didn't totally change my life, it came pretty close.

What were the benefits for me? First, it allows much better management and control under a wide range of circumstances and situations. With a continuous supply of precisely determined basal insulin, I feel much better on a daily basis. This is more natural, and there are fewer swings during the day. If my blood sugar rises above my target limit, it is easy to take an additional unit to bring the level down. I am currently using lispro, the fast acting, short duration analog insulin released in August, 1996. Although it has not yet been specifically indicated for pump use by the FDA, several studies are nearing completion at the time of this writing and I expect that pump use will become an FDA approved use. Just like all of diabetes care, I'm sure we will learn over time when and how it is best used.

Another benefit is that the timing of meals is much less critical, because there isn't any long or intermediate acting insulin present to cause low blood sugar. In fact, for the first time in 41 years, I actually missed a meal! (Our friends, with whom we often cook dinner together at their house, love my pump because they no longer have to worry about delays!) When I travel across time zones or take "red eye" flights, my blood sugar and insulin adjustments are no longer a challenge. In short, my control is substantially improved and my freedom is enhanced. The testimonials were true, at least for me!

What about the downside? Well, you are attached to the pump 24 hours a day. However, for me, my heightened awareness of the pump disappeared after about a week. The new tubing connectors make temporary detachment quite easy, and do not necessitate a new needle stick. Furthermore, the pump books provide instructions and tips on what to do with the pump during swimming, showering, sleeping, sexual intercourse, strenuous exercise, and other activities where a pump would be awkward or inconvenient. The negatives of testing are still present, since the pump does not yet test your blood sugar for you! Although you do a lot of blood sugar testing initially, this can taper off a bit after fine tuning your pump use. Also, if your eating and activity pattern is stable, tests are used mainly to confirm that all is well, or identify a need for more insulin. It is also important to make sure that you are not developing ketoacidosis, often due to an inadvertently crimped or kinked tube. This is no longer common, but it does happen. The pumps have good alarms that are triggered if flow is impaired. Another potential negative: some people have skin reactions at the insertion site, but there are many different tapes, skin preps, and hints to help minimize this (see the Walsh and Roberts book noted above, or a booklet available from Minimed). The pump and supplies are fairly expensive, but more and more insurance companies are covering some or all of these costs, recognizing the pump's potential to reduce short term hospitalization costs and long term costs associated with complications.

For me, the benefits far outweigh the negatives.

If you choose to use a pump, it is critical that you work with a physician and diabetes educator (ideally a team) who are experienced in initiating and maintaining pump therapy. In addition to the technical and practical instruction, you will determine three specific ratios or numbers: your basal insulin rate or rates, your carbohydrate/insulin ratio, and your blood sugar/insulin ratio. Although there are rules of thumb that will get you started, these are specific to your metabolism.

The basal rate is how many units of insulin you need per hour to maintain normal blood sugar levels. Because this can vary depending on time of day, activity level, and other factors, you may have several different basal rates programmed during the day. You can also program temporary basal rates, for example during heavy exercise.

The carbo/insulin ratio is used for boluses when you eat. Because our blood sugar level is affected primarily by how much carbohydrate we eat, rather than protein or fat (see Chapter 11), you will determine how many grams of carbohydrate one unit of insulin will metabolize. Typically, they range between 7 and 15 grams per unit of insulin.

The blood sugar/insulin ratio is used for boluses when you want to lower your blood sugar with insulin. It is the amount by which one unit of insulin will lower your blood sugar level. For example, suppose your blood sugar is 200 mg/dl (11.1 mmol/ L) when you test, and you want to lower it to 100 (5.6 mmol/L). You will need a bolus of two units. This is because in pump training you determined that for you one unit of insulin will lower your blood sugar by 50 (2.8 mmol/L).

Now the art of medicine comes into play. There is no formula for pre-scribing an insulin regimen. This is a highly individualized process that takes into account your test records, personal preferences, daily schedule, and even your physician. Over the course of several weeks, you and your physician or diabetes educator will work together, most likely with a phone consultation every few days, to adjust the initial dosage. Your test results and insulin reactions will provide the feedback needed to fine-tune the regimen and achieve blood sugar levels within the limits you have established. (If you are loosely controlled to begin with, these levels may be higher for the first months and gradually brought down.) For doctors and patients alike, the teamwork that develops at this stage is rewarding. However, if your doctor gives little guidance at this stage, you will need to find one who is either more knowledgeable or more cooperative.

The general guidelines for adjusting insulin regimen include the fol-lowing:

1. Normalize the fasting blood sugar level by adjusting the overnight insulin. Increase it only after determining that nighttime reactions are not the cause of high fasting blood glucose tests. (See "Somogyi Reactions" in Chapter 9.)

2. When changes in dosage are needed, change only one type of insulin given at a particular time of day. (Determine the overall impact of changing morning NPH, for instance, before changing morning rapid-acting, or dosage at other times.)

3. Wait two to three days to see the effect of a change before making any further changes. (Wait three to four days with Ultralente insulin.)

4. Dosage should not be changed more than one unit at a time for any-one under 90 pounds.

5. For those over 90 pounds, increases of insulin should generally occur one to two units at a time, although changes of two to six units can be made if your doctor advises.

6. Adjustments in dosage should be made on the basis of a pattern documented over several days of testing, not because of one high test or reaction.

7. Check for Somogyi reactions if the results of changes oppose what you would expect. If insulin is increased (or food decreased) and

blood sugar goes up, high tests might indicate a rebound from too much insulin.

By the time you have established your insulin regimen, you will understand the timing of each insulin component—when it peaks and what meal it covers. The timing of reactions will help you understand your schedule. You will also be able to make adjustments in dosage to keep your tests within the target range you have established.

If your activity level changes significantly from weekday to weekend, you will need to adjust dosage to account for the change. Women will need to make adjustments when menstruation affects blood sugar levels. Workers with swing or graveyard shifts will also have to adjust their insulin. In the beginning, check with your physician before making such changes. As you become experienced, you will probably be encouraged to take the initiative.

If you experience a major improvement in control at this stage, and the majority of your tests are in the target range, you might feel uncomfortable for a short time. You may even have symptoms of hypoglycemia when your blood sugar levels are normal. This is natural while you adjust to the new level of control. The discomfort can last up to two weeks. When your system adjusts to the new level, you will feel better than you ever did when blood sugar was chronically high.

If it is difficult to bring your tests within your target range, or if there is a great fluctuation in readings, don't despair. There can be many reasons for the frustration you experience, and there are just as many solutions. Determine the cause and define what has to be done to correct the problem. Skip to Step 9 for help in clarifying your difficulty and solutions to overcome it.

Step 7: Observe the variations in blood sugar level caused by changes in food, exercise, stress, illness, and other factors.

You will begin to observe the causes of blood sugar variations as soon as you begin testing. But now it will be easier to determine what is causing a particular high or low reading. In Step 3, you reviewed the influences at work here; this information will now prove very useful. Your doctor may want you to spend some time observing before you begin making changes to compensate for levels outside your target range. Or you may begin making changes right away, in which case you will be doing the two parts of Step 7 at the same time.

Look through the sample logs that follow and see how many of the high tests or reactions you can explain. Then read the discussion of each log.

Daily Diabetes Log II

Susan is on insulin regimen 1, with a regular dose of 15 NPH & 4 rapid-acting before breakfast, 10 NPH & 5 rapid-acting before dinner.

Date Time	Blood Test & Reactions	Insulin Dosage	Activity & Exercise	Food	Comments: stress illness, etc.
8-15					
7 am	110	15 NPH 4 rapid-acting	walk 30 min.	2 bread 1 oz. cheese orange	
10:00 am	240 Ⓐ				My boss blew up at me for losing an important account. I felt guilty & angry, and kept it inside.
11:45 am	#2 react Ⓑ			green salad & ham	Cut the carbo for lunch
4 pm				pack of chocolate cookies	
5:30 pm	200	10 NPH 7 rapid-acting		3 oz. hamburger yellow squash cup rice 3 plums	
10:00 pm	120 Ⓒ		walk 30 min.		Quiet evening

Before reading on, analyze the high tests at (**A**) and (**C**) and the reaction at (**B**) and try to figure out what caused them. What, if anything, could Susan have done to avoid them? What did she do to compensate?

Susan's high blood sugar level at lunch was probably caused by the emotional stress of being disciplined by her boss, and not being able to express her feelings. Nothing short of extreme inner peace could have prevented this high test. She then overcompensated for the high reading by avoiding carbohydrates altogether at lunch, rather than just reducing them. Her roller coaster went from high to low, resulting in the reaction at 4:00 P.M. Rebound from the reaction (and probably an overdose of chocolate cookies) caused another high blood sugar level at 5:30. One can do nothing to avoid rebound, but not overtreating reactions help lessen the rise in blood sugar. An additional two units of rapid-acting insulin (over her usual five units) and a thirty-minute walk enabled Susan to return to a blood sugar level within her target range by bedtime.

Daily Diabetes Log

George is on regimen 3. His standard dosage is eight units of Ultralente and seven units of rapid-acting before breakfast and dinner, and seven units of rapid-acting before lunch.

Date Time	Blood Test & Reactions	Insulin Dosage	Activity & Exercise	Food	Comments: stress illness, etc.
8-15					
6:30 am	90	8 ultra 7 rapid-acting	walk 30 min.	2 bread 1 oz. cheese orange	
7:30 am			jogging 45 min.		
11 am	mild reaction Ⓐ			orange juice	
noon	140 Ⓑ	8 rapid-acting		egg salad sand. medium apple	Headache, sore muscles, Flu??
3:30 pm				1 oz. nuts & raisins	Feeling worse. Going home early
4:30 pm	240 Ⓒ	8 ultra 11 rapid acting		split pea soup muffin	
5 pm				banana	
8 pm	150 Ⓓ			6 oz. apple juice	Vomiting

Date Time	Blood Test & Reactions	Insulin Dosage	Activity & Exercise	Food	Comments: stress illness, etc.
11 pm	100			6 oz. apple juice	
2 am	120				Vomiting
7 am	150	8 ultra 9 rapid-acting		6 oz. orange juice	

You probably already know the reasons for the reaction at 11:00 A.M. and the high blood sugar levels later. In addition to jogging in the morning, George missed his midmorning snack. It was a mild reaction because the action of the morning rapid-acting insulin was almost over. The slightly high test at noon might have been caused by rebound from the reaction, but it is more likely that the developing illness was responsible. He took an extra unit of rapid-acting insulin before lunch, but by the time he tested at 4:30, his blood sugar had climbed to a fairly high level. Knowing that this was caused by the physical stress of the flu, he took four extra units of rapid-acting before dinner and reduced the amount of carbohydrate eaten by 100 calories. Dinner was vomited by 8:00, so George tested to see how much more food seemed advisable. Blood sugar at 150 mg/dl (mmol/L), with the extra rapid-acting still working, told him that more carbohydrate was needed. The rest of the record shows him using frequent tests to maintain relative balance, despite the effects of the flu.

As you work with your own logs, you will learn to interpret the results and understand the reasons for high tests and reactions. You will also learn the effects of the actions you take to bring blood sugar levels back to normal.

7a. Learn to vary insulin dosage, diet, and exercise in order to compensate for high or low tests and with changes in routine

The skills you learn in this step are central to improving blood sugar levels while maintaining a flexible lifestyle. When you are able to vary the ingredients of your regimen, you are able to live with a level of freedom previously associated with a lack of control for people with diabetes. You can bring blood sugar levels back to normal within a few hours when they are high, and the effects of illness or emotional stress are easily handled.

You can change schedules, diet, and activity and still maintain your target levels. The decisions you make are part of a balancing act that used to take place automatically before you had diabetes.

There are two types of changes you will be making on a daily basis: those that compensate for tests that are too high or too low, and those necessary to prepare for a change in routine. We can offer some general guidelines for making these alterations in regimen, but the feedback from your tests will teach you exactly how much you should adjust insulin, food, or exercise to produce a change in blood sugar level. At first, change only one element at a time so you can determine what effect the change has. Later, you will be able to change more than one aspect at a time.

Use these target levels, or those you and your physician have agreed upon, to determine the need for short-term changes in insulin, diet, or exercise. These target levels can be difficult to achieve. You may need to begin with less demanding goals if stress or other factors make it difficult to achieve this level of control. Determine a level that you can attain.

A Menu of Adjustments

If blood sugar is too high

▷ Increase insulin (rapid-acting), or

▷ Increase exercise, or

▷ Decrease carbohydrates

To prepare for extra activity or exercise

▷ Decrease insulin (rapid-acting or intermediate), or

▷ Increase carbohydrates

Changing insulin dosage is the easiest way to compensate for high test levels. Extra insulin taken for this reason is called supplemental. In general, if you are an adult of average weight, take one additional unit of rapid-acting for each 30 mg/dl (1.6 mmol/L) above 120 (6.6) that your premeal test shows. (If you are a child, or an adult under 100 pounds, take one unit for every 50 mg/dl [2.7 mmol/L] above 150 [8.3].) If you are on a pump, you will have already determined your specific ratio. Thus, if your usual dose of rapid-acting is five units before dinner, take seven units (two supplemental units) to compensate for a test of 180 mg/dl (10 mmol/L), or nine units (four supplemental units) for a test of 240 (13.3). If a high test occurs at a premeal time when you don't usually take a shot, take a supplement, as long as you eat your usual meal. Don't compensate for high tests after a meal; wait to see what the next premeal test is. Testing 2 hours after you have eaten will give you an idea of the maximum effect of the meal. If the test is beyond your post-meal target, perhaps over 180 mg/dl (10 mmol/L), you might want to take a bolus, and adjust your pre-meal insulin for the next day.

It is best not to take supplements before going to bed. (When Ernest was a teenager, he woke up in the hospital after trying to balance a hot fudge sundae with a midnight injection of rapid-acting insulin. He overestimated the impact of the sundae because blood glucose testing wasn't available then.)

In most cases, no more than two to five extra units of rapid-acting insulin should be taken at one time, even if blood sugar is very high. It is best to lower your blood sugar in stages, thus reducing the risk of severe reactions. Children and lightweight adults should supplement no more than three units at a time.

Similarly, you can take a supplement of insulin before a large meal or snack to prevent the extra food from increasing your blood glucose too much. Be cautious and increase rapid-acting by only one or two units. It is better to have a high reading than a serious insulin reaction caused by too large a supplement. Also, don't take the rapid-acting insulin more than half an hour before eating, or you may need to ask for dessert before dinner. Lispro insulin should be taken at mealtime, or only a few minutes before.

Feedback from your blood tests (especially tests taken 1-2 hours after eating) will tell you if you need larger or smaller supplements of rapid-acting insulin than those indicated here. This is a matter that has to be determined individually.

You can also decrease your insulin dose to accommodate a period of strenuous exercise. Rapid-acting should be reduced for a shorter exercise period occurring two to three hours after injection. Intermediate insulin should also be reduced if you engage in an extended period of exercise, such as working in the garden or hiking all day. An approximate reduction should be one unit for every thirty minutes of moderate exercise, or one unit for every fifteen minutes of strenuous exercise. But do not decrease your dose by more than one-third of the total that you would normally take. Your test results and reactions will indicate whether your reductions need to be smaller or larger.

If supplementing your insulin was the only thing you did to keep blood sugar normal, you would soon encounter a serious side effect: You would gain weight because the blood sugar that used to be excreted in the urine would be stored as fat. Extra insulin is the easiest way to compensate for high tests, but it should not be the only one you use if you want to avoid gaining weight.

After working with insulin supplements long enough to know how to use them, begin using the other two methods that decrease high blood sugar levels: exercise and reducing meal size. When your tests are high, decrease your carbohydrate intake (especially rapidly absorbed carbohydrates, such as fruit and white potatoes). Eat one slice of toast instead of two, and don't eat fruit if your morning blood sugar is between 150 and 200 mg/dl (8.3 and 11.1 mmol/L). Test an hour after the breakfast and before lunch to see if this change was enough to bring you within your target levels. Through trial and error, you will know how much of a reduction is needed to normalize blood sugar and avoid a reaction.

Eating additional food to compensate for exercise is a good practice. In general, add 10 to 15 grams of carbohydrate (such as a medium orange, a half-pint of milk, or a half-ounce of raisins) for every thirty to forty-five minutes of moderate activity. If the exercise continues for an extended period, you might need additional, rapidly absorbed carbohydrates as you go along (such as dried fruit or juices). Reactions occurring during exercise and a blood test following exercise will indicate how much extra food you need for the activities you engage in.

Exercise is the third method you can use to reduce blood sugar when it is too high. If the fasting test is between 150 and 240 mg/dl (8.3 and 13.3 mmol/L), a brisk walk or a half-hour of dancing between your insulin injection and breakfast may be enough to make blood sugar levels normal. There are so many levels of exercise that it doesn't seem wise to set guidelines here. Again, you have the feedback system necessary to determine how exercise works to reduce your blood sugar. Test an hour after a meal and see if your blood sugar is within acceptable limits. After a few trials, you will understand how much a particular activity reduces blood sugar.

The ability of exercise to lower blood sugar is limited. In fact, at levels over 300 mg/dl (16.6 mmol/L), exercise can actually increase blood sugar levels and produce ketones in your blood and urine (see Chapter 11). When your blood sugar is this high, insulin supplements and moderation in diet are the only ways to reduce it. When you deal with tests this high, it is important not to be excessive in treatment. Serious reactions can result from dramatic insulin supplements and decreases of food intake. It is best to lower your blood sugar in stages, taking no more than three or five additional units of insulin at a time (three units for a child or adult under 100 pounds), and never decreasing food intake by more than half. It is a good idea to monitor your progress by testing between meals when lowering blood sugar.

Record keeping will hasten the process of learning to make these daily alterations in regimen. On the basis of your logs, you will be able to determine what changes need to be made. For example, for every 30-50 mg/dl (1.6-2.7 mmol/L) above 120 (6.6), take one extra unit of insulin, or eat fewer grams of carbohydrate, or engage in moderate activity (using the values that work for you). You will be able to prepare for changes and deal with the results of changes after they occur.

Remember, you are an individual and these are only guidelines. You and your physician have the information needed to tailor these guidelines according to your needs. You are a pioneer in a generation of those with diabetes who for the first time are able to live a flexible life and still maintain blood sugar control.

Step 8: Have new lab tests done to measure the effect of your new regimen and establish an ongoing regimen

After you have been on the intensive regimen for two to three months, your physician will order new hemoglobin A1c and blood lipid (fats) tests and will probably want to review your daily logs. (See Chapter 13 for guidelines on monitoring diabetes on a regular basis.) The logs provide objective information concerning your level of control. With it, you and your doctor can determine if any further changes in regimen are needed.

At this point, you will establish how often to continue blood glucose testing and the level of record keeping to maintain. One study found that control suffered if subjects tested fewer than three or four times a day. Some doctors recommend testing each time insulin is taken, and at bedtime. Others suggest at least two tests a day, one of them upon arising. One day a week, test before every meal and at bedtime. Whatever the recommendation, many of us want to test three to four times a day because the feedback is so valuable. Discuss testing and the question of records with your physician or diabetes educator.

Step 9: Assess your progress and determine what (if anything) is needed to further improve control

You may have made great progress, having most tests within your target range. Or perhaps you have made significant improvements but are still testing higher than you would like. It's possible that your tests show little improvement, even though you have devoted yourself to the intensive regimen. Your blood sugar level may vary greatly with frequent insulin reactions. Possibly you have been struggling just to follow the regimen.

No matter what you have achieved at this point, it is a time to pause and congratulate yourself. Even if you are out of control and fighting against everything you know is good for you, it is time to reward yourself. Whether you have much or little to accomplish, take time to define your progress, what you need to learn, what obstacles are holding you back, and what you can do to overcome them.

Assessing Your Progress

Give Yourself Some Credit

1. No matter what you have achieved so far, the fact that you are still at work earns points for you. If you feel like it, create a "hanging-in-there" award and give yourself a special treat.

2. Go through the list of eleven steps that you have been working on (at the beginning of this chapter); see which ones you have completed and which ones need more work. Make sure you haven't missed any. Again, give yourself credit for what you have done and don't blame yourself for what needs to be done. (If you are one who was able to gain optimal control quickly, you are fortunate.)

If You Choose to Make Further Improvements in Control, Go Through the Following Checklist to Determine What You Still Need to Learn

1. Do you understand your insulin regimen—what type of insulin you are supposed to take and when each of them peaks? If not, review this with your doctor and read the section in Step 6 describing it.

▷ Do you understand how the different factors determining blood sugar work? If not, go back to Step 3 and review this information.

2. Is your blood glucose testing accurate? If you haven't taken a class or been instructed in the technique, ask your doctor or diabetes educator to help you, and review Step 3.

3. Is your life filled with stress, or are you especially sensitive to stress? If so, read Chapter 12, and consider taking a stress-management class.

4. Are you finding it difficult to regularize diet, activity, and schedule for this learning period? Use Chapter 3 to help you discover the obstacles.

5. Do you understand and follow your diet? Do you need some tips? Read Chapter 10 and see a dietitian or nutritionist if you need more information.

6. Do you notice any signs of nighttime reactions or Somogyi effects? (See Chapter 9.) Have you tested blood sugar during the night (around 2:00 or 3:00 A.M.) to be sure you are not having reactions?

7. Are there any irregularities or imbalances in endocrine hormones other than insulin? Your doctor can determine whether this is possible and order tests.

8. Is any other physical condition affecting your control? Discuss this with your doctor.

9. Do you have strong doubts that optimal control is worth the effort it takes to achieve it? Do you believe that the intensive regimen intrudes on your life too much or creates too many inconveniences?

▷ Review the section of Chapter 4 on the benefits of the intensive regimen and review your answers to the guide to decision making at the end of that chapter.

▷ Do the work in the next step: Maintaining Motivation.

▷ Do you doubt yourself—either your ability to learn, or your worth as a person? See Chapter 15.

10. Are your learning the intensive regimen at a time when too many other demands are being made on you? It's possible that problems with school, work, family, relationships, or emotional difficulties are competing with your need to manage your diabetes. If so, can you put any of the other challenges on hold? You may decide now to work with a moderate regimen. (See Chapter 7.)

11. Do you have enough support and guidance from your physician and others?

▷ Let your doctor and other health professionals know what you need. If your requests are legitimate and they are unwilling to meet them, consider changing doctors. (See Chapter 13.)

▷ Have you enlisted the support of others with diabetes? (See Chapter 14.)

12. Is there anything else that could cause your difficulty?

If you are tempted to quit because you're having difficulties gaining the level of control you want, you may need a short break. Remove yourself from all of the details you are trying to learn and look at your whole situation. Even if your tests are not yet on target, you might find that you have made progress by mastering some of the tasks of the intensive regimen. You haven't failed; there is just more to be learned.

You may need to accept higher blood sugar levels while you work on motivation, reducing your stress level, or other issues outside diabetes. There may also be physical conditions that make control more difficult to attain. You may need to find a physician who is better informed or more sympathetic to your goals. If you want a referral to a different diabetes educator or diabetes education program, call the American Association of Diabetes Educators— 1-800-TEAM-UP-4 or the American Diabetes Association—1-800-DIABETES.

If, after determining the reasons for your frustration, you decide to take a break from the intensive regimen, don't punish yourself. Make a commitment to re-evaluate your decision at a scheduled date in the future. Understand the reasons for your decision, and let them guide you to your next step in diabetes education. Follow the moderate regimen, and work on the issues that have prevented you from succeeding with the intensive regimen. There may be negative beliefs or self-image issues (see Chapter 15) that must be cleared up before you can achieve optimal control. Perhaps there are too many concerns aside from health that you are dealing with. Whatever the reason, if you discontinue the intensive regimen without blaming yourself, you will find it much easier to begin again later.

You may also decide, on the basis of this experience with the intensive regimen, that you do not want to manage diabetes at this level. As we have said before, you are the only one who can balance the questions of physical health and quality of life involved in this decision. Living well with diabetes is finding the balance that works for you.

Step 10: Maintain motivation for continuing with the intensive regimen

The intensive regimen becomes easier to manage once you know the basics. The testing schedule is not as demanding, you can be flexible in lifestyle and still maintain good control, and you have a new set of habits that help you live well with diabetes. Your regimen is easier, but it is not what most people would call easy. You have assumed a position of responsibility, one calling for daily awareness and decision making. It is advisable that you remain motivated so that this responsibility does not become a burden.

The immediate rewards of following the intensive regimen reinforce your motivation. When you have immediate feedback regarding blood sugar levels and the ability to do something about it, you enjoy a sense of power and control. (Those who have lived with diabetes for many years know the frustration and sense of powerlessness that often accompanies attempts to gain control.) This emotional benefit is reinforced by the feeling of physical well-being that accompanies optimal control. Don't take these improvements for granted. Remember that you have worked hard to achieve them and that you will continue to enjoy them by maintaining your regimen.

You can also use the long-term benefits of optimal control as motivation to adhere to regimen. You are increasing your chances of living a long and healthful life. You are maintaining a body that functions like that of someone without diabetes. If you have children, you are more likely to be an active parent throughout their childhood. If you are a woman who wants to become pregnant, you can be more assured of having a safe pregnancy and healthy baby. Periodically, review what your personal reasons for living well are, and keep in mind how the intensive regimen will help you get what you want in your life.

Contact with others following the same regimen can also reinforce your motivation. Participation in a support group, or having friends with diabetes you can talk to when you need understanding and encouragement, helps in a special way. You are talking with people who know what you are dealing with. You can get practical tips from experienced people and you will soon be giving advice to beginners. It is easier to stay involved with quality self-care when you know you are not alone.

Earlier, we described the role of brief vacations from intensive management as a way of relieving the sense of burden. With the skills you have learned in varying insulin, diet, and exercise, you can relax for a day or two and not end up with severely elevated blood sugar levels. When doing this, don't create conditions that can cause severe insulin reactions such as too much additional rapid-acting insulin, late meals, or meals of sweets unaccompanied by more slowly absorbed carbohydrates. It is much easier to continue with the intensive regimen if you do not think of it as a straitjacket that labels any departure as cheating. Living well includes brief periods of relaxed control as part of the regimen.

If you feel resistance toward continuing with the intensive regimen, you can explore the causes and deal with them. Be aware of the rationalizations or denials that you use to justify resistance. Don't accept "I'm really too busy," or "I don't need to be so careful," "I'm all right now," or "It won't do any good anyway." Use Chapter 3 to gain awareness of what is happening, and ask for help if you need to.

Step 11: Celebrate!

When you finish learning the intensive regimen, you understand the most demanding body of information medicine has to offer its patients. Celebrate your accomplishment; let your family and friends know what it means to you. After all, most of what you are doing to live well with diabetes would also help them live more healthful lives. Share the joy of reaching your goal; it will help you to continue your new level of self-care. You can take this task literally and have a party or a special dinner to announce your "graduation." It can be as subtle or as exuberant as you want.

If you have a reward system, now is the time to collect whatever prize you contracted for. Even if you haven't been working with this idea in mind, you might want to give yourself something special, beyond the rewards of good control. It doesn't have to be something you buy. It might be an experience you have been postponing, a relationship you have not felt ready for, or even time alone, away from all other demands. You will know what is right for you.

Next Steps

You will also know what you still need to learn about diabetes. Mastering the intensive regimen does not mean that you have finished your diabetes education. Look through the other sections of the book to see what you need to study next. The pace will be easier and you will have the basis of the learning you have just completed.

Fortunately, you are engaged in a lifelong learning process, as there will always be new research and techniques for diabetes care. Let us hope that the self-care in this book is made obsolete by technological breakthroughs. To keep up with new developments, you can subscribe to publications such as *Diabetes Interview,* published by King Publishing in San Francisco; *Diabetes Forecast,* published by the American Diabetes Association; or *Diabetes Self-Management.* (See the Appendix at the end of the book for addresses.)

If you are willing to deal with medical jargon, two excellent journals, *Diabetes Care* and *Diabetes Spectrum,* are available in medical libraries. Your local ADA chapter is another source of excellent diabetes information.

Chapter Six

Living Well
With Type 2
Diabetes

"Type 2 diabetes is not the result of a character flaw. Do not judge yourself. They say people with Type 2 diabetes are all older, overweight, and sedentary. I say, my friends are mostly older, overweight, and sedentary, but they don't have diabetes. This is definitely not a glamorous disease." —Nancy

Previous editions of this book focused primarily on Type 1 diabetes, but they were also helpful to people with Type 2 diabetes who used insulin. Even those who didn't use insulin found many chapters helpful. Still, for this edition, we revised all the chapters to make them as relevant as possible to all people with diabetes. We even added this chapter specifically for those with Type 2 diabetes, placing it right after the intensive regimen discussion to reflect its importance.

It is natural to discuss both types of diabetes because Type 2 is just as serious a condition as Type 1. The same complications can develop; in fact, some may already be present when Type 2 diabetes is diagnosed. Furthermore, although the DCCT found that tighter blood glucose control has many benefits for people with Type 1 diabetes, it is believed that the same applies to people with Type 2 diabetes. (This is being confirmed by results such as those from the Japanese Kumamoto study.)

It is time for everyone—you as well as your physician— to take Type 2 diabetes seriously. You can choose how intensive an effort you wish to make to manage your blood sugar. So many new tools are now available (primarily medications) that it is possible for almost anyone with Type 2 diabetes to bring his or her blood sugars into the near normal range. The goals for blood glucose management, as recommended by the American Diabetes Association, are the same for both Type 1 and Type 2 diabetes (see Chapter 5). The goal for overnight (fasting) or before meal (preprandial) blood sugars is less than 120 mg/dl (6.6 mmol/L) and an HbA1c reading of less than 7% (based on a nondiabetic range of 4 to 6%). Of course, these goals may need adjusting depending the person's age, capability and willingness to carry out a regimen, his or her risk of low blood sugar, the presence of other chronic illnesses, and other factors.

To achieve your goals, you may need to lose weight (and keep it off) and increase the amount of regular physical activity. The good news is that losing 10 to 20 pounds (5 to 10% of body weight) or walking 15 to 30 minutes every day may be enough to make a significant difference. In addition, you may need to take a combination of glucose-lowering pills, pills plus insulin, or insulin alone. Because those with Type 2 diabetes still make some insulin, the goal is to increase secretion of your own insulin, make the insulin you do have work more efficiently, or accomplish both, which is what most treatment plans aim to do. In general, lean people with Type 2 diabetes have more of a problem with impaired insulin secretion while overweight people tend to have a greater problem with insulin resistance or decreased sensitivity.

Defining Type 2 Diabetes

Approximately 85 to 90 percent of Americans with diabetes have Type 2 diabetes, yet researchers estimate that half (7 to 8 million) do not know they have Type 2 diabetes and have not been diagnosed. While many are older, overweight, and sedentary, age alone is not a distinguishing characteristic. Whether you are in your thirties or fifties, you can develop Type 2 diabetes. Even teenagers are being diagnosed with it.

Until recently, Type 2 diabetes was also called adult-onset diabetes or noninsulin-dependent diabetes. However, these terms are misleading. After all, an estimated 40 percent of people with Type 2 diabetes use insulin. In June 1997, the American Diabetes Association released new definitions and terminology for diabetes. The terms insulin-dependent and noninsulin dependent (as well as juvenile-onset and adult-onset) were dropped and replaced by Type 1 and Type 2 diabetes. It is believed that a disease should not be defined according to its treatment or age of onset. The point at which Type 2 diabetes is diagnosed has also been lowered from a fasting blood sugar of 140 mg/dl to 126 mg/dl (7.7 mmol/L to 7.0 mmol/L).

In those with Type 1 diabetes, the pancreas produces no insulin at all, so self-administered injections of insulin are necessary. In Type 2 diabetes, either the pancreas doesn't produce enough insulin to meet the body's needs or the body's cells aren't able to use insulin properly (insulin resistance). Treatment plans vary according to the person's need, but may include healthful food choices and regular physical activity, weight loss, oral medication, combinations of oral medications, oral medication plus insulin, or insulin alone.

Because treatments are influenced by the underlying causes, it is important to understand the three basic changes (the pathophysiology) that can occur in diabetes: decreased use of blood sugar primarily by muscle cells; increased production of glucose by the liver; and insufficient insulin secretion by the pancreas to overcome the other defects. Treatments now can be directed at each of these specific deficiencies, as detailed in the "Medications" section later in this chapter.

Your overnight, pre-breakfast fasting blood sugar is a measure of your basal level of insulin, the insulin produced to keep cells functioning when not stimulated by energy from food. If it's too high, it is primarily the result of increased production of glucose by the liver. Furthermore, because this is the blood sugar level above which your blood sugar will vary during the day, it is critical to bring this level into the target range. If your overnight levels are in the target range, your postprandial sugars (1 to 2 hours after a meal) are primarily a measure of how well your pancreas responds to food, or how well your medications are stimulating the pancreas to produce more insulin or cells to take up more glucose.

What are Possible Causes of Type 2 Diabetes?

Heredity plays a major but not exclusive factor. Type 2 diabetes may skip generations or occur in every one. Immediate family members may not have Type 2 diabetes but aunts, uncles, or cousins may. Or there may be no obvious family history at all.

Lifestyle has a significant impact on the development of Type 2 diabetes. Statistics show that 90 percent of people newly diagnosed with Type 2 diabetes are overweight. Other risk factors include being 65 or older; having a baby who weighed more than 9 pounds at birth; or being African American, Hispanic/Latino American, or Native American. Whatever the cause, there is much you can do to be more healthy, improve blood sugar control, and delay or avoid possible complications.

How It is Usually Diagnosed

While the onset of Type 1 diabetes can be very dramatic and even require a stay in the hospital, the onset of Type 2 is usually much more subtle. The large number of people with undiagnosed diabetes points to this fact. In fact, most people who develop Type 2 diabetes probably have had some degree of impaired glucose tolerance (IGT) for years. IGT is the inability to burn or use sugar normally, but not enough to reach the criterion for the diagnosis of diabetes.

You might have had some but not all of the signs and symptoms that often point to the development of Type 2: frequent urination, unusual thirst, extreme hunger, unusual weight loss, extreme fatigue, irritability, frequent or recurring infections (especially yeast infections), blurred vision, cuts or bruises that are slow to heal, and tingling or numbness in the hands and feet.

Sophie remembers

"It was a very hot summer in the valley and I was moaning even more than usual about how thirsty and tired I was. I thought it was just that—the usual. What finally got me to the doctor was a very uncomfortable vaginal infection. The gynecologist, as part of the exam, took a urine and blood sample and returned to say 'You have a blood sugar of 190. You have diabetes.' I couldn't believe it, but she sent me the same day to another doctor in the clinic who started me on oral medication. It didn't take long for me to feel a lot better."

Any diagnosis of a serious, lifelong condition comes as a shock. We almost always go through a series of responses such as denial, anger, fear, bargaining, and testing limits before coming to terms with reality. If you find yourself on this continuum, read the first three chapters to get you going. And then go on to Chapter 15, Living Well With Yourself.

Managing Your Type 2 Diabetes

How to choose your health care team

Chapter 13, Living Well With Your Medical Team, covers the needs of people with Type 2 diabetes as well as those with Type 1. It also includes recommended guidelines for the important blood tests and other health checks that you and your health care team should be tracking.

Take note of the many professionals you may need to be in touch with from time to time. As with people with Type 1 diabetes, you will want to

be an active member of your own team. Simply knowing which qu[e]
to ask can assure you of good care. You'll find a wealth of informatio[n]
magazines specially published for people with diabetes, and at semina[r]
and conferences. Many of us have found that we can even help to educate
some health care providers in the details of our management requirements. Management of Type 2 diabetes, with all the new treatment
options, is becoming more sophisticated than just prescribing one pill.
You have more choices than ever before for shaping your life, and your
physician has many more tools to help you achieve near-normal blood
sugar levels. And if you are not comfortable with the care you are getting,
it's your right to change providers.

"I had an MD who refused to take my diabetes seriously. He said it really didn't
matter what my blood sugars were, and he was sure that if I just lost 10 pounds
I wouldn't need to take any pills. On the other hand, my ophthalmologist was
screaming I'd go blind if I didn't get my sugars down. I would carry messages
back and forth from them but they wouldn't speak to each other. I finally got
rid of both of them and started to build a real team."—Myra

"I really liked my doctor, but he just didn't keep up with the latest diabetes
research. It was frustrating that I was the one who had to initiate discussions on
new studies and recommendations. I felt like I was carrying the whole load. I
found a diabetes specialist and I'm much happier."—Jack

Nutrition Therapy and Physical Activity

The three major components for controlling diabetes are the right medication or combination of medications, eating a healthful meal plan, and
following a physical activity program. The latter two are particularly
important for managing Type 2 diabetes because nine out of ten people
with Type 2 diabetes have a weight problem at the time of diagnosis. If
you are overweight, losing weight will help your blood sugar. A lower
weight will also help decrease your insulin resistance, allowing insulin to
more effectively move glucose into cells and decrease the excessive production of glucose by the liver.

Yes, it can be difficult to break a lifetime of routines and change how
and what we eat and become more physically active, but you don't have
to do it alone. The advice and guidance of a diabetes educator, dietitian
or nutritionist, or participation in an organized weight loss program can
be invaluable. You'll also find help in Chapters 10 and 11.

ok people are buying lots of fresh fruit and vegetables and read-
packages. And it seems like more and more people are out
treets or in the park. I've recently started working with an
gist to recover from a broken leg. I have been amazed and
to see women who are 10 to 20 years older than I am who are lifting
heavier weights than I can and bicycling longer and harder than I do. It makes
me feel great to see them. I do believe it's never too late to get going."—Sophie

Two measurements related to your weight are important: your body mass index (BMI) and waist/hip ratio (WHR).

Body Mass Index. This measurement defines how overweight or obese you may be. More experts are using this instead of the traditional percentage above your "ideal body weight" (IBW), largely because BMI can predict more precisely the risk of other abnormal conditions, primarily heart disease, high blood pressure, and Type 2 diabetes. If your BMI is over 25, you are considered overweight; over 27, mildly obese; over 30, moderately obese; and over 40, very severely (morbidly) obese. If your BMI is over 27 for men and 28 for women, you are at increased risk for the conditions noted above because you already have diabetes, itself a risk factor.

The BMI is calculated by dividing your weight in kilograms by your height in meters squared (or your weight in pounds multiplied by 704, divided by your height in inches squared). This sounds complicated, but with a calculator it is fairly easy to determine. Or you can use the following formula.

For example, take a man who is 5'10" and weighs 225 pounds. First, multiply his weight by 704 (225 x 704 = 158,400). Then, convert his height into inches and square it (5'10" divided by 12 = 70 inches; 70 x 70 = 4,900.) Finally, to get his BMI, take the first number and divide it by the second (158,400 divided by 4,900 = 32.3 BMI). He needs to lose weight. (If you want to use the other equivalent formula, you must convert pounds to kilograms by multiplying pounds by 0.45, and height in inches times 0.0254, then square the height.)

Waist/Hip Ratio (WHR). This measurement reflects whether body fat is distributed in such a way as to make someone pear or apple shaped. A pear shaped body, which is more common in women, comes from thigh fat and has a lower health risk than abdominal (or visceral) fat around the waist, which is more common in men. WHR is calculated by measuring your waist at the narrowest part between the bottom of your ribs and your navel, and the hip measure at the maximum place around your buttocks. Then divide your waist measurement by your hip measurement. You are at increased risk of other diseases if you're a man with a WHR greater than 0.90 or a woman with a WHR greater than 0.80.

What options are available if you choose to lose weight? If you're like most, you might first try dieting. The basic principle is to consume fewer calories than you normally would. If you diet on your own, you might find some success, especially at first. But for long-lasting weight loss, your best bet is to work out a personalized program with a physician, diabetes educator, dietitian, or nutritionist. Beyond limiting your calorie intake to a reasonable level, you should also increase your physical activity and adopt proven behavior modification strategies such as shopping when you're not hungry, resisting buying foods you shouldn't eat, putting your fork down between bites, chewing more slowly, taking smaller bites, charting your progress, and rewarding your successes.

Another weight loss option is the newly popular appetite suppressants, "Fen-Phen" (short for fenfluramine and phentermine) and dexfenfluramine (Redux). Although there are no studies on their long term safety, and dexfenfluramine is currently only approved by the FDA for use up to one year, they can help produce an average 10 to 20 pound weight loss when used in conjunction with the above weight loss strategies.

A 10 to 20 pound weight loss may be very helpful in controlling blood sugar and reducing the risk of complications. The concern is that once the medication is stopped, the weight returns. In a sense, this means they are medications for a chronic condition, obesity, and need to be taken indefinitely. There is also a known but very slight risk of a serious condition called pulmonary hypertension.

In May 1997, an FDA advisory panel recommended approval of a new drug called orlistat (Xenical). It works by preventing absorption of up to 30 percent of the fat you eat, resulting in an average weight loss of about 9 percent over one year. Further data are not available at the time of this writing. The FDA itself has not yet actually approved the drug's release, although this is expected.

Finally, if you are extremely overweight (morbidly obese with a BMI over 40—about 100 pounds overweight), you might be a candidate for gastric reduction or gastric bypass surgery. This dramatic intervention has had good long-term results in those with diabetes. The main risks are those of the surgery itself, which you should discuss with your physician or surgeon.

Medications

Managing Type 2 diabetes is a stepwise process. If weight loss and regular physical activity do not bring your diabetes under control, it's time for the next step, medication. There is now a much larger toolbox available than there was at the time of our last edition. These Type 2 medications are used singly or in combination—basically starting simply and progressing depending on how much your blood sugars decrease and their pattern. There are four major types of oral medications, each with a different action, plus insulin. The four types are sulfonylureas, biguanides, alpha-glucosidase inhibitors, and thiazolidinediones (pronounced thigh-a-zole-adine-die-own).

Sulfonylureas. These have been used for many years and, in fact, now include a "2nd generation" of medications. The first generation includes acetohexamide (Dymelor), chlorpropamide (Diabinese), tolazamide (Tolinase), and tolbutamide (Orinase). The second generation includes glimiperide (Amaryl), glipizide and glipizide extended release (Glucotrol and Glucotrol XL), and glyburide (DiaBeta, Glynase, and Micronase). All of the sulfonylureas work primarily by stimulating the pancreas to secrete more insulin. They do not directly affect the other two pathophysiologic defects, increased liver glucose production and decreased muscle glucose utilization. One of these medications is typically the first choice of drugs, particularly for the thin or non-overweight person with Type 2 diabetes.

Biguanides. Metformin (Glucophage) was approved by the FDA in 1995, although it had been used for years in Europe and elsewhere. This drug lowers blood sugar by decreasing liver glucose production and increasing muscle utilization, without stimulating insulin secretion. If your overnight blood sugar is too high, it is primarily because of increased liver production. Thus, metformin may be a good choice if this your main problem. (Also see troglitazone, below.) Metformin by itself is about as effective in lowering blood sugar as the sulfonylureas, but tends not to cause weight gain and may even be associated with weight loss. For this reason, it is useful as the initial medication in those who are overweight. Another advantage is that, by itself, it will not cause low blood sugar because it does not stimulate insulin secretion.

If you are already taking the maximum dose of a sulfonylurea without reaching the desired blood sugar, the addition of metformin is likely to lower the HbA1c by an additional 2 percentage points, thereby improving control. Similarly, if originally taking only metformin without meeting blood sugar goals, a sulfonylurea could be added to further lower blood sugar. To minimize the most common side effects, nausea and diarrhea, the dose should be started at a low level and gradually increased, even though these side effects are usually mild and short-lived. Metformin should not be used if there are kidney problems (serum creatinine greater than 1.5 in men or 1.4 in women). And it should be temporarily stopped if the you are undergoing major surgery or having any IV X-Ray contrast studies.

Alpha-Glucosidase Inhibitors. Acarbose (Precose) was also recently approved by the FDA. It works by a different action from any of the others, by inhibiting the ability of the gut to absorb sugars and starches. As you would expect, its primary effect is to reduce the aftermeal (postprandial) rise in blood sugars. It has relatively little effect on the fasting or overnight blood sugars. It's been shown to be effective in lowering HbA1c's in patients on diet alone, diet and sulfonylureas, diet and metformin, and diet and insulin. In the first three groups, it lowered HbA1c's by almost 1 percentage point; in the insulin group, it only lowered it by an average of 0.4 percentage points. The main side effects are excessive gas. If acarbose is started at a low dose and gradually increased, the side effects (primarily gas) can be avoided or minimized.

Thiazolidinediones. Troglitazone (Rezulin) was released in the spring of 1997. It is likely that other medications in the same class will be approved and released within the next year or so. These medications are called "insulin sensitizers" because they improve insulin action, primarily by increasing glucose uptake by muscle and decreasing glucose production by the liver. Thus, it may be particularly helpful if your overnight blood sugars are too high (see Defining Type 2 Diabetes section, page 120, and metformin above). Because of the increased muscle uptake, which makes it easier for the insulin to send sugar from your blood into your cells, thiazolidinediones can also help if your aftermeal (postprandial) blood sugars are too high.

Insulin. If oral medications, either alone or in combination, are not effective in bringing your sugars into your target range, insulin should be considered. Various options are available. Typically, a bedtime injection of intermediate (NPH or Lente) or long-acting (Ultralente) insulin is begun, often in addition to the oral meds. The bedtime insulin is directed at high pre-breakfast overnight fasting sugars, providing a better basal level of insulin to start the day. Similarly, bedtime insulin is used in combination with daytime sulfonylureas, which boost the insulin secretion after meals. Alternatively, two daily doses of NPH or Lente could be taken, usually before breakfast and before dinner, without any oral meds. The premixed 70/30 NPH/Regular is an option here as well. Troglitazone or acarbose can also be added to an insulin regimen.

A more intensive insulin regimen might be used, particularly if it has been difficult to bring blood sugars under control. Using NPH, Lente, or Ultralente as a basal insulin, regular or the very fast acting insulin analog lispro, could be used with meals to control the post-meal peaks in blood sugar. Often, once the blood sugar has come down substantially, it is possible to reduce or even eliminate the regular or lispro, because the lower blood sugars themselves can lead to improved insulin secretion and decreased insulin resistance. Because of lispro's quick action and shorter duration (2 hours) compared to regular (4 to 6 hours), it is somewhat easier to precisely regulate it. An insulin pump can also be used, either temporarily to bring sugars under control, or on a more permanent basis.

Combinations. Combination therapy is recommended if a single drug (monotherapy) is not adequate to bring your sugars into the target range. Several combinations have already been mentioned, particularly sulfonylureas and metformin, and insulin and sulfonylureas. It is possible to add acarbose or troglitazone to any of the other medications, which may result in lower blood sugars, or decrease or eliminate insulin. It is generally accepted that if monotherapy with a sulfonylurea or metformin is not sufficient, adding the other is a good step before adding insulin, acarbose, or troglitazone (triple therapy). If you are taking a sulfonylurea and metformin, and add insulin, you may be able to decrease the dose of one of the oral meds.

Thus, you can see that there are many more choices available now than a few years ago. It is critical to work with your health care providers to work out a regimen that will bring your blood sugars to the target level. Once you reach good control, it is just as important to monitor it and maintain it. Your body's metabolism is likely to change over time, and what is now your optimal regimen will change as well.

Support Groups

The final key to living well with Type 2 diabetes is seeking and nurturing support for your efforts. One of the best ways to receive this is through support groups. Read Chapter 14, Living Well With Others With Diabetes, for where to find support groups or even how to set one up and run it yourself.

"Two years ago I was looking through the local paper when I saw a story saying that a local college was looking for people with Type 2 diabetes to participate in a year-long study. I signed up for it. There was a monthly meeting, with two lay-leaders and a specific topic for each meeting. We also had our HbA1c tested every three months. The purpose of the study was to see if being part of a group helped to lower blood sugars.

"It was an amazing experience. We started out with about 15 folks, meeting at a local HMO. There were people on insulin, people on oral medications, and people taking nothing at all. We were tall and short, thin and fat, black, brown, and white, loud and quiet. And did we have a lot to teach each other! I had expected most of the people to be pretty much like me. But the diversity turned out to be the most important aspect for me. We struggled with the same problems, but seeing the way different people solve problems opened up a world of possibilities.

"We talked about food. More than one person had scoped out the lowest fat, non-sugared foods on the grocery shelves, others knew doctors who listened. We talked about insurance and some of the problems people were having getting their supplies covered and where they might go for care and supplies if they didn't have insurance. We also discussed what it was like being a diabetic in the real world. How to react to a present of a box of chocolate from a relative that should know you are a diabetic. We discovered some of us would never eat something that we shouldn't, while others would occasionally have a bite or two or even a small piece of something usually forbidden and not feel the least bit guilty. We shared much and we laughed a lot. So, this is why I think support groups are a great thing and that everyone should find one." —Grace

Become aware of the choices you have for shaping your life. It is not pleasing to learn that you have developed a condition that, as yet, has no cure and that calls for constant awareness. Just as dental work has become easier and less painful than thirty years ago, it is better to receive the diagnosis of Type 2 today than it was thirty years ago. Medical advances have made it much easier to have diabetes today. Because of the number of different medications available it is possible to find the one or the combination that works best for you. More and more people will avoid or delay complications because of these new medications and the knowledge of how diabetes affects us and how to live a lifestyle that will keep us healthy.

Chapter Seven

The Moderate Regimen

Learning the Moderate Regimen

The moderate regimen for Type 1 diabetes is part of a continuum of diabetes care and blood sugar control. This chapter is about finding a place on the continuum that is right for you at this time. The DCCT showed a direct relationship between risk of complications and level of blood sugar as measured by HbA1c. What this means is that every bit of improvement in blood sugar helps. Moreover, there is some evidence that an HbA1c of less than 8.1% provides the best chance to avoid complications. This convincing evidence makes it all the more important to attain the best control possible. Still, we know that not everyone is ready for the intensive regimen. We believe that it's critical for people to choose their level of care themselves, weighing the positives and negatives for them. That is why we have included guidelines for moderate and even loose regimens (see Chapter 8).

The moderate regimen can begin to improve your blood sugars; however, for it to be most effective, you'll need to:

1. Be sure you have a positive setting for your diabetes learning, a physician who agrees with your goals, and support from family, friends, and other people with diabetes.
2. Get lab tests of HbA1c, kidney function, and blood lipids (triglycerides and cholesterol) to indicate your present level of control.
3. Learn the skills and information needed for managing your diabetic control through the moderate regimen.

    a. Learn how to test blood sugar and urine. Understand the meaning of lab tests relevant to control. Know the criteria of control.

    b. Review Chapter 9, on recognizing and treating insulin reactions.

c. Survey the basics of diabetic metabolism (how your system processes food and liquids to produce energy and growth).

    d. Understand all the factors that determine blood sugar level.

4. Determine the level of regularity of diet, activity, and schedule you are willing to follow. Establish a schedule of blood and urine testing that is acceptable to you.

5. With your doctor's guidance, establish your ongoing insulin regimen (no more than two injections of insulin per day; use of the insulin pump is not recommended for the moderate regimen). Set target levels for your tests and action steps to take when blood sugar is high.

6. Observe how blood sugar levels are affected by stress, illness, changes in food and exercise, and other factors. Learn to vary insulin dosage, diet, and exercise cautiously to compensate for high or low tests and to deal with changes in your daily routine.

7. Have new lab tests done after two or three months to determine the effect of your new regimen.

8. Assess your progress. Find out how to further improve your control or maintain the level you have achieved. If you have not achieved all of your goals, determine the obstacles and how to overcome them.

9. Take steps to maintain your motivation for continuing to work on improving control.

10. Celebrate!

Step 1: Be sure you have a positive setting for your diabetes learning

There are many different reasons for choosing a moderate level of control. It may be the level that best balances the whole spectrum of needs in your life. For some, following the moderate regimen represents an enormous improvement in management. For others, it is a fall-back position chosen after attempting the intensive regimen and finding too many obstacles in the way. Some will be comfortable with this level of control until their motivation is boosted by an event like the onset of complications. Some will see it as only a temporary treatment plan until they have time and energy for learning the more disciplined approach.

    Whatever your reasons for selecting the moderate regimen, it is important that you allow yourself the most basic ingredient of living well—accepting your decision. The intensive regimen is praised so highly that you may feel a bit anxious, perhaps even guilty about choosing "second-best." Feelings like these are not good for your health.

Your decision to follow the moderate regimen was not made in isolation. You weighed your needs as a person and as a person with diabetes, your motivation, and the support available to you. The moderate regimen seems to you to be the wisest choice. Live well with it. (Plus, know that we have built into the regimen a periodic review of this choice—Step 8.)

As you work with this regimen, you may find your interest in care of diabetes growing, or other concerns may diminish, allowing you to devote more time to diabetes care. Simply having the immediate feedback of blood glucose testing may improve your control and increase your motivation to manage your diabetes. Gradually you may find yourself moving toward improved control, learning the information and skills needed at a pace that is right for you.

You may feel anxious because you are not ready or willing to gain optimal control right away. Many of us have experienced a degree of anxiety concerning the possibility of developing complications. It was just something we lived with, consciously or unconsciously. It is natural to experience it, and there are positive things you can do to handle it (see Chapter 16). The moderate regimen is likely to reduce your risks of complications, though not as much as the intensive regimen.

All of the suggestions made in Step 1 of the intensive regimen (page 57) apply to those working with the moderate regiment, so you can continue by reviewing that information. See what you need to do to be sure you have adequate support: a physician (and ideally a diabetes educator and other diabetes care providers) you can work with effectively, family and friends acquainted with your goals, and others with diabetes with whom you can compare notes.

Step 2: Have lab tests done to determine your present level of control

HbA1c, kidney function tests, and the blood lipids (fats) tests will allow you to see how effective your regimen has been to this point. You and your physician can set goals for these tests that are reasonable, given the moderate regimen. Then, new lab tests every three months, along with your own feelings of well-being, will be the best cue to how you are doing. You will find that the feedback from the tests will be very helpful, although at first you may need guidance from your doctor or diabetes educator in interpreting them. See Step 2 of the intensive regimen (page 60) for details.

Step 3: Learn the skills and information needed for managing your diabetic control through the moderate regimen

3a. Learn how to test blood sugar and urine

A major difference from the intensive regimen emerges in this step. Although you will still be using home blood glucose testing, you will not do it as often and you will also test for glucose in your urine. (Possibly, one of the reasons you chose a moderate regimen was that you did not want to test your blood several times a day. However, blood testing technology has improved substantially in the last few years, providing finer, gentler lancets, and very user friendly meters. The more often you test your blood rather than your urine, the better information you'll have to help better manage your diabetes.)

The best testing schedule for this moderate level of control is to test your blood glucose before taking your morning insulin and to test your urine before meals and at bedtime. The daily fasting blood sugar test allows you to supplement your morning shot with regular insulin to compensate for high readings when they occur. Starting the day in control helps you stay controlled throughout the day. The later urine tests give a very rough idea of how well you maintain control throughout the day. (Specifically, they tell whether blood sugar is staying over 180 mg/dl (10 mmol/L) or so before meals. More on this later.) You may also find yourself more willing to test your blood a second time than to test your urine at all. If so, fine!

If this is more testing than you are willing to do, determine a minimal schedule of testing that you feel able to follow consistently. Blood tests two or three times a week and urine tests once or twice a day are better than none. Schedule the urine tests at different times each day so you can see the pattern of results throughout the day—before and after meals—when you look at your log for several days.

By starting to test regularly, you will create a habit that you can expand on later. Even a few blood tests each week can help you improve control to some extent. Some people find it helpful to make a contract with themselves or their doctor, stating the number of tests they will do. Then a report is regularly filed with the results.

You should do additional blood glucose tests when illness upsets your control and to check your perception of insulin reactions. Sometimes you may mistake symptoms of anxiety and stress for those of an insulin reaction or even a rebound from a reaction (the Somogyi effect). This special form of insulin reaction usually occurs during sleep as a result of too much insulin in the bloodstream. Low blood sugar levels trigger the release of glucose and hormones, which lead to high blood sugar levels which in turn may mistakenly be treated by an increased insulin dose. If you show any signs of Somogyi reactions during the night, you can find out whether blood sugar is low by testing around 2:00 or 3:00 in the morning. In fact, whenever insulin dosage is more than 35 units a day, and morning blood sugar tests are high, you should check for low blood sugar during the night. It might also be the "dawn phenomenon." (See Chapter 8 for a full discussion of Somogyi reactions.)

To become more comfortable with blood glucose testing, it helps to take a class on the topic if one is available, or to have your doctor or diabetes educator instruct you in the correct testing procedures. A number of suggestions on home testing are given in Chapter 5, Step 3a (page 60). Also, read the previous sections on laboratory tests and record keeping.

With the moderate regimen, a different set of target values is necessary for evaluating your blood tests and urine tests than with the intensive program.

Moderate Regimen Target Glucose Levels

Fasting blood sugar test	70-150 mg/dl (3.8-8.3 mmol/L)
Before meal blood sugar test	70-180 mg/dl (3.8-10 mmol/L)
1-2 hr after meal blood sugar test	140-250 mg/dl (7.7-13.8 mmol/L)
Before-meal urine test	Negative
Bedtime urine test	Negative or 1/4%

We need to redeem the value of urine sugar testing. Blood sugar testing offers such improved accuracy that there is a tendency to dismiss the old urine test. This is a mistake for anyone who has not yet chosen the intensive level of diabetes management. Although limited, the traditional urine test still provides useful information. It tells you if your blood sugar since you last urinated has been higher than about 180 mg/dl (10 mmol/L) (the exact level varies from person to person). This information is not precise enough for optimal control, but it can help you keep to a moderate level of control. If your tests are usually negative, you know that your blood sugar has been below 180 mg/dl (10 mmol/L) or so.

Your average blood sugar over the past 2-3 months can also be corroborated by a HbA1c test. For example, if your HbA1c is around 9%, your average blood sugar is about 210 mg/dl (11.6 mmol/L); if it's 10%, your average is about 240 mg/dl (13.3 mmol/L); and if it's 14%, your average is 360 mg/dl (20 mmol/L). Under this regimen, your HbA1c should be under 9%. Of course, the goal under the intensive regimen is below 7%.

One of the shortcomings of urine testing is that the sample tested may reflect earlier blood glucose values. For instance, it is possible to have a positive test (indicating a blood sugar higher than 180 mg/dl [10 mmol/L]) while undergoing an insulin reaction. For this reason, to get a current reading, you should empty your bladder completely and then take the test when you urinate again in 10 or 20 minutes. Testing this second sample gives a more up-to-date reading. (Testing the first sample gives you an idea of how much sugar was spilled during the whole time since you last urinated.)

Another problem with urine tests is the varying level at which blood sugar spills into the urine from person to person. This level is called the renal threshold. Someone with a low renal threshold will show a positive urine test when the blood sugar is 140 mg/dl (7.7 mmol/L) or lower. Another person, with a high threshold, will not have a positive test until blood sugar is 200 mg/dl (11.1 mmol/L) or higher. (The average level at which sugar spills into the urine is 160 to 180 mg/dl [8.8 to 10 mmol/L].) Even in the same person, the renal threshold may change over time, usually becoming higher with age or as kidney function declines. Pregnancy also affects the renal threshold.

Finding Your Renal Threshold

The variability of renal thresholds makes it important for you to determine your specific blood sugar spilling point. This knowledge makes urine testing a much more effective tool. You can identify your renal threshold by testing both blood sugar and urine sugar at the same time. Probably the easiest way to do this is to test every 30 to 45 minutes, beginning when urine sugar is positive and continuing until it is negative. Empty your bladder, test your blood sugar, and then urinate again a few minutes later and test this sample. Drinking a glass of water each time you urinate will help. Record results of both tests until you can see the threshold level. A sample log illustrates this process:

Time A.M.	Blood Sugar Test mg/dl (mmol/L)	Urine Test (%)
9:00	240 (13.3)	
9:10		2
9:45	200 (11.1)	
9:50		1
10:30	160 (8.8)	
10:35		1/4
11:00	140 (7.7)	
11:05		Negative

The person above has a low renal threshold. A positive urine test here indicates that blood sugar is over 150. Another example shows a high threshold:

Time P.M.	Blood Sugar Test mg/dl (mmol/L)	Urine Test (%)
6:00	300 (16.6)	
6:05		1
6:45	260 (14.4)	
6:50		1/4
7:30	220 (12.2)	
7:35		1/10
8:00	200 (11.1)	
8:05		Negative

In the second example, the threshold is between 200 and 220 mg/dl (11.1 and 12.2 mmol/L) blood sugar. A negative test indicates only that blood sugar level is less than that; it may be anywhere from very low (40 mg/dl [2.2 mmol/L]) to fairly high (200 mg/dl [11.1 mmol/L]) and still be negative.

There is a variety of products, from tablets to strips, for testing urine sugar. Tests results can be affected seriously by large doses of vitamin C and some medications; so be sure to read the manufacturer's instructions to see if this is true with your product.

A second type of urine test, for urinary ketones, provides very important feedback on certain occasions. Ketones in your urine indicate that your diabetes is getting out of control due to insufficient insulin (too much food, not enough insulin, or too much physical or emotional stress). Strips are commonly available. It is especially important to check for ketones if you are ill (even with a bad cold) or experiencing high blood sugars (greater than 240 mg/dl [13.3 mmol/L]) or have four positive urine tests in a row. (See end of this book for more information on ketoacidosis.)

3b. Review the chapter on recognizing and treating insulin reactions

Anyone working to improve their control of diabetes runs the risk of having more insulin reactions while establishing the new level of regimen. You may feel comfortable handling reactions, but you will find some new approaches in Chapter 9.

3c. Survey the basics of diabetic metabolism

Go to Chapter 5, Step 3c.

3d. Understand the different factors that determine blood sugar level

The previous information on these subjects will help you gain a general understanding of the ups and downs of your blood sugar level, even though you won't be working intensively to keep it close to normal range at this point. Later, if you decide to move to the intensive regimen, you can review it in more detail.

Go to Chapter 5, Step 3d.

Step 4: Determine the level of regularity of diet, activity, and schedule you are willing to follow

With this step, we reach one of the contradictions of the moderate regimen. On this treatment plan, you have a wider range of acceptable blood sugar levels than on the intensive program, but you also have less capacity for adapting to irregularities. Without several blood tests a day to guide you, you are more likely to have reactions or high blood sugar levels if you do not follow a fairly regular diet, activity plan, and schedule. (Some people prefer to keep blood sugar level a bit high to avoid reactions.) The intensive regimen, on the other hand, allows much more flexibility, especially once you are past the first two or three months needed to learn it.

Ideally, your choice of moderate regimen means that you will stick to a fairly consistent healthful meal plan, either using exchanges, carbohydrate counting, or calorie count, and eat according to a fairly consistent schedule (not more than an hour off schedule unless you know your blood sugar is high). When a meal must be delayed, you should eat a snack and deduct the calories or exchanges from the meal. Similarly, physical activities should be fairly regular from day to day, adjusting your insulin dosage or food when there is an increase or decrease in the amount of exercise. As you gain experience with such adjustments, you may find it possible to increase the flexibility of this regimen.

It is up to you to decide the level of regularity you are willing to follow in your management of diabetes. Fortunately, the combination of your home blood and urine tests and the HbA1c test in the lab will tell you if your decision allows you to maintain a moderate level of control over a two- or three-month period. If the hemoglobin test is too high, you will know that you need greater regularity. Work with your doctor or diabetes educator to find the places where your regimen needs to be tightened up.

Step 5: With your doctor's guidance, establish your ongoing insulin regimen

Your insulin regimen is the overall dosage of one or two types of insulin taken in a single morning injection, or a dose split between morning and predinner injections. To be successful, you need to know the pattern of insulin activity—when it begins, when it peaks, and how long it is effective. Four insulin plans are available for the moderate regimen. (We do not recommend that people on the moderate regimen use more than two injections a day, nor should they use an insulin pump. This would require more frequent blood sugar tests and a stricter control program to be effective and safe.)

The Regimens

Plan 1: A single daily dose of intermediate-acting insulin (NPH or Lente), taken 20 to 60 minutes before the first meal of the day.

Plan 2: A single daily dose of intermediate- and rapid-acting insulin mixed, taken 20 to 60 minutes before the first meal. Pre-mixed intermediate- and rapid-acting insulins are available in 70/30 or 50/50 ratios and may work for you, either in this plan or Plan 4.

Plan 3: A split dose of intermediate-acting insulin, part taken before breakfast, part before dinner.

Plan 4: A split dose, mixing intermediate- and rapid-acting insulin before breakfast and dinner.

Plan 1

The single daily shot of NPH or Lente insulin was the standard insulin regimen for many years. This was a convenient breakthrough in the beginning, compared to the earlier multiple-dose plans using regular alone. Only one injection a day! It must have felt like an enormous improvement, especially because we had only urine testing to show our level of control each day.

Unfortunately, for most people with Type 1 diabetes, convenience is the only strength of this regimen. One shot of intermediate insulin has an extended peak, usually not beginning until the afternoon and lasting through early evening. (Thus, morning high blood sugar levels and afternoon reactions are common.) By evening, the insulin action is waning and often there is insufficient insulin to prevent high blood sugar levels overnight. Because there is only one long peak of activity, it is difficult to make adjustments to keep blood sugar within the moderate target range. Probably only a person whose pancreas still produces a substantial amount of insulin can maintain a moderate level of control on this treatment plan. A single dose of long-acting Ultralente insulin may also work for you. See page 98 for Gary's Ultralente anecdote.

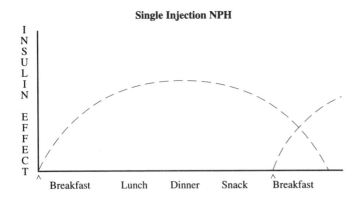

Single Injection NPH

INSULIN EFFECT

Breakfast   Lunch   Dinner   Snack   Breakfast

Plan 2

The single injection shown on page 141 mixes rapid-acting insulin with intermediate to cover the need for insulin between breakfast and lunch. The regular dosage can be increased to reduce high blood sugar or decreased if there will be added exercise in the morning. Control in the morning is improved, but care is necessary to avoid afternoon reactions. For most people, it is still likely that blood sugar will rise during the night.

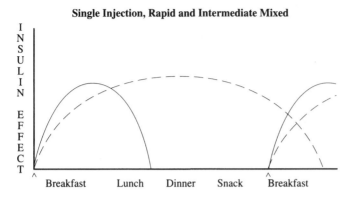

Single Injection, Rapid and Intermediate Mixed

Plan 3

By taking intermediate insulin (NPH or Lente) twice a day, there is a better overall distribution of insulin activity, with peaks in the early afternoon and around bedtime. Overnight coverage is improved, and you are more likely to arise with blood sugar within your target range. Small doses of rapid-acting insulin can be added to the intermediate when tests show high blood sugar. Because each of the NPH injections is smaller, the effective duration of action is shorter. The overlap between the two shots helps to handle the need for insulin following breakfast and dinner.

Still, if you are taking two shots of insulin a day, Plan 4 provides much better coverage and flexibility than this plan.

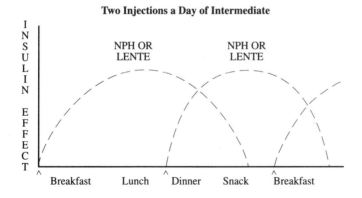

Two Injections a Day of Intermediate

Two injections of rapid- and intermediate-acting insulin, one before breakfast and one before dinner, provide the most effective distribution of insulin activity available under the moderate regimen.

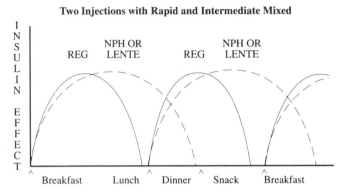

Two Injections with Rapid and Intermediate Mixed

With this plan, a peak of insulin activity follows each meal and an adequate supply continues through the night. (The same schedule is used in the intensive regimen. Combined with frequent blood glucose testing, it allows normal or near-normal blood sugar levels for some.) It is possible for you to learn to vary the amounts of either kind of insulin cautiously to prepare for changes in routine and to vary the regular insulin to correct high blood sugar levels. In this way you gain more flexibility than the other moderate insulin regimens offer. You may also be able to use a premixed fixed ratio of intermediate to rapid-acting (70/30 or 50/50).

These four insulin regimens are described in terms of idealized patterns of insulin activity. In you, each type of insulin may have a pattern of activity that is very different from the averages. This is why you should work closely with your physician or diabetes educator at this stage, identifying patterns by studying your test logs. Your physician may recommend a variation on one of these plans, or even a plan not mentioned, so that insulin activity matches your lifestyle and physical needs.

Step 6: Observe the variations in blood sugar level caused by stress, illness, changes in food and exercise, and other factors

Earlier you studied the different influences on blood sugar level—insulin, diet, exercise, and physical and emotional stress. Now you can use that information to understand your daily and weekly diabetes records. Seeing your blood or urine glucose levels swing up and down and not knowing why they change can be frustrating. But if you keep thorough records for

Diabetes: A Guide to Living Well

a few weeks, you can quickly learn to recognize the reasons for your fluctuations. With understanding, you gain more power to control your blood sugar levels.

We will illustrate this process by looking at several sample logs of people on the moderate regimen.

Daily Diabetes Log I

Bill takes two shots of NPH insulin daily, 20 units before breakfast and 12 units before dinner. He records only carbohydrates under the "Food" heading and usually eats snacks midmorning, in the afternoon, and at bedtime. His urine tests begin to show sugar when his blood sugar is around 200 mg/dl (11.1 mmol/L).

Date Time	Blood Test & Reactions	Insulin Dosage	Activity & Exercise	Food	Comments: stress illness, etc.
5-12					
7 am	150 mg/dl (8.3 mmol/L)	20 NPH	30 min bike	2 toast grapefruit	
11 am	strong react. **A**			roll of hard candies	
12 noon	2% urine gl **B**			cut 1 bread & fruit	
3 pm				cut snack **C**	
5:30 pm	neg	12 NPH		normal din	
8 pm					Big fight with Sue. She yelled. I bit my tongue.
10 pm	300 mg/dl (16.6 mmol/L) **D**			no snack	
5-13					
7 am	180 **E**	20 NPH	30 min bike	2 toast	
10 am				crackers	

Date Time	Blood Test & Reactions	Insulin Dosage	Activity & Exercise	Food	Comments: stress illness, etc.
12 noon	neg			normal lunch	
5 pm	neg			nuts & raisins	Knew dinner would be late
7:30 pm	1% (F)	12 NPH		Mexican din	Extra carbos & 2 beers
10 pm	150				
5-14					
7 am		20 NPH		usual breakfast	

First, go through this log and explain the blood or urine sugar readings or reactions followed by a letter (A-F). Then read the following paragraphs.

Bill's reaction at 11:00 a.m. (a) on May 12 occurred because he missed his midmorning snack, which was especially important given the bike ride earlier. The strength of the reaction caused him to overtreat it with an entire pack of hard candies. This, plus blood sugar rebound caused by the stress of the reaction, produced a 2 percent urine glucose test at noon (b). Since he starts spilling sugar into his urine only at 200 mg/dl (11.1 mmol/L), the 2 percent reading meant his blood sugar may have been as high as 300 mg/dl. He reduced carbohydrates at lunch to compensate and eliminated his snack (c) when urine still tested positively at 3:00. His urine test before dinner was negative (which only shows that it was under 200 mg/dl [11.1 mmol/L]) but the upsetting fight with his girlfriend caused another blood sugar peak by bedtime (d). He used a blood sugar test when he normally would have tested urine so he could see the impact of the strong emotional stress. He eliminated his evening snack.

His fasting blood test the next morning (e) was down to 180 mg/dl (10 mmol/L), 30 mg/dl (1.6 mmol/L) above his target range for fasting tests, so he compensated by omitting fruit from breakfast and riding his bike more energetically than usual. (Note: A urine test would have been negative for him because of his slightly high renal threshold.)

These changes in diet and activity balanced blood sugar enough so that urine tests were negative at lunch and at 5:00 p.m. Knowing that dinner would be late, he ate an extra snack to avoid reactions. Bill overate at dinner, which produced a 1 percent urine test at 10:00 (f). This probably indicated that his blood sugar was over 240 mg/dl (13.3 mmol/L). By omitting his late night snack on the basis of this test, he was able to return to his target range for fasting tests by the next morning.

Daily Diabetes Log II

Sandra, a working mother with two children, takes 40 units of NPH before breakfast. She records only carbohydrates in the food column and usually snacks in the afternoon and before bed. Her urine tests begin to show sugar when her blood sugar is around 160 mg/dl (8.8 mmol/L).

Date Time	Blood Test & Reactions	Insulin Dosage	Activity & Exercise	Food	Comments: stress illness, etc.
6:30 am	180 mg/dl (10 mmol/L)	40 NPH		cut 1 bread no fruit **Ⓐ**	Kids wild!
11:30 am	reaction **Ⓑ**		missed jazz dance class	2 donuts	Too much, but I've got to be sharp for noon meeting
12:15 pm				2 rolls bean soup 1/2 piece cake	Client insisted I share cake
3:00 pm	peeing a lot thirsty **Ⓒ**			skip snack	Must be high
5:30 pm	4+ urine 1+ ketones **Ⓓ**		took kids for 40 min walk	raw veggie salad & broth	
9:30 pm	still peeing xtra **Ⓔ**			skipped snack	
6:30 am	4+ urine but 150 mg/dl (8.3 mmol/L)	40 NPH **Ⓕ**		2 toast, 1/2 orange	

Again, see how you would explain the test results and symptoms marked by a letter (**A-F**), and then read the following.

By skipping too much carbohydrate at breakfast (**A**), Sandra found herself with low blood sugar before lunch (**B**). Lunch was an important meeting with a business client, so she knowingly overtreated the insulin reaction to be sure she wouldn't have another one. Too many doughnuts, a usual amount of lunch, a missed exercise session, and the stress of the meeting conspired to increase her blood sugar to a symptomatic level (**C**) and (**D**). She knew from the excess urination and thirst that her blood sugar was fairly high, so she skipped her afternoon snack. Then, finding ketones in her urine, she ate a very light dinner. Sandra's blood sugar stayed high in spite of reduced carbohydrates and an evening walk with the kids (**E**). (Remember, when blood sugar is high, each unit of insulin is less effective at lowering it, and exercise may even cause it to increase.) Using frequent urination as a signal that her blood sugar level was high, she skipped her bedtime snack. Her morning urine test was high (reflecting earlier high blood sugar), but her blood sugar test indicated she was within her target range (**F**). By cutting back on food, she had been able to cut the high blood sugar down to size.

Learn to vary insulin dosage, diet, and exercise cautiously to compensate for high or low tests and to deal with changes in routine.

Begin this step by reviewing Chapter 5, Step 7a (page 108). The basic kinds of changes you can make are described there, although the amount of change advised is for the person on intensive regimen only. With fewer blood sugar tests to guide changes, you will have to work much more cautiously. After you read that material, come back to this point.

Supplementary insulin can be used when tests are high or to prepare for a larger-than-usual meal. Supplements are always taken as rapid-acting insulin, so the impact is over a limited period of time. Do not take extra insulin on the basis of tests of urine that has been in your bladder for more than 15 or 20 minutes. (It may represent high blood sugar levels from hours ago.) Use urine samples collected a few minutes after you have completely emptied your bladder. Also, consider what you have discovered about your renal threshold, the level at which you spill glucose from bloodstream into urine. If you have done the tests comparing urine and blood sugar readings described earlier in "Finding Your Renal Threshold" (Step 3a in this chapter), you will better interpret your urine tests.

You can make such supplements of insulin more accurate (and safer) if you base them on blood sugar tests rather than urine tests. More and more people on the moderate regimen are using blood sugar tests when they feel a need to, even though they use urine tests on a daily basis.

When your blood sugar control is upset by physical illness, emotional stress, or other factors, you may want to do more blood sugar tests than usual. The greater accuracy will help you deal with the unusual conditions.

A rule of thumb for supplementing insulin on the basis of urine tests is to use 5 percent of your daily dose if the reading is 1 to 2 percent, and 10 percent of your daily dose if the reading is over 2 percent.

Urine Test (%)	Daily Total Dose	Extra Rapid-Acting Units to Take	% of Total Dose
1-2	20	1	5
2+	20	2	10
1-2	50	2-3	5
2-5	50	5	10

If your supplement is based on a blood sugar test, take one unit of rapid-acting insulin for every 30 mg/dl (1.6 mmol/L) over 120 mg/dl (6.6 mmol/L) your test shows, up to five units. It is wise not to take more than five extra units of rapid-acting at a time (2 to 3 units if you are a child or small adult). If your blood sugar level is still high at the next test, you can take another supplement then. Avoid taking supplemental insulin at bedtime unless your doctor advises it because of severe illness and very high blood sugar.

If you are consistently spilling sugar into your urine (revealed in more than one test a day or even one test at the same time every day), you should discuss this with your doctor. You may need a larger standard dose of insulin or an adjustment in your diet.

Supplements of rapid-acting insulin can also be taken before a special meal that you know will be larger or richer than usual. How much extra to take depends, of course, on the size of the meal. At first, don't take more than one or two extra units before seeing your next test. By trial and error, you will learn how much to add, but it is better to err by adding too little rather than too much. Be sure not to take the supplement too early. Special meals have a way of being delayed. If you are using the very fast acting lispro insulin, you can take the insulin within a few minutes of starting the meal.

When you plan to be more active than usual, compensate by taking less insulin or eating more. If you take only NPH, reduce insulin only if the extra activity will last for an hour or more, or if you know it will be occurring around the time of your insulin peak (roughly 6 to 12 hours after injections). Otherwise it is better to eat extra food to cover the exercise period. Generally one extra serving of carbohydrate (a slice of bread, for instance) should be eaten for every 30 minutes of hard exercise.

Do not rely only on increases in insulin to correct for high blood or urine sugar tests. You should also bring down blood sugar by adjusting exercise and food. This is especially important in the moderate regimen, because you are likely to have more high blood sugar levels than someone on the intensive plan. If you use only insulin supplements to reduce these highs you will gain weight.

Remember that when blood sugar is quite high (over 250 or 300 mg/dl [13.8 or 16.6 mmol/L]), exercise is not likely to reduce it and may even cause an increase. Meals may be reduced by one or two carbohydrate servings, but you should not fast because of the risk of severe reactions if there is no food in your system. The safest way of reducing a very high blood sugar level is to take a series of small injections of rapid-acting insulin (10% of daily dose), four to six hours apart until urine tests show less than 1 percent glucose or until blood sugar tests are under 200 mg/dl (11.1 mmol/L). (Someone with a total daily dose of 40 units should take no more than four units at a time.) When you are reducing an extra-high blood sugar level in this way, it is wise to rely on the greater precision of the blood glucose tests to guide you. Urine tests can still be positive when blood sugar has already reached normal range. If you have high blood sugar and ketones in your urine or are ill, it's best to contact your physician for guidance.

Step 7: Have lab tests done after two or three months
to determine the effect of your new regimen

At this point, you will have solid feedback on the effectiveness of your regimen. Tests for HbA1c and blood lipids, together with your home test records, will let you know if you have found the right balance in your program of self-care. As you review the results with your physician, be objective. You have certain target levels you want to achieve. If you haven't reached them, suspend all judgments of yourself and simply look for the reasons. The next step will help you do this.

Step 8: Assess your progress and determine what (if anything) is needed to improve control further

Again, you can use the same step in the intensive regimen (page 112), with just a few changes (like substituting the word moderate for intensive). Then instead of the 11 steps mentioned in the intensive plan, go to the beginning of this chapter where the learning steps of the moderate regimen are listed.

If you find that you have learned all you need to achieve a moderate level of control, we suggest you take a moment to review the decision you made on regimens. When you consider all factors, is a moderate regimen still your choice? You may feel content with the improvements in control you have achieved and prefer to give attention to other aspects of your life.

Or you may choose to move on to the intensive regimen. If so, you have already studied a major portion of what you need to learn, so it will be much easier to make the transition. Probably the main changes will be testing blood more frequently, possibly changing insulin regimen, and giving more attention to compensating for the variations you observe. Discuss the necessary changes with your doctor and review each step of the intensive regimen.

Step 9: Maintain motivation for continuing to work on improving control

If you choose to continue managing your diabetes at the moderate level, or if you still have more to learn about this level, keeping your motivation high is important. It may have been an easy process so far, or it may have been intensely frustrating. Either way, you will need to take steps to ensure that you remain willing to continue.

Rereading Step 1 at the beginning of this chapter may be useful. Building a positive foundation for this endeavor continues to be relevant now. You might find elements you neglected the first time around but now feel like putting into effect.

Support from other people with diabetes who are also working on improving control is one of the most important ways of keeping motivation strong. If you have not yet found ways of obtaining this, it may be time to do so. Support groups or individual contacts can give valuable emotional support and encouragement. You can receive practical guidance from people who have overcome the obstacles you may still be struggling with. You may also be able to help others with problems you have already solved. Serving someone else in this way keeps your motivation high. (See Chapter 14, "Living Well With Others With Diabetes.")

Living on a regimen is easier if you do not feel you are serving on "active duty" every day of the year. Occasional leaves or vacations should be part of your regimen; don't feel that you are cheating at these times. A day or two of relaxed management can make it much easier for you to continue with your usual level of control. If you take supplements of rapid-acting insulin to handle any feasts, keep them moderate to avoid severe reactions. (Such vacations are not advisable if you have any infection or a complication that could be made worse by higher blood sugar levels.)

If you have significantly improved your control, you are probably feeling better, both physically and mentally. This immediate payoff makes it easier to continue following your regimen. It also becomes an inspiration for continued learning. This is reinforced by the blood testing process itself. When you can see exactly what your blood glucose level is—and do something about it—you gain power over diabetes, instead of feeling controlled by it. It is natural to want to extend this sense of power by learning more about managing your condition well.

If you ever feel a strong resistance to continuing with your regimen, remember that there are steps you can take to explore and neutralize the issues that are getting in the way. Be aware of any rationalizations or denials that you use to justify the resistance. Don't accept "I'm really too busy" or "I don't need to be so careful, I'm all right now," or "It won't do any good anyway." Use the help processes in Chapter 3 to gain awareness of what is happening and ask for personal help if needed.

Step 10: Celebrate!

When you understand the moderate regimen, you have completed a challenging assignment. You may feel like honoring yourself for your achievement, privately or even publicly, with a party, dinner, or picnic. Whether you invite a small group or a large one, give yourself credit for the many things you have learned. What you are doing to live well with diabetes can be generalized. Other than taking insulin and testing blood, the basics of your regimen would give good health to anyone. So share the health.

Now is the time to collect a reward if you promised yourself one to build motivation at the beginning. In fact, even if you haven't made an agreement with yourself, go ahead and treat yourself to some special thing, event, or experience. Living well is its own reward, but there is nothing wrong with a bonus from time to time.

Next Steps

You may have chosen to stay at a moderate level of control while you dealt with other aspects of having diabetes. Review the Table of Contents to see what else you would like to work on now. You may find that you have learned enough to continue gradually improving your blood sugar management while you focus on other issues.

Possibly, there are problems or challenges in your life that you need to handle while you take a break in your diabetes learning (perhaps applying in other areas what you have learned about yourself here). If so, make a date with yourself to reopen the subject in three months or so. Mark the calendar: Time To Start Learning More About Diabetes? Diabetes is a lifelong companion, so you will benefit from also seeing it as a lifelong teacher.

On the other hand, now that you have mastered the moderate regimen, you may be eager to go right on to the intensive program. You have a solid foundation of knowledge, so it will be much easier than it would have been a few months ago.

Whatever your next steps, you might consider a subscription to the publications *Diabetes Interview* published by King Publishing, *Diabetes Forecast,* published by the American Diabetes Association, or *Diabetes Self-Management.* They are good sources for news on the latest developments in diabetes research and care. (See Appendix Two, Resources.)

Chapter Eight

The Loose Regimen

"It sure would have helped if someone had told me I was in control, even though my diabetes was out of control. I never saw that I was the one who went on binges or 'forgot' my shot. It just happened, like somebody else was doing it to me." —Ernest

Learning The Loose Regimen

1. Review the survival issues at the end of the book—insulin reactions, diabetic coma, and infections.

2. Learn to do home blood and urine glucose testing. Do tests occasionally, especially when you are ill or have an infection. Do urine ketone tests when you are ill or are experiencing high stress.

3. Take one or two insulin injections daily. (More injections or the insulin pump are not recommended without regular blood sugar testing.) HbA1c's will likely be over 3 percentage points above normal. People with Type 2 diabetes will take a combination of pills and/or insulin on a schedule prescribed by their physicians. If taking a combination of pills and/or insulin, you are already very close to an intensive or moderate regimen. Work with your diabetes educator or physician to explore improving your blood sugar levels.

4. Eat healthfully, and in moderation. Learn how to increase the pleasure of eating without increasing the sugar and fat content.

5. Observe great caution in adjusting insulin dosage. If you have Type 2 diabetes, consult your physician before making any changes in your medication.

6. Make a commitment to continuing diabetes learning, maintain your motivation, and review obstacles to improving control.

We assume in this book that all people who have diabetes are on a controlled regimen, no matter how wildly their blood sugar levels rise and fall. We make a series of self-care choices every day; together, they are the regimen we live by. Not taking insulin or oral meds, missing meals, overeating, and keeping an irregular schedule are some of the ingredients in regimens that are usually considered rebellion against a treatment plan.

We prefer to acknowledge the power you have if you are at this level of management. If we believe that we control our diabetes management, we are more likely to realize there are other choices. We can live well while finding an approach that matches our physical needs as people with diabetes.

We have outlined a loose regimen, with recommendations for certain minimal self-care standards. It is a fairly simple approach without elaborate tasks. The loose regimen is far from the standards of control recommended for diabetes today, but we can still live well by doing what we can (or will) and not condemning ourselves for what we can't (or won't) do. We can live well by finding whatever it is we are willing to do to achieve control. This is the heart of our philosophy of diabetes care.

Step 1. Review the survival issues at the end of the book

The highest priorities in your diabetes education are low blood sugar, diabetic coma, and infections. Ignorance of these could cost you your life.

If you often have low blood sugar levels (more than a couple of times a week), you may need information on avoiding them. Chapter 9 deals with reactions and could be a lifesaver for you.

Step 2. Learn to do home blood and urine glucose testing

We suggest that you learn to do home blood glucose tests. Even if you use these infrequently, they are one of the most valuable things you can learn. As few as two tests a week have proven effective in helping people with diabetes improve their metabolic control. Keep the test strips available so you can easily test when you want to know how changes in diet, activity, or stress have affected your blood sugar levels. If you think your blood sugar has become high, check it and validate your perception. When you become ill, home blood testing makes it much easier to prevent blood sugar levels from skyrocketing. This can promote quick recovery.

If you wish to learn more about home blood glucose testing, see Chapter 5, Step 3a. You may also find it useful to take a class, or ask your doctor or diabetes educator to show you test techniques.

If you have not been doing urine glucose testing, you might also consider this as part of your regimen. Although not particularly useful for intensive management, urine tests give useful feedback with less strict regimens. You can determine when your blood sugar is more or less controlled, and when it is quite high, you can take action to bring it down.

The test for ketones in the urine is especially important because it indicates when your control is significantly off, due to physical illness, emotional stress, or very high blood sugar levels. For information on making the feedback from urine tests more meaningful, see Chapter 7, Step 3a.

Step 3. Take one or two insulin injections daily

(More injections or the insulin pump are not recommended without blood sugar testing.) HbA1c will likely be 3 percentage points above normal. People with Type 2 diabetics will take a combination of pills and/or insulin on the schedule prescribed by their physicians. If taking multiple pills, or pills and insulin, you are already very close to an intensive or moderate regimen. Work with your diabetes educator or physician to explore improving your blood sugar levels.

If you have Type 1 diabetes, without frequent blood sugar testing, you should not take more than one or two injections of insulin a day. Your physician will help you determine the types of insulin and dosage that will best suit your schedule. Chapter 7, Step 5 describes several one or two injection schedules.

If you have Type 2 and do not check your blood sugar regularly, it is necessary that you take the prescribed medications on a schedule outlined by your doctor.

Step 4. Eat healthfully, and in moderation

If you overeat, binge eat, and ignore your meal plan, you might find Chapter 10 helpful. It contains tips on ways to enjoy food while eating more healthfully.

Step 5. Observe great caution in adjusting insulin dosage

Be cautious in adjusting insulin dosage to compensate for changes in diet and level of activity. You need the feedback of regular blood sugar and urine tests to do this safely. If blood sugar is high because you are ill, consult with your doctor on any changes in the amount of insulin you take.

Because the medications prescribed for Type 2 diabetes come in pills of different types and dosages, it is difficult to determine the effects of changes. Consult your doctor if you feel changes are needed. In this instance Type 1's have somewhat more flexibility than Type 2's.

Step 6. Make a commitment to continue diabetes learning, maintain your motivation and review obstacles to improve control

Explore what commitment you are prepared to make to continue learning about diabetes self-care. Determine the aspects of diabetes management that you are willing to work on. By proceeding this way, you are likely to learn more quickly.

Scan the sections of the moderate and intensive regimens to see if you are interested in learning about them. Look again through the Table of Contents and find what you are now willing to learn about. A conversation with your physician or diabetes educator might help you define your next steps. (Call 1-800-TEAM-UP- 4 to obtain a list of diabetes educators in your area.)

Who Chooses the Loose Regimen?

A variety of people choose this level of diabetes management. The loose regimen may be your choice if you are someone:

▷ Whose life is in turmoil or filled with external demands.
▷ Who values quality of lifestyle in the present over the possible reduction of future risks.
▷ Who feels rebellious and unwilling, or weak and unable to change.
▷ Who has a poor self-image.
▷ Who has little money and cannot afford necessary supplies.

We can offer specific guidance to people in each of these groups.

1. If your life is filled with external demands or is in turmoil, set aside some minimum amount of time for learning to manage your diabetes more effectively. As little as ten or twenty minutes a day can be a good beginning. The important thing is to make a commitment in spite of a challenging schedule or an overwhelming set of problems. Once you have begun, it may be easier for you to give diabetes care a higher priority and give more time to it. You may find that some of those other tasks can be scaled down or put on hold for a while. If not, you will at least learn information and skills vital to your well-being. You also are likely to find that you feel better physically. This can give you more strength to deal with your other life demands.

2. If you have chosen the loose regimen because you tend to live for the moment, valuing present pleasures over future risks, you may be surprised. Many people following more intensive regimens report no shortage of enjoyable experiences. For them, greater control is equal to greater freedom. Regular blood glucose testing and the ability to adjust insulin, diet, and exercise allow great flexibility in lifestyle, at a relatively small cost in time. (Those with Type 2 diabetes, of course, do not have the same freedom in adjusting medications.) This freedom in living carries with it less anxiety about the future. People who are actively controlling diabetes are doing the best they can to reduce the risk of complications later in life. Physically, you will be amazed at how much better you feel when your blood sugar levels are close to normal.

You will find it useful to review the leading pleasures in your life and ask yourself how they can be reconciled with improved diabetes care. There are relatively few absolute contradictions, so long as you are not attached to excess itself as a pleasure. It might help you to talk with others who are following more intensive regimens but who have found ways to respect the pleasure principle.

Although you may feel set in your habits, you should remember that human beings are very adaptable. You can probably think of changes that have occurred in your own life that at first seemed very negative but soon proved to be definite improvements.

3. If rebelliousness or a sense of weakness and incapacity are what you feel, you may want to work on issues of power. Diabetes regimens are followed with greater ease when you find the source of authority within yourself, rather than in the medical system. You are the one who ultimately decides what you will or will not do, no matter what your doctor says. If you see doctors as authorities who give orders, and you then act against their advice, your rebellion is hardly freedom. If you feel weak and unable to do what your doctor says, this too is a form of rebellion though more subtle. Either way you lose.

Real freedom and power come from consciously deciding what you will do in each situation you face. Even if your doctor does tend to give commands, hear them as intelligent advice. Make conscious decisions of what you will or will not do and give yourself room to make new decisions. (See Chapters 3 and 15.)

The Loose Regimen

4. Some of us feel that we don't deserve first-class care. If this is your reason for choosing loose regimen, you may need to work on developing a more positive self-image. Unfortunately, negative beliefs about yourself tend to produce behavior that reinforces them. Escape from this cycle can take place through changes in the beliefs themselves or in the behavior. In some cases the assistance of a trained therapist is advisable, but many people have made changes at this level solely through their own efforts. (See the sections on self-image and beliefs in Chapter 15. Chapter 3 also contains information you may find helpful.)

5. If you lack the money for home blood glucose testing or other diabetes care supplies, seek help from your local American Diabetes Association chapter. A staff person there can help you search for community resources that may provide you with essential supplies. Some health insurance companies now cover testing supplies and equipment, as well as diabetes education. Several states have also passed laws requiring health insurance companies to pay for necessary equipment, supplies, and education. If your state has not passed such legislation, it is likely that your advocacy help will be welcomed by the American Diabetes Association's Delegates for Diabetes program. Also, see Appendix Two for discount mail-order supply houses offering significant savings.

Chapter Nine

Living Well
With Insulin Reactions

"There's nothing that makes me feel more anxious than the idea that I may just lose it if I don't eat enough or if I jog too far. I've had one reaction I didn't wake up from and one where I got so confused I forgot I was looking for food. My son finally came home and had to tell me what to do. I don't ever want to go through that again!"

—Jan, a 35-year-old woman

When psychologists ask what bothers us about having diabetes, we usually cite insulin reactions as our top concern. If we don't respond adequately to this short-term complication of diabetes, we can find ourselves in embarrassing situations because of things we did in a less-than-coherent state. We could even find ourselves waking up in the hospital or in jail. Simply stated, very low blood sugar levels result in unclear thinking and emotional outbursts. And if blood sugar levels fall too far, we can lose consciousness. Is there any wonder we feel bothered by this?

Because proper response to insulin reactions is so vital, this chapter reviews the traditional ways of treating these reactions. We have added new approaches to help people change emotional and behavioral patterns that can cause insulin reactions. There is also a section for those working with optimal control, since hypoglycemia (low blood sugar) tends to work differently when blood sugar levels are usually near normal than when they are usually high. While you are gaining optimal control, the risk of having reactions is greater than usual, and you need to know what to expect. This is true for people on the insulin pump as well as for those on multiple-injection regimens. This can happen in both Type 1 and in Type 2 diabetes, especially if you are taking sulfonylurea drugs, with or without insulin. Metformin (Glucophage) alone does not cause hypoglycemia.

The Action Of Reaction

When blood sugar falls below a certain level (usually around 60–70 mg/dl [3.3–3.8 mmol/L]) our body signals red alert. The resulting stress reaction releases adrenal hormones that produce the racing pulse, nervousness, and sweating indicative of an insulin reaction. This is our involuntary (or autonomic) nervous system going to work. The response is appropriate, because the situation is serious. If our blood sugar levels become too low, we lose consciousness—our brain and central nervous system need glucose to function properly. If it stays too low for too long we risk brain damage, though our bodies usually respond if we lose consciousness. One of the hormones released in a serious reaction is glucagon, which is stored in the liver and helps raise blood sugar levels. However, repeated insulin reactions can lower the amount of glycogen or glucose available to deal with hypoglycemia.

(High blood sugar levels that can follow a moderate to severe reaction are often caused by glucagon stimulating more glucose release than necessary. This is known as the rebound effect. The effect is multiplied when the person with diabetes eats more than necessary to compensate for the reaction. More about the rebound effect can be found later in the chapter under "Somogyi Reactions.")

Insulin reactions are caused by several different factors, such as a delayed meal or missed snack, an unexpected period of strenuous activity, too much insulin because of a mistake in measuring dosage, a period of strong emotional expression, or even a time of relaxation after a week of high tension. It's a matter of eating too little or too late, or an excess of activity, insulin, or emotional stress. (However, stress can lower or raise blood sugar, depending on the circumstances.)

Well managed diabetes depends on balancing the different factors affecting blood sugar level. Reactions occur because food, exercise, insulin (or oral hypoglycemic medications such as sulfonylureas) and stress levels are out of balance. As we learn to regulate these factors, we learn to avoid reactions. We discover how different activities affect blood sugar, and how to adjust food intake or medication dosage to compensate for increased activity. We learn what kind of stress is likely to lower blood sugar for us and when to compensate.

The symptoms of a hypoglycemic reaction vary by person and type of reaction. Fortunately, blood glucose testing provides a solution: If blood glucose is below 60 to 70 mg/dl (3.3 to 3.8 mmol/L), it's time to eat a snack that will be rapidly absorbed. Testing whenever a reaction is suspected is excellent practice for a person newly diagnosed, as well as the individual who is tightening metabolic control. The feedback of the test helps you develop and sharpen awareness of the symptoms that signal the onset of a reaction for you.

Other than blood sugar levels, the particular symptoms of a reaction depend upon the severity of the reaction, the rapidity of onset, and other individual factors. The particular symptoms are the result of low blood sugar levels on the autonomic nervous system (the ANS) and the central nervous system (the CNS—primarily the brain). The typical symptoms of a mild to moderate reaction include lightheadedness, dizziness, shakiness, sweating, increase in heart rate, and hunger. As the reaction progresses, vision may become blurry and the mind fuzzy (related to the CNS). There can be mental confusion, emotional outbursts, numbness and tingling in the lips, tongue, or fingers, or extreme anxiety (related to the ANS). A person can forget that he or she is looking for candy, or become distracted in their search. (If it's a nocturnal reaction, the person may dream or imagine that the candy has been eaten.) In some cases, one may even become angry or resistant if anyone else suggests eating something sweet. Anger and change of personality are signs often recognized by those close to us.

Finally, if nothing is eaten, the person loses consciousness and can experience convulsions. (The muscular movements can be imagined as the body's attempt to squeeze out any sugar the muscles might be storing.) If someone else knows what is happening, treatment can usually revive the person immediately. Otherwise, a visit to the emergency room will be necessary.

This sequence isn't always the same. Sometimes a reaction will approach very quietly, especially if the decrease in blood sugar has been slow. The first sign may be confusion or irritability. There may be a sense of unease or difficulty getting to sleep. However, in times otherwise marked by anxiety, it can be difficult to determine that shakiness is indicating a reaction rather than stress. Later, we will describe ways of increasing your sensitivity to these signs so you can treat reactions early.

Symptoms of Insulin Reactions

You will experience some, but not necessarily all, of these symptoms, and you may find a few unique to your body.

A mild reaction—Tiredness or weakness, hunger, sweatiness, chills, cold hands, increased heart rate, shakiness (or shaky feeling), dizziness, lightheadedness, headache, pallor, and difficulty getting to sleep.

A moderate reaction—An increase in any of the above, anxiety, confusion, anger, unclear thinking, loss of emotional control, strange behavior, poor coordination, speech difficulties, and blurred, spotty, or double vision.

A severe reaction—Stupor, loss of consciousness, and convulsions. Both you and those close to you should be familiar with these symptoms.

Some people with diabetes do not experience the typical reaction symptoms. Because of reduced production of the hormones that signal a reaction, blood sugar can fall very low without producing symptoms. If you are not experiencing the usual symptoms of a reaction, discuss this with your physician or diabetes educator. "Hypoglycemic unawareness" is becoming more recognized, and its causes appear to be more numerous and complex than previously thought. (If you have developed diabetic neuropathy or are taking prescription drugs like beta blockers, you might also not be experiencing some of the typical symptoms such as rapid pulse, shakiness, or sweatiness.)

To a large extent, the symptoms of a reaction and those of other conditions overlap. Anxiety or fear can cause a quickened pulse, cold hands, and shaking. Too many cups of coffee can produce a nervousness like that of a reaction. The hot flashes of menopause or other hormonal changes can mimic hypoglycemia. And rapidly falling blood sugar levels can produce symptoms of a reaction long before blood sugar really is low. Treating a reaction when your symptoms are actually caused by anxiety can result in high blood sugar levels. It is best to test your blood whenever possible to verify that glucose levels are too low. However, any time you are in doubt and cannot test, it is better to eat some rapidly absorbed carbohydrate than risk a severe reaction. If the symptoms begin to decrease, it's likely your blood sugar was too low. (Some diabetes educators are finding people with all the symptoms of a reaction whose blood sugar is normal or high. Usually they have had high blood sugar for a long time. If this is the case for you, discuss it with your physician. However, you should still eat some carbohydrates to relieve your symptoms.)

The symptoms of hypoglycemia can also be masked by the effects of alcohol or other drugs. Someone who becomes even moderately intoxicated or high may not notice a reaction until blood sugar levels are quite low. The need for caution is compounded by alcohol, because this drug lowers blood sugar when one has not eaten for some time. It also blocks the liver's ability to release glucose into the blood. A couple of drinks before dinner can generate a severe insulin reaction that may not be discovered until the process has already advanced. If you choose to drink or use other drugs, it is best to check your blood sugar level and eat a moderate snack (unless your tests are high—over 180 mg/dl [10 mmol/L]).

Somogyi Reactions

The Somogyi reaction (named for its discoverer, Dr. I. M. Somogyi), is a prolonged insulin reaction that usually occurs during sleep as a result of too much insulin in the bloodstream. During this unique type of reaction, the symptoms are usually not strong enough to wake you, however, blood sugar does not continue to go down. (Somogyi reactions are different from typical nighttime insulin reactions in which you either wake up in a sweat or don't wake up until the medics administer glucose to you.)

Low blood sugar levels trigger the body's defense system, and glucose is released along with hormones to slow the burning of glucose. A side effect of this process is the burning of fat, resulting in ketosis (indicated by a positive test for ketones in the urine). Because of the rebound effect, one may find ketones in the urine and blood sugar at a relatively high level in the morning. If the doctor responds by giving you more insulin, a vicious cycle is started that leads to more severe Somogyi reactions. The appropriate response is either a reduction in total insulin dosage or an adjustment in the type of insulin action.

Signs of a Somogyi reaction:
1. Ketones in the urine, with blood sugar under 250 mg/dl (13.8 mmol/L).
2. Evidence of night sweating (wet bedclothes).
3. Low temperature in the morning (body temperature may be low for as long as six hours after an insulin reaction).

4. Bad dreams or nightmares.

5. Irritability, abdominal pain, or headache upon awakening.

6. An apparent need for high insulin dosage (more than 50-60 units a day).

If you suspect that you are having Somogyi reactions, discuss your symptoms with your doctor. However, do some research beforehand by setting an alarm to wake you midway through your sleep period. Test your blood on several different nights to see if your blood sugar is at hypo-glycemic levels (below 60 mg/dl [3.3 mmol/L]). If so, the component of your insulin dose active during the night will need to be decreased. Usually only a few units are cut, however, if your overall insulin dose is excessive, larger cuts might be needed. (Normal bedtime sugars with low 3:00 a.m. levels and high prebreakfast levels suggest the Somogyi reaction.) Do not make changes in your insulin dosage without talking to your physician.

Reactions and Optimal Control

In people who manage diabetes with moderate or loose control, reactions might represent large and rapid decreases in blood sugar levels. The symptoms are usually strong and easily recognized. When tighter control is gained on the intensive regimen, a decrease in blood sugar of only 20 or 30 mg/dl (1.1 or 1.6 mmol/L), can be enough to cause a reaction, and the change can take place very gradually. As a result, the symptoms are often much subtler. Slight confusion or unclear vision could be the only signs that blood sugar has dropped to 50 or 60 mg/dl (2.7 or 3.3 mmol/L). Those of us who maintain this level of management need to heighten our awareness and not expect all reactions to sound a strong alarm. One of the early findings from the Diabetes Control and Complications Trial (DCCT) is that those on intensive regimen had significantly more reactions than those on the loose regimen. Again, the ability to check blood sugar levels allows verification of hypoglycemia. By doing this, we can learn what our new and subtle signals are.

While adjusting to the intensive regimen, reactions are also likely to occur more frequently. The protection against hypoglycemia provided by high blood sugar levels is gone, and it takes time to gain the skills and knowledge necessary to stay in balance. Keep schedules, diet, and exercise regular during this time. Once you've learned to manage diabetes, you can make changes easily and still maintain balance.

Those gaining optimal control may find that normal blood sugar levels feel rather uncomfortable and trigger symptoms of hypoglycemia. This is especially true if earlier blood sugar levels were consistently high. This is a brief occurrence, usually lasting no more than a week or two. The symptoms fade after adjusting to a more normal metabolism.

Treating Insulin Reactions

You now have a choice between making diabetes care a "treat" or a treatment. When blood sugar is too low, the sweets you usually avoid are prescribed medicine. Some of us use this opportunity to satisfy our craving for candy, cookies, and ice cream. Eating these foods is perfectly acceptable as long as you are able to control the amount you eat and do not end up bingeing. Pharmaceutical companies are now making products designed to treat insulin reactions. These are made of straight glucose—sugar in its most rapidly absorbed form. The advantage of using glucose lies in its quick absorption rate, having a precisely measured dose, and that it is less likely to lead to overdose or indiscriminate use when blood sugar is not low. The disadvantages are that the flavor is rather bland, they cost more than candy, and they're difficult to carry in the pocket.

Assuming the sugar can be absorbed quickly, the amount used is more important than the type. The usual recommendation is to eat a food containing 10 to 15 grams of simple carbohydrate. Some foods that satisfy this requirement are listed in the accompanying table. For comparison, we also list some dessert servings that would be too much if taken for a moderate reaction.

Some Appropriate Treats for Insulin Reactions

One-half cup (4 ounces) orange juice—13 grams carbohydrate

One-half cup apple juice—15 grams carbohydrate

Six ounces (1/2 can) cola—15 grams carbohydrate

One fig bar—10 grams carbohydrate

Two 2-inch chocolate chip cookies—12 grams carbohydrate

One tablespoon of granulated sugar—12 grams carbohydrate

Two teaspoons jam—14 grams carbohydrate

One-half-ounce raisins (2 tablespoons or half a small bag)—10 grams carbohydrate

One-half-ounce caramel or peanut brittle—12 grams carbohydrate

Five Life Savers—10 gram carbohydrate

(Always carry a couple of servings of these items, and keep some in your glove compartment, desk, or locker. A role of Life Savers is especially convenient and inconspicuous.)

Some Excessive Treats

One slice apple pie—60 grams carbohydrate (four times as much as you need)

One piece of cake with frosting—60 grams carbohydrate

Twelve ounces of cola (a full can or bottle)—30 grams carbohydrate (twice times the necessary amount)

One jelly doughnut—48 grams carbohydrate (three times as much as you need)

When you are dealing with a severe insulin reaction, the temptation to over compensate can be powerful. (This is especially true in the middle of the night, when blood sugar can fall to very low levels before you wake up.) However, if you want to avoid leaps in blood sugar levels, you need to eat moderately. Treat reactions in stages, first eating 10 to 15 grams of carbohydrate, waiting ten or fifteen minutes, and then eating another 10 to 15 grams if the symptoms have not subsided. (The exception to this practice would be when you are experiencing a very severe reaction following strenuous exercise or a missed meal. At such a time, you may need to double the amount of sugar to bring blood glucose back to normal.) Remember that you are likely to have a rebound effect, with the glucose from your liver increasing blood sugar along with the sugar you use to treat the reaction. If you overeat, your next blood test could be in the 300s.

Unless a reaction occurs within an hour of mealtime, you should have a moderate snack of carbohydrate along with some protein or fat (such as crackers and cheese, or nuts) after you have eaten a sweet. This will tide you over to the next meal and prevent another reaction.

If you are take insulin or sulfonylureas, you run the risk of not waking up when a reaction occurs, or of becoming unconscious because hypoglycemia is not treated in time. This is not common with sulfonylureas alone, but it can and does happen. The people close to you should know what to do if they find you unconscious, so ask them to read this next section and take notes.

If you cannot awaken your sleeping beauty, it is most likely that he or she is in insulin shock (severe hypoglycemia or insulin reaction, the result of very low blood sugar). The accompanying table compares the outward symptoms of insulin shock and diabetic coma (the result of very high blood sugar), so you can know for sure what is happening.

If your friend is in a diabetic coma, the only treatment you can administer is to call a physician and get them to a hospital immediately. If a doctor is not available, get your friend to an emergency room. Most likely, he or she will not have been feeling well for the last half-day or more. Diabetic coma is gradual in onset, and usually one feels ill, is thirsty, and has to urinate frequently as the condition progresses.

Outward Signs of Insulin Shock and Diabetic Coma

Shock	Coma
Sudden onset (minutes to hours)	Gradual onset (days)
Pale, moist, sweaty skin	Flushed, dry skin
Shallow breathing	Deep, labored breathing
Normal breath	Fruity smell on breath
Rapid pulse	Usually rapid pulse
Low blood sugar	Very high blood sugar

If the patient is in insulin shock, you might be able to help them regain consciousness on your own by providing sugar in a form that they won't choke on. The best possible treatment is glucagon, a substance injected like insulin. If you're lucky, there is a kit available and you have been instructed in its use. There are two vials—one containing dry glucagon and the other sterile water. Mix the two to create a liquid solution of water and glucagon; using the syringe, inject the solution under the skin in a fleshy spot such as the thigh or back of the arm. The glucagon promotes the release of glucose from the liver.

If there is no glucagon, jam, jelly, or frosting is the treatment of choice. Jellied glucose products such as Glutose or Monojel are also recommended. Place some of the product on their lips and in their mouth. Encourage ingesting the product by massaging the mouth, cheeks, and throat. Provide a couple of tablespoons or more. (Ernest's wife, Grace, revived him once with an appropriately named preserve—Hero's Jam.)

If nothing is available in jellied form, have your friend swallow small sips of fruit juice or soda pop (not diet soda). Be cautious—you don't want to cause choking. Avoid solids unless you can be sure they will be chewed and swallowed and not cause gagging.

The lack of blood sugar reaching the person's brain may produce antagonism and uncooperativeness as they begin to revive. It may seem like poor thanks for all you've been through, but don't be alarmed, it's the result of a serious insulin reaction.

If you're not sure whether it's diabetic coma or insulin shock, it's best to try giving a sweet (as above) to see what happens. Low blood sugar can cause harm more quickly than high blood sugar.

If your patient doesn't recover consciousness within five minutes, call the paramedics or get him or her to an emergency room. You've done everything you can. Thank you for your loving care.

To the Person with Diabetes...

Show your love for the people close to you by not putting them through the process just described. It is one of the most terrifying events one can experience. Study the next section on preventing reactions, and practice what you learn. If you have had more than one reaction in recent years that you did not awaken from, we suggest that you do the exercise on page 170.

Preventing Insulin Reactions

The best way to avoid reactions is to maintain an awareness of your diabetes. Don't obsess about it, but acknowledge that it is a companion who refuses to be left behind. People who frequently suffer from insulin reactions are often the ones who pretend they do not have diabetes. This lack of management doesn't work, and they often end up with vivid reminders of their illness.

You are more likely to have an insulin reaction in certain situations. If you have been more active, delayed a meal, or eaten lightly, hypoglycemia will occur if you don't compensate for the change in routine. If these situations heighten your awareness, you will find that you automatically take the appropriate action. The light meal or the delay becomes a signal to eat a snack (unless blood sugar tests are high).

To adjust to an increase in activity level, take less insulin (cutting dose by two or three units or up to one-third the total dose, depending on the increase in exercise), or increase your food intake. In general, eat an additional 10 to 15 grams of carbohydrate for every thirty minutes of extra physical activity (a slice of bread, a whole graham cracker, one-half ounce of raisins, or a medium orange).

Through trial and error you will find the amount that's right for the kind of activities you are involved in. You will be able to hike or work in the garden all afternoon and maintain balance, avoiding both reactions and high blood sugar. The chart of calorie expenditures in Chapter 11, gives you an idea of how much energy you burn with different activities. Note that vigorous activities such as digging with a shovel, playing tennis, or hiking uphill can use nearly an entire meal's worth of calories in one hour.

Remember that vigorous exercise continues to lower blood sugar for as much as six hours after you stop; you may need an extra snack or a larger meal after a period of prolonged or intense activity. This happens because well-exercised muscles absorb more sugar from the bloodstream, even after the activity stops. Exercising regularly helps you avoid reactions; because glucose stored in the muscles can be utilized when blood sugar levels go down.

Diet is another factor that helps stabilize blood sugar levels and prevent hypoglycemia. If you eat slower-burning foods, you will have a more continuous supply of glucose entering the bloodstream. This is one reason that high complex-carbohydrate, high-fiber diets are being recommended by many nutritionists. Protein burns even slower, but it is usually accompanied by more fat than we need.

As you become more aware of the physical sensations that precede an insulin reaction, you will be able to determine how much simple carbohydrate you need to maintain normal blood sugar levels. You gain a sense of "dosage" with foods such as raisins, prunes, and fresh fruit. ("There's that feeling. I could test, but there's no reason to think that I have anything but normal or low blood sugar. Let's see, four prunes should see me through to lunch.") Sometimes this becomes a matter of shifting the order of a meal, eating the fruit or other simple carbohydrate at the beginning of the meal rather than at the end. Anyone who has experienced a reaction that occurs while eating a meal that won't be absorbed for an hour knows the value of this practice.

Sensitivity to the symptoms of insulin reactions varies greatly from person to person. One may be very aware of bodily states, noting the onset of hypoglycemia at a very early stage. Another may be so absorbed in day-to-day activities that they recognize a reaction only when sweat is pouring down their brow and speech is slurred. You can take steps to increase your awareness and thereby your chances for survival. Be aware that diabetic neuropathy (see Chapter 18) and certain prescription drugs (such as beta blockers prescribed for high blood pressure or heart disease) can block the typical symptoms. Again, "hypoglycemic unawareness" is now becoming more widely recognized.

Some people with diabetes have rare hormone deficiencies that mask or even eliminate the symptoms of hypoglycemia. Blood sugar can fall to very low levels before any symptoms are experienced. Unfortunately, the symptoms that do occur are likely to be confusion or emotional instability caused by the brain receiving too little glucose. Frequent blood testing and meticulous adherence to regimen is especially important for anyone in this category.

Many of us can recognize an insulin reaction before blood sugar levels reach a hypoglycemic level. It is possible to create sensitivity to the subtle cues your body gives that indicate you are about to bottom out. This requires heightening physical awareness, something many people avoid. When blood sugar is continually high (over 200 mg/dl [11.1 mmol/L]), we tend to be mildly uncomfortable. (Ernest describes his discomfort as the feeling of having fine sand or granules of sugar in his muscles.) Rather than deal with this distress, many of us ignore our bodies; reactions have to be more serious before we notice them. If you are out of touch with your body, there are ways you can increase your level of awareness.

One way is to make routine physical activities like brushing your teeth, shaving, or showering occasions for feeling your body rather than thinking about other things. Become aware of the sensation of temperature in various body parts, muscle tensions, the texture of whatever surface is in contact with your skin, or the feeling of your breath or pulse. (When you are still you can sense the pulsing of your whole circulatory system.) A good time for observing is when you are waiting for something to happen. Your body is always happening—no waiting necessary!

A more direct way of heightening physical awareness is to focus on everything you experience as you become hypoglycemic (and, of course, as you eat something). See how many different sensations you can notice and make mental notes; the sensations may differ from time to time. This is also a good time to identify the more subtle changes that may be present during hypoglycemic unawareness. (More techniques are described in Chapter 12.)

Along with increasing body awareness, you can use blood testing to help determine when a reaction is near. When you note a physical change that might be signaling the approach of low blood sugar, check to see what your level actually is. If you are in the normal range (70-120 mg/dl[3.8-6.6 mmol/L]) wait a few minutes and see if more distinct symptoms develop. (A reaction is more likely to follow a normal blood sugar reading of 80 rather than 120mg/dl [4.4 rather than 6.6 mmol/L].) If you write down the symptoms that are followed by a reaction, you will soon be able to bring blood sugar levels up before the stronger symptoms have developed. This enables you to avoid rebounding to high blood sugar levels produced by the stress of a serious reaction.

If you have difficulty waking up at night when blood sugar plummets, there are two solutions, one mental and one medical. The first is a matter of learning to pay attention to your body's signals, no matter what time they appear. This can be accomplished through a dialogue with yourself as you relax into sleep, a time when your mind is open to suggestion. Find your own words to express thoughts such as: "Body, I know you send me signals when a reaction is happening and I want you to know I am willing to hear them, no matter how deeply I am sleeping. I don't want to put you through the stress that occurs when I fail to wake up. I want to live well with you and our special needs. I'm willing to hear your call for help." Reinforce the message by remembering the sensations that tell you a reaction is beginning. Visualize yourself awakening, getting out of bed, and going to the kitchen for a 3:00 a.m. snack. You can also use this process to reinforce your awareness of daytime hypoglycemia.

The medical solution to not waking up when reactions occur is based on wet bedclothes. The sweat of a serious reaction triggers a moisture sensor under the bedding that sets off an alarm. There is also a sweat sensor called The Sleep Sentry that is worn on the wrist. (Ask your pharmacist or the diabetic supply firms listed in the Appendix about these products.)

As we mentioned earlier, certain types of stress can have a hypoglycemic effect. Relatively little is known about stress and diabetes, but it is possible that actively expressing emotions, especially anger, can lower blood sugar. (The opposite—suppressing and withholding emotions—appears to raise blood sugar.) Study the effects that different kinds of stress have on you so you can determine which ones might cause insulin reactions. This way you will know when you need to take preventive steps.

With a Little Help...

There is a social side to preventing insulin reactions. People close to you and those with whom you work need to know that you have diabetes and what the outward signs of hypoglycemia are for you. Don't risk a situation dangerous for you—and difficult for others—because of pride. There are times when one is concentrating on an activity, or when confusion is the first symptom to appear. At such times, someone else may notice the signs of hypoglycemia long before you do. If someone close to you thinks you are having a reaction, make it easy for them to approach you.

Another social aspect of reactions is that some of us feel embarrassed or bothersome to others when we need food fast, especially if it interrupts or changes planned activities. It can be difficult to say, "I can't wait until we get to the beach to eat. Can we stop now? I'm having a reaction." However, you will be putting your friends to much greater bother if you pass out on them while trying to remain "inconspicuous." If you state your needs directly, most people will be understanding. Don't feel self-conscious about eating in front of others who are not eating, even if they think of you as someone who shouldn't eat sweets.

If you are about to engage in a public performance, such as giving a speech or making a long sales call, you may feel anxious about becoming hypoglycemic. The anxiety may even feel like a reaction. If possible, test your blood sugar beforehand and, if needed, eat enough to get you through your engagement. If you can't test, go ahead and have a moderate snack. The risk of one high test is certainly less than the risk of having a reaction at an important moment. (The precaution here is especially important when the performance involves physical activity.)

Wearing a diabetes I.D. bracelet or necklace and carrying a card with details of medication dosage is often taken for granted. Unfortunately, some of us are afraid to be recognized as having diabetes and neglect to carry this important information. In an accident or episode of insulin shock, it could save your life.

Some Questionable Benefits Of Reactions

If you resist doing anything to reduce the number of reactions you have, you might be gaining hidden benefits. A simple example of this is when you are hypoglycemic and it is medically prescribed to eat something you are normally discouraged from eating ("Oh boy, a sweet treat! This is a pretty strong one. I must need a hot fudge sundae or apple pie a la mode"). Children are not the only ones to use reactions as an excuse to indulge. As we mentioned before, the sugar of the food combined with the rebound effect, produces blood sugar levels much higher than if you had eaten the candy without having a reaction.

The solution is simple: Don't use the reaction to gain something you can already do. In this case, reward yourself once in a while and eat something sweet. It is best to do it when your blood sugar level is near normal or when you are planning to be more active than usual. If you're going to be really outrageous (hot fudge sundae level), take an extra unit or two of rapid-acting insulin just before you gorge (but not at bedtime). Your control will be much steadier if you avoid having reactions in order to eat sweets. Don't substitute a big dessert for a well-balanced meal with the same amount of calories or carbohydrates. You could experience a serious reaction because the simple carbohydrate is absorbed rapidly and there is no continuous source of glucose.

Some of us use hypoglycemia as permission to express hostility we normally keep inside. Some of the nicest people rant and rage when their blood sugar levels fall too low; anyone who suggests that they may need a few chocolate chip cookies becomes a target for their abuse. When it is all over, the insulin reaction is blamed. If this is your approach, learning to express your anger directly is the key to living well.

There are other ways some people with diabetes use reactions to escape responsibility. Not waking up from a nighttime reaction practically guarantees that someone else will take care of you; when you are knocked out by hypoglycemia, someone else has to bring you out of it. It can become a way of testing a mate or a parent: "If you really love me, you'll save my life." It can also be a form of revenge, given the amount of stress the rescuer must go through to revive you. Ironically, the person who fails to wake up at night may be the very one who fights off all assistance when they are hypoglycemic during the day, saying, "Don't you think I can take care of myself?"

Two couples in one of Ernest's support groups played identical games around reactions. Each of the two men had experienced repeated nighttime hypoglycemia that had to be treated by their wives or the paramedics. The men insisted they couldn't do anything about it and their wives were growing increasingly frustrated and angry.

When reactions occurred during the day, the men insisted on their independence and ability to take care of themselves. They were very reluctant to pay attention to the symptoms their wives would point out in the evening, often waiting until they were hypoglycemic before they would eat. It took the feedback of the support group to help the men see the pattern of dependence they were caught in. They and their wives had to work to form a more balanced relationship.

This is a delicate issue to work with. We want to be independent, yet we depend on food, medications, regularity of meals, family and friends, and doctors to help us handle our condition and its complications. And worst of all, in a very fundamental way, we cannot depend on our own bodies as others do. No wonder we declare our independence and act very dependent.

If you suspect that a desire to be taken care of is at the root of your difficulties with insulin reactions, you might explore the question with those who are important to you. In what ways can you be more direct in asking for care and support? What can you give in return? And most important, what can you give yourself to increase your sense of being well cared for?

Reactions And Sex

One of the frustrations in the life of a person with diabetes occurs when the passion drains away just before or while making love, and an insulin reaction takes the place of an orgasm. The body makes the wise choice of preservation over reproduction and pleasure, but sometimes that's not easy to explain to your partner. This is another time when a pre-event blood test and extra food may be in order, especially if you tend to be an athletic lover.

Section Three
Living Well With
The Keys To Control

Chapter Ten

Living Well
With Your Food Choices

"Tell me what you eat, and I shall tell you what you are," wrote Brillat-Savarin in 1825. But beyond the individual, food and eating are an inextricable part of our culture, from daily activities (the coffee break) to major events (Thanksgiving feast). Edward Espe Brown, a Zen priest, poet, chef and cookbook writer wrote in 1991 that "food is not just food, something 'out there;' food is our body, the body of the world, the way the body of the world becomes our body...Eating with awareness, we know that life is delicious...We join again the ageless dance of life—and rejoice."

These words are especially meaningful to those with diabetes; food and eating are very important parts of our lives. Most of us are very conscious of how particular foods—as well as how much and when we eat them—affect how we feel. Nutritional research has increased our understanding of the effects of various foods on our metabolism.

In this chapter, we highlight how the recommended "diabetic diet" has changed over the years. In fact, there is no longer a diabetic diet but rather an individualized meal plan. We will describe new findings, and integrate them into guidelines for healthy, appealing meals. We will also share tips on ways to enjoy food and eat within these guidelines. During this process, old nutritional beliefs will become myth.

The So-Called Diabetic Diet

Before insulin was discovered, people with diabetes were instructed to completely avoid carbohydrates (starches and sugars). After insulin was discovered, those with diabetes were usually put on low-carbohydrate diets with moderately high fat and protein. (In the 1920s and 1930s, some research showed that high-carbohydrate diets may be more advantageous than low-carbohydrate diets, but this work was largely ignored.)

The exchange system, based on the number of grams (weight) of carbohydrate, protein, and fat in each food, became the basis for determining the proper diet for individuals with diabetes. Usually a physician would determine how many calories seemed appropriate and refer the patient to a dietitian. Patients would learn about exchange groups, create a diet prescription tailored to their preferences, and learn about which foods to avoid.

By the 1960s and 1970s, many physicians were recommending less rigid diets, based on the experiences of their patients. New research was scarce, and doctors were conveying different truths—and myths—to their patients. By the mid-seventies Americans were becoming more food conscious, and the effects of various foods on health were becoming more widely known. Along with growing interest in nutrition, research was adding new and better data, which was widely advertised to the general public.

Recommendations included decreasing cholesterol, total fat, and saturated fat in our diets, increasing the proportion of polyunsaturated and monounsaturated fats such as olive oil and canola oil to saturated fats, and increasing the amount of fruit, vegetables, and fiber in our daily meals. Not surprisingly, these guidelines are totally appropriate for people with diabetes.

Research on the effects that specific foods have on blood sugar levels produced surprising findings for those with diabetes. Certain foods that we were taught to avoid, such as ice cream, raised blood sugar levels half as much as "good" foods such as whole wheat bread. Nutritionists were finding the glycemic effect (impact on blood sugar level) of a particular food was determined by a variety of factors, not simply by the number of grams of carbohydrate. The physical form of the food and the amount of fat eaten with it appeared to make a difference in the effects, although the quantity eaten was still the most important factor.

Before we look at these recommendations in more detail, answer the following questions.

1. Among the foods you eat regularly, which do you enjoy most?

_____

_____

2. Which of the foods mentioned above do you consider healthy? Which do you consider unhealthy?

_____

_____

3. What foods would you like to eat more of, but don't, because you feel they are unhealthy?

_____

_____

4. What foods do you eat too much of?

_____

_____

Review your answers to these questions. You may change some of your judgments about "good" and "bad" foods as you learn new information in this chapter.

New Facts About Food

The New American Diabetes Association Nutrition Guidelines

The most important change is that meal plan recommendations should be individualized, based on an assessment of weight, lifestyle, ethnic background, blood sugar control, blood pressure, and lipid (fat) levels in the blood. Insulin, oral medications, activity, and other lifestyle factors, such as working the night shift, should be integrated into the individual's daily schedule. While some of this may not be new, there is now more freedom and fewer restrictions. It is helpful to work with your physician and a registered dietitian (RD) or diabetes educator considering these guidelines.

Fat, Cholesterol, Protein, and Carbohydrate

Most scientists and health professionals agree that we would benefit from decreasing the total fat and cholesterol in our diets and increasing the ratio of polyunsaturated and monounsaturated fats to saturated fats.

Living Well With Your Food Choices

Total fat, especially saturated fat, is the major factor affecting our cholesterol levels, more so than the amount of cholesterol we eat. (Polyunsaturated fats include most liquid vegetable oils; monounsaturated fats include olive oil and canola oil; saturated fats include all animal fats, dairy products, and coconut and palm oil.) These changes have been linked to a reduced risk of heart disease in those without diabetes. Because people with diabetes have two to four times the risk of heart disease as the general population, these dietary guidelines are especially important.

The American Diabetes Association, as well as the British and Canadian diabetes associations and the American Heart Association, with few exceptions, have recommended lowering the fat content of diabetic diets from 40 to 45 percent to less than 30 percent of total calories. The gap needs to be filled with more calories from either carbohydrate or protein. Evidence does not support higher or lower protein levels than what is appropriate for the general public. (The minimum amount that most of us need is between 45 and 65 grams per day, much less than most of us eat.)This means that 10 to 20% of total daily calories should come from protein. Fewer than 10% of calories should come from saturated fats and no more than 10% from polyunsaturated fats, which leaves 60 to 70% from monounsaturated fats and carbohydrates. Recent studies indicate no adverse effects from high carbohydrate diets, especially when most of the calories come from complex carbohydrates (starches) and fiber. (More about carbohydrates when we discuss the glycemic index.) However, this is a controversial area with some who recommend increasing monounsaturated fats and decreasing carbohydrates. This is applicable to those who have high triglyceride levels. Nonetheless, if obesity and weight loss are primary concerns, decreasing the overall calories in the meal plan is most important. Even a 10-20 pound weight loss can be enough to improve blood sugar and lipid levels significantly.

What about cholesterol? Doctors are increasingly recommending moderate intake of cholesterol. The "Lipid Research Clinics Coronary Primary Prevention Trial" studied middle-aged men who had no evidence of heart disease but did have cholesterol levels of 265 mg/dl or higher. The study showed that a low cholesterol diet along with the drug cholestyramine not only lowered cholesterol levels, but also reduced the risk of heart attack. This research provided strong evidence, for the first time, that decreasing cholesterol may prevent the development of coronary heart disease.

Total cholesterol is made up of the "good" HDL cholesterol and the "bad" cholesterols, LDL and VLDL. Many experts believe it is important to know your HDL level, especially if your total cholesterol is high. It appears that the ratio of total cholesterol to HDL cholesterol is the most significant number for determining risk. For example, if your total cholesterol is 200 and your HDL is 50, your ratio is 200/50, or four-to-one. (Any ratio under 4.5-to-one is considered good.) Current recommendations for people with diabetes are total cholesterol and triglycerides of less than 200 mg/dl, LDL less than 130 mg/dl (unless you already have evidence of coronary heart disease, in which case, less than 100) and HDL greater that 35mg/dl.

What does all this mean for us? It means we have to be more aware of the food we eat. Fortunately, food labeling regulations have made it easier for people with diabetes to determine the nutrient content of particular foods. This applies only to prepackaged and fast foods; we have to calculate this information for foods we prepare ourselves in the old-fashioned way. Furthermore, manufacturers and restaurants are offering more low-fat and sugar-free products. Support for these practices is growing among the general population. The diabetic diet is good for everyone. However, just because a food is low-fat or fat-free or sugar-free does not mean you can eat more or unlimited amounts. Calories still count and these foods usually are not calorie free.

There have been special news items recently that seemingly cast doubt on the benefits of eating healthy. However, for people with diabetes, the benefits far outweigh the costs. For example, some of you may have heard about the French paradox, where the French apparently eat more fat than we do, yet have a lower rate of heart disease. Or you may have read about the study that calculated the average American would live only three to four months longer by following a 30 percent fat diet. Years ago the French had a diet much lower in fat than they currently do, and the rate of heart disease is likely to increase as those currently eating a high-fat diet age. And the mathematical study averaged the benefits over all individuals, rather than those who might benefit the most. Some also attribute the lower heart disease rate among the French to a more relaxed lifestyle and greater consumption of fruits and vegetables. Researchers will probably find that some of us have genes that will protect us no matter what we eat. However, today we know that those with diabetes are at high risk for heart disease, and the odds are that following a low-fat diet will benefit us.

Fiber

Food scientists and health professionals have increasing evidence that dietary fiber is good for those with diabetes. High fiber intake improves lipid levels and can lower the usual rise in blood sugar following meals, decreasing insulin requirements. However, the effect of fiber on blood sugar control is probably insignificant, according to the ADA nutrition recommendations. Therefore, people with diabetes should follow the same recommendations as everyone else, eating about 20-35 grams of fiber daily from a variety of foods.

The fiber we are talking about is plant fiber, found in vegetables, fruits, grains, and legumes (beans). It is useful to divide fiber into two types, soluble (guar and pectin) and insoluble. Soluble fiber is found in fruits, dried beans, and oat products (or in a pure form extracted from them); insoluble fiber is in grains, wheat (cereal) bran, and vegetables. Soluble fiber lowers cholesterol.

How does fiber work? In general, the water-soluble fiber decreases the time required for food, particularly glucose, to leave the stomach, pass through the intestine, and be absorbed into the bloodstream. Soluble fiber increases the thickness of food in the digestive tract. However, insoluble fiber acts like roughage and increases the bulk of our stool. Soluble fiber has an acute effect on our blood sugar, balancing the response to food, whereas insoluble fiber has a more long-term effect (two to three weeks) on glucose tolerance. Thus, it's wise to eat both kinds of fiber.

We can increase our fiber intake by eating more fresh fruits and vegetables, beans, bran, and whole grain. (See Table 2 at the end of this chapter.) Many health-food products are available to add purified fiber to the diet, but these must be mixed into the food in order to affect the glycemic response. We favor the fiber found in natural plant sources rather than these supplements.

The Glycemic Effect

Traditionally, carbohydrates have been divided into simple and complex groups. Simple carbohydrates consist of refined sugar and unprocessed sugar found in fruits and vegetables; complex carbohydrates consist of starches found in potatoes, rice, grains, and beans. People with diabetes have been taught to avoid simple sugars, in the belief that they were absorbed more quickly and raised the blood sugar higher and faster than starches. However, there is little scientific research to support this, despite the years this belief was held and taught. Recent research has shown that the biologic effect of food on blood sugar is much more complex. It is clear, however, that proteins and fats will not raise blood sugar substantially, unless eaten in large amounts. The ADA guidelines recommend that the first priority should be to the total amount of carbohydrates eaten, rather than source of the carbohydrate (simple or complex).

One method of figuring your carbohydrate intake is called "Carbohydrate Counting." This is a technique one of us (Gary) has been using since he was a teen, although it wasn't called carbohydrate counting then.

Gary Counting Carbohydrates

As a teen, I had been following a typical diabetic diet based on food exchanges. However, I had been taught how much carbohydrate, fat, and protein were in each exchange. I had also been given a book of food values similar to the one by Pennington referenced at the end of this chapter. Therefore, I had the tools to do some creative exchanging. If I were supposed to eat 4 bread exchanges at lunch, I knew that this was 60 grams of carbohydrate(15 grams per bread exchange). So I knew that I could eat any sort of carbohydrates that totaled about 60 grams. Furthermore, my physician told me that the carbohydrates were the main food that would affect my blood sugar, and that I didn't really need to consider fat and protein as far as my blood sugar was concerned. Ever since, I have been basing my diet on counting carbohydrates, and moderating my fat and protein intake.

In recent years, carbohydrate counting has become a main tool used by dietitians for teaching meal planning. If you take insulin before meals, you can adjust the amount of insulin you take based on how much carbohydrate you expect to eat. You need to learn to estimate the amount of carbohydrates in the foods you eat (the new food labels help tremendously). Also, you need to learn how much insulin you need (either what you produce or what you inject) to utilize the amount of carbohydrates you eat. There are general guidelines, but each individual is different. Your physician, dietitian, or diabetes educator will need to work with you to determine the correct ratio (or ratios—some people vary depending on the time of day). The Pennington, Netzer, Ulene, and Kraus books at the end of this chapter give carbohydrate counts for foods; books are also available that can help with carbohydrate counting.

Researchers have found that foods thought to have less rapid effects on blood sugar, such as potatoes, raise blood sugar as rapidly as a Mars candy bar. And other foods, such as yogurt, raise blood sugar half as fast as a starchy staple like bread. Various foods have been studied and compared to the effect of pure glucose on blood sugar. Glucose was assigned a glycemic index of 100, and all other foods received a score proportional to the pure glucose effect. More recently, the standard has been changed to one slice of white bread equal to 100, and the scores adjusted appropriately (see Table 1 at the end of this chapter). Foods with a low glycemic index are called slow releasers.

What have these studies taught us? First, that pure sugars have a high glycemic index, but table sugar (sucrose) is less than bread at 92, and fructose (fruit sugar) a low 32. You still need to limit them, however, because of their high concentration. They should not be added to your meal plan, but rather they should be substituted for other carbohydrates. Again, this should be done in moderation, because the sugars in high concentration tend to be found in foods with "empty" calories. High-fat foods, such as whole milk and pastry, have relatively low indexes, whether they are simple or complex carbohydrates. (Fat is thought to slow absorption of carbohydrates.) Grain products vary, but there is little difference between whole grain and white bread, or whole grain and white pasta. The difference between pasta and bread is considerable. Pasta is a slow releaser, raising blood sugar levels much less than other grain products.

Physical form appears to explain the differences between pasta and bread. The starch in pasta is more compact and perhaps less accessible to digestive enzymes. Similarly, rice ground into flour is more accessible and results in higher glycemic levels than does whole grain rice. Legumes (beans and peas), as a food group, have the lowest index. Presumably, their soluble fiber increases food thickness, slows movement through the digestive system, and slows absorption. Finally, cooked root vegetables, such as white potatoes, beets, and carrots, have a very high index as a group. However, an average serving of cooked carrots has only 5 grams of carbohydrate. Surprisingly, sweet potatoes and yams (not candied) have relatively low glycemic indexes.

An interesting observation we have made, and confirmed with others (although we have seen no published studies), is the high glycemic effect of Indian and Chinese food. This is independent of the obvious sources of carbohydrate such as rice and flour products. Many of us have experienced a similar effect with pizza; perhaps the effect was the result of eating more pizza than we thought! However, a study testing the effects of pizza on blood sugar showed that in a controlled setting, pizza raised blood sugars significantly greater than an equal amount of carbohydrate and fats in other foods. There was no obvious explanation for this effect.

Although practical application of the glycemic index for meal planning has been de-emphasized, we believe that we can offer reasonable guidelines based on experience. Suggestions on how to use the glycemic index are incorporated into the next section.

Nutrition Guidelines

These guidelines are based on the preceding information, current ADA recommendations, and experiences of ourselves and others. Under each guideline, are tips that make the recommendation easier to follow. We recommend that you work with your physician, dietitian, or diabetes educator to tailor a meal plan that works for you, and continue to adjust it as necessary. Remember, you are what you eat! (Your physician can help with a referral, or you can call 1-800-366-1655 for a dietitian referral or 1-800-TEAMUP4 for a referral to a diabetes educator. Calling 1-800-DIABETES will reach DIAL, the Diabetes Information and Action Line of the American Diabetes Association.)

Work with your physician, dietitian, or diabetes educator to establish a general plan for total calories, distributed as mentioned earlier among carbohydrates, monounsaturated, polyunsaturated, and saturated fat, protein, and alcohol (if desired). One gram of carbohydrate or protein equals 4 calories, one gram of fat equals 9 calories, and one gram of alcohol about 7 calories. The calorie conversion will greatly assist you in reading labels and calculating the percentage of calories from fat and other food groups. For example, if the label says one serving is 150 calories and the amount of fat is 10 grams, multiply the number of grams of fat (10) by 9 calories per gram of fat. This equates to 90 of the 150 calories (60%) coming from fat.

Use Moderation

This principle is a guiding rule that will usually keep you out of trouble. What you typically or habitually eat (for example, every day for breakfast, 3 days a week at work, every night while watching television) is what will have the most impact. What you eat only occasionally is far less important. It won't poison you!

1. Become a taster. Eat just a bite or two of a food that would greatly raise your blood sugar if you ate the whole thing.

2. Slowly absorbed foods such as pasta should be eaten in moderate amounts. Too large a serving will produce high blood sugar tests later in the day. Be moderate with high-fat foods as well, such as nuts and nut butters or potato chips. One ounce of peanuts has 165 calories, or more if cooked in oil.

3. Share sweet desserts with friends when you want a treat. Satisfy your craving without overloading your system. (You may have to explain that small servings of dessert are not poison to you.)

4. You may fear that sugar lust will overcome you, and one bite will lead to a binge. Since binges are usually a secret activity, you can control this urge by eating sweets only when you are with other people. Say, "I'm going to eat three bites of this pie and then it's all yours."

Ernie and the Microchips

I managed to acquire a taste for Swiss chocolate in the last few years, in spite of its high fat content. Bittersweet, especially, doesn't have that much sugar, I told myself. And traditionally I'd worried more about sugar than fats. Then I decided to break with tradition and cut the fat content fairly drastically. Give up chocolate? Well, how about less? And I find the flavor is so intense that I can now thoroughly enjoy eating two or three microchips—a half inch square weighing a few grams—where before I would have eaten a whole section of a bar. Principle: moderation enables us to enjoy.

Lose Weight if You Are Overweight

This is easier said than done. However, there are many benefits of weight loss if you have diabetes. Over 85% of those with Type 2 diabetes are overweight when diagnosed. Losing just 10–20 pounds (and keeping it off) can make your body more responsive to the insulin you produce, help lower your blood pressure if it is high, and can improve your blood lipid levels.

Work with your physician, dietitian, or diabetes educator to develop a balanced plan of food intake and physical activity. For those who want to lose weight, a general rule is to eat 10 calories per pound of desired body weight. So if you want to reach 180 pounds, an 1800 calorie diet would be appropriate (you are likely eating many more calories than this). For maintaining a particular weight, the general rule is 13 to15 calories per pound. If you want to maintain 150 pounds, you could eat approximately 1,950 to 2,250 calories per day.

Since most of us don't know our caloric intake, the first step is to keep a diary of all the food you eat in a typical week. Be brutally honest, and include everything—snacks, nibbles, and drinks, too. Share this information with your dietitian, who will help you calculate the calories.

Decrease Total Fat, Saturated Fat, and Cholesterol

1. Eat less red meat. When you do eat it, choose cuts that have little fat. Limit your consumption of fast-food hamburgers. Many fast food chains now offer low-fat items. Most will provide the nutritional information of their foods upon request. *Fast Food Facts* is a useful compendium of nutritional values for fast food restaurants (see the references section at the end of this chapter).

2. Eat more poultry, but don't eat the skin and fat. You can broil or grill chicken with the skin removed if you baste it with vegetable oil or an oily marinade.

3. Substitute turkey or chicken products for beef, pork, hot dogs, regular bologna (non-fat bologna is now available and tastes pretty good) and ground meats. But don't always assume that poultry is lower in fat— do the calculations. Also, try Morningstar Farm products, made from soy. It may take some time to get accustomed to soy products, but they are worth the effort. Taste preferences are surprisingly changeable.

4. Use low-fat or nondairy products. Certain cheeses, such as hoop or farmer cheese, low-fat feta and skim milk mozzarella, are lower in fat than others. Fat-free sour cream and low-fat and nonfat cream cheese are widely available and taste very similar to their high-fat counterparts. In earlier editions of this book, we had recipes for low-fat sour cream, cream cheese, and mayonnaise. The commercial products are now so widely available that we have removed them!

5. Substitute fish, beans, or tofu for fatty red meat. Fish oil, contained in all fish, is the most unsaturated oil you can eat; it's about twice as beneficial as vegetable oils.

   A word of advice: Don't take fish oil capsules. They are expensive, they offer no obvious benefit, and they may be harmful. Eat fatty cold-water fish such as salmon, trout, haddock, and mackerel. They contain the largest quantity of the oils known as omega-3 fatty acids, which help lower cholesterol and triglycerides and prevent blood clots by thinning the blood.

Most seafood is believed to be relatively low in cholesterol. Although most researchers believe what was thought to be cholesterol also includes similar appearing fish sterols, it is still unclear how much cholesterol is in shellfish such as shrimp, lobster, and crab. Because they are low in saturated fats, most researchers believe they are fine to eat in moderation. Mollusks, such as scallops, clams, and oysters, are even lower in cholesterol.

Tofu is rapidly becoming a staple of delicious, healthy cooking. This soybean product is itself quite bland, so you can bestow many different flavors on it by your choice of recipes. With the water pressed out, tofu can be grilled (prepared in your favorite marinade first) or crumbled, sauteed, and substituted for ground beef in Mexican and Italian recipes. It is high in protein and contains no cholesterol, but does get about 50 percent of its calories from fat; consider this in your meal plan.

To reduce the fat in ground meat, crumble, simmer in water, wine, and garlic powder or cumin for about 15 minutes, and drain. The meat can then be used in other recipes or frozen for later use (see references for *Health Smart Gourmet Cooking*, at the end of this chapter). Very low fat ground beef is also available in the meat or frozen sections of your supermarket. Sometimes the fat is replaced by water bound to a food product such as carrageenan, a naturally occurring carbohydrate extracted from seaweed.

6. Eat egg yolks and organ meats such as liver, kidneys, and sweetbreads no more than once a week. They are extremely high in cholesterol. However, the yolk of the egg contains all the cholesterol so you can safely eat egg whites, which are all protein. There are cholesterol-free egg substitutes, but we prefer throwing away the yolks; it's less expensive. See the recipe below:

Yolkless Eggs

Although these eggs should be made without whole yolks, you can add a small amount of yolk to give the dish a yellow color and improve its texture.

Omelets and fried eggs can be made with yolkless eggs. Eggs can also be fried, boiled, or shirred, and the firm yolk removed after cooking. For fried egg whites, separate the whites and fry them as you would a whole egg. For an omelet, separate the whites into a mixing bowl, season with garlic, pepper, and herbs to taste, and mix gently (do not beat them). The pan should be hot enough that a drop of water vaporizes immediately. Use a nonstick pan that is large enough so that the white will cover the bottom and cook through almost immediately. A fat-free nonstick cooking spray can also be used.

For more elaborate scrambled eggs or omelets, you can use the whites and replace each yolk with 1 teaspoon olive or polyunsaturated vegetable oil and 1/2 teaspoon low-fat dry milk. Yellow food coloring can be added if desired.

Bon appetit!

7. The recommendations concerning butter and margarine are mixed. Some feel that margarine is more harmful than helpful, because of its saturated fats. However, you can choose a diet or imitation margarine that lists liquid vegetable oil as the first ingredient. (Ingredients are listed on product labels in order of amount, with the highest quantity ingredient listed first. Liquid is better than partially hydrogenated oil.) Some recommend butter instead of margarine. If you prefer to use butter on some foods, use whipped butter in moderate amounts, or mix butter and margarine together.

8. Use noncaloric sprays and non-stick pans when you sauté or fry foods. You can even purchase olive oil spray. You can also use 1 teaspoon of canola or olive oil (combined with 1 teaspoon of butter if you want the butter flavor). The good browned flavor that fat adds to sauces can be duplicated by repeated pan reductions of vegetables, sauteed and deglazed with broth or wine.

9. Try Butter Buds, Best O' Butter, or similar products. Sprinkle on dry or dissolved in water to add a buttery flavor to vegetables or popcorn. They have no fat or cholesterol. Low-fat or nonfat buttermilk adds a wonderful buttery flavor to sauces and mashed potatoes.

10. Use olive or canola oil in salad dressings and for sauteing. Nutritionists once considered monounsaturated fats such as olive oil to be "neutral" compared to polyunsaturated (good) and saturated (bad) fats. Newer research has determined that monounsaturated oils are good fats, particularly in terms of lowering the bad cholesterol (LDL) and raising the good cholesterol (HDL). Canola oil is healthier and is

now comparable in price to other vegetable oils.

11. Eat less total fat. The total fat you eat—particularly saturated fat—is the major dietary factor determining your cholesterol level. Remember, even if a particular food has a high percentage of its calories from fat, it can be offset by a food low in fat percentage. The daily total of calories from fat is what counts. If you are on an 1,800 calorie diet, 20–30 percent of the calories is 360–540; this is the maximum amount of fat you should eat each day. Divide this by 9 calories per gram, which amounts to 40–60 grams maximum for the day. (Another way to calculate the 30 percent maximum is to drop the last number from your total calories, so 1800 becomes 180. Divide by 3 to get your maximum grams of fat per day.) The amount of fat grams per serving is listed on food labels, or you can calculate it by using the food tables in the references at the end of the chapter. If you eat foods that are less than 5 grams of fat per serving, you will be able to stay within your limit relatively easily. However, many foods have 20–25 grams of fat per serving, and it is easy to see how quickly you can exceed your daily total of 40–60.

12. Limit your intake of saturated vegetable fats such as palm and coconut oil. These are used in preparing canned nuts, cookies, candy, and other processed foods. Many manufacturers are eliminating their use in response to public concern, but be sure to check the labels.

13. Look for low-fat, low-calorie frozen meals or meals-in-a-cup. Also look for low-fat, low-calorie frozen desserts (Weight Watchers makes several varieties). Be sure to do the percentage of fat calculations, and confirm the amount of carbohydrate (sometimes the carbohydrate remains very high even in foods sweetened with NutraSweet). Check the effects of these new foods on your blood sugar levels by testing one or two hours after eating.

14. Now available on your grocery shelves are a selection of nonfat salad dressings, mayonnaise, cheeses, and even potato chips! Some taste great, others are OK. The cheeses are particularly good for adding texture or consistency to food or for melting onto chili. The fat replacers are usually carbohydrate or protein based, so check the amounts to determine how they fit into your meal plan. Also, the FDA recently approved a new fat replacer called olestra (trade name Olean) that contains vegetable oil and table sugar, but is not absorbed and thus does not add any calories. Currently, it is being

used in snack foods such as potato chips, corn chips, and cheese puffs. Foods with olestra, if eaten in large quantities, may cause digestive symptoms such as loose stool and cramps. We have not yet tried olestra, but those we've talked with say the chips are as good as regular potato chips.

Eat Foods with High Fiber and Low Glycemic Index

Don't eliminate foods solely because of their high glycemic index, but do shift the balance. Eat pasta, beans, and fresh fruit more often than potatoes, rice, and bread.

As you increase the carbohydrate in your diet, it is important to increase the fiber as well. High fiber may be more beneficial when eaten in a high-carbohydrate diet (see Table 2 at the end of this chapter).

Finally, by using home blood glucose testing you can determine glycemic responses to various foods by measuring your blood glucose one or two hours after eating. Let your home tests and blood lipid (fat) levels, as determined by your physician, be your guide in balancing your diet.

Here are some ideas on using fiber and the glycemic index in your diet:

1. Begin to eat more pasta and beans; choose a slow-release over a fast-release carbohydrate.
2. Eat more fresh fruit and cut down on fruit juices, particularly frozen ones. Many people with Type 2 diabetes drink large quantities of fruit juice because they don't think of them as food with calories, but simply as a drink. You can add many calories and raise your blood sugar substantially with such drinks.
3. Popcorn is a wonderful high-fiber, low-calorie food, especially without butter or margarine. To season it, use herbs or spices instead of salt.
4. Look for packaged or processed foods that use fructose instead of sugar or corn syrup. Fructose has a lower glycemic effect. However, people with abnormal lipids should avoid large amounts of fructose, which can increase total cholesterol and LDL cholesterol.
5. Use nonnutritive sweeteners and products that contain them in moderation. Instead of powdered sugar, sprinkle powdered sweeteners very lightly on berries or pancakes, for instance. Some sweeteners recently approved by the FDA can also be used in cooking.
6. Try tofu ice cream (Tofutti) or low-fat frozen yogurt. These have little fat or cholesterol and contain less sugar than ice cream. Several

frozen desserts are sweetened with NutraSweet instead of sugar. HaagenDazs makes low-fat and nonfat frozen bars that are delicious. The low-fat products may have a higher glycemic index than ice cream.

7. Eat more whole grain breads, cereals, crackers, and pasta.
8. Use the glycemic index only to choose between one carbohydrate and another, not between carbohydrates and fats or proteins. Don't substitute ice cream for potatoes, or sausage for toast.

Moderate Alcohol Use

Alcohol is no longer prohibited for people with diabetes and can be used in moderation, with a few precautions. (Alcohol does not need insulin to be metabolized.) The ADA now approves limited alcohol use.

Alcohol can lower blood sugar. Drinking before dinner can cause insulin reactions and at the same time mask the signs of low blood sugar.

The consequences of intoxication are more significant for those with diabetes, since getting drunk might lead to skipping a meal or an insulin injection.

On the positive side, in a study of 480 randomly selected Italian and Italian-American adults, 73 had overt or borderline diabetes. All 73 were total abstainers or drank wine in small amounts. The remaining 407 drank wine on a regular basis. Other studies have suggested that 1 to 2 ounces of alcohol daily protects against heart disease. (Abstainers and heavy drinkers had higher incidence of heart disease than moderate drinkers.) Many scientists agree that this effect is real, although few recommend beginning drinking just to protect your heart. Adding to this good news, a more recent study concluded that "low to moderate amounts of alcohol, when taken on a regular basis, improve insulin sensitivity." This means that less insulin is needed by the body to utilize a given amount of glucose.

Needless to say, the consequences of alcohol abuse are just as serious for those with diabetes as those without. Follow these guidelines when you drink:

1. Remember to figure the calories of the carbohydrate as well as the alcohol in your drink.
2. Dry wines (most table wines, not dessert wines) have very little carbohydrate in them.

3. Avoid sweet mixers. Use diet soft drinks and diet tonic. Regular tonic water has more carbohydrate than most soft drinks.
4. Check the effects of different alcoholic beverages on your metabolism by testing your blood sugar one to two hours after drinking.

Moderate Salt Use

Evidence shows that avoiding salt will lower high blood pressure after it develops. However, no research has proven that minimizing salt intake will decrease your risk of becoming hypertensive if you do not already have high blood pressure. Salt is an important ingredient in cooking and food preparation. It helps bring out and blend flavors. Salt can be used judiciously in cooking, if there are no medical reasons to avoid it. Still, hypertension greatly increases the risk of other complications for those with diabetes, so prudence argues for restraint with the salt shaker at the table. Less than 2,000 mg a day is low (see Table 3 at end of this chapter for a table listing the salt content of various foods). You can decrease your craving for salt. Begin at home by following these suggestions:

1. Learn to appreciate the flavors of fresh foods without additives.
2. Add only a small amount of salt to the foods you cook, enough to bring out the flavors.
3. Avoid canned vegetables and other processed foods; they are usually very high in salt.
4. Use alternative seasonings, such as lemon juice, garlic, and onion as well as flavored powders (not salts), herbs, spices, and wine or flavored vinegars.
5. Limit your use of soy sauce. Even the low-salt lite soy sauce has a lot of salt.

Eating Well With Diabetes

Both of the authors of this book love good food. With creativity and moderation, and using the ideas in this chapter, we have healthfully eaten our way through a variety of restaurants and cuisines. In addition to reading the tips in this chapter, we suggest that you find a nutritionist or dietitian who can tailor some specific diets or menus to your needs and preferences (see above for toll-free referral numbers). At the end of this chapter, we have listed books and other references we have found useful. If you don't have a book that lists food values, we recommend you get one.

Gary's Invisible Diet

I now use an insulin pump, and do not need to adjust for late or missed meals. (I take extra lispro insulin based on the food I am eating at the moment.) However, before the pump, my friends were generally not aware that I was continuously monitoring my food and drink intake. For years I counted only carbohydrates, but then I watched my fat intake as well. If my schedule of meals differed from my routine, I usually adjusted my intake in advance or delay or took extra insulin (for example, Superbowl Sunday, a big dinner dance, or a late afternoon movie). A delayed, hearty breakfast on Superbowl Sunday held me over until the midafternoon party, with its abundant snack foods (eaten mindfully and in moderation) that became both lunch and supper. The late dinner dance was taken care of with a later lunch and perhaps some cocktail time appetizers. Popcorn (and maybe chili or a hot dog) in the movie took care of a potentially very late dinner. Of course, being able to check blood sugar levels easily is a big help.

Finally, remember that the best way to determine how different foods affect you is to try them and measure their effect on your blood sugar one or two hours after you've eaten. This feedback helps you change your diet when tests are high. And it helps you know the types and amounts of food that are appropriate for you.

Table 1:
Glycemic Index

Grain Foods
White bread 100
Whole meal bread 99
White rice 81
Brown rice 79
Sweet corn 78
Whole grain rye bread 66
White spaghetti 59
Whole wheat spaghetti 53

Breakfast cereals
Corn Flakes 119
Wheetabix 100
Shredded Wheat 99
All-Bran 60

Root vegetables
Baked potato (russet) 121
Instant potato 118
Boiled potato (new) 81
Sweet potato 77

Dried peas and beans
Baked beans (canned) 56
Chickpeas 47
Kidney beans 42
Soy beans (canned) 20

Fruits
Raisins 91
Banana 76
Orange juice 74
Grapes 62
Apple 52
Pear 51
Peach 40
Plum 34

Sugar
Maltose 150
Glucose 138
Honey 104
Sucrose 92
Fructose 32

Dairy products
Ice cream 87
Yogurt 51
Whole milk 39
Skim milk............. 46

Note: All foods in this table are standardized against one slice of white bread, assigned a value of 100. In most cases, the stated glycemic index represents a mean average of published data.

A low index is good, because the food is absorbed more slowly.

Adapted from Kay Foster-Powell and Janette Brand Miller, "International Tables of Glycemic Index," *The American Journal of Clinical Nutrition* (October 1995), The American Society for Clinical Nutrition, Inc.

Table 2:
Fiber Content Of Selected Foods

Food	Portion Size	Plant Fiber (grams)
Breads, Cereals, and Starchy Vegetables (cooked/prepared)		
Beans, kidney	1/2 cup	3.0
Bran (100 percent), cereal	1/3 cup	8.0
Bread		
Pumpernickel	1 slice	3.0
White	1 slice	<1
Whole grain wheat	1 slice	2.0
Corn, kernels	1/3 cup	2.1
Parsnips	2/3 cup	5.9
Peas	1/2 cup	5.2
Potatoes, white	1 small	3.8
Rice, brown	1/2 cup	1.3
Rice, white	1/2 cup	0.5
Squash, winter	1/2 cup	3.6
Sweet potatoes	1/4 cup	2.9
Fruit (uncooked)		
Apples	1 medium	3.0
Banana	1 medium	2.0
Blueberries	1/2 cup	2.0
Cantaloupe	1 cup	1.0
Orange	1 medium	3.0
Peach	1 medium	1.0
Prunes, dried	3	2.0
Strawberries	1 cup	4.0
Vegetables (cooked unless indicated by plus sign)		
Baked Beans	1/2 cup	3.0
Beans, string	1/2 cup	1.7
Broccoli	1/2 cup	2.0
Carrots +	1 medium	2.0
Cucumbers +	1/2 cup	<1
Lettuce, romaine +	1 cup	1.0
Spinach	1/2 cup	2.0
Tomato +	1 medium	2.0

Sources: *Bowes & Church's Food Values of Portions Commonly Used, 16th Edition*, 1994; *Plant Fiber in Foods, 2nd Edition*; and manufacturer data.

Table 3:
Salt Content Of Common Foods

Fresh/Minimally Processed Foods

1 cup orange juice . . . . 2 mg.

1 cup apple juice . . . . 2 mg.

1 c. long-cooking oatmeal . 10 mg.

3 ounces ground beef . . . 60 mg.

3 ounces pork . . . . 65 mg.

1 cup fresh green beans. . . 5 mg.

1 cup frozen green beans . 2 mg.

1 cup whole milk . . . . . 120 mg.

1 large egg . . . . 70 mg.

1 lemon . . . . 1 mg.

1 head Boston lettuce . . . 15 mg.

1 peach . . . . 1 mg.

8 ounces bluefish. . . . . . 170 mg.

3 apricots . . . . 1 mg.

1 banana . . . . 1 mg.

1 carrot . . . . 35 mg.

Prepared Foods

1 cup tomato juice . . . . 640 mg.

1 cup Puffed Rice . . . . 1 mg.

1 cup Corn Flakes. . . . . 305 mg.

3 ounces corned beef . 1500 mg.

1 c. canned green beans . 320 mg.

1 c. chicken noodle soup. 1050 mg.

3 ounces bacon . . . . . . 1400 mg.

1 dill pickle . . . . 1930 mg.

1 slice white bread . . . . 100 mg.

cooking oil . . . . 0 mg.

1 cinnamon roll . . . . . . 630 mg.

1 tablespoon ketchup . . 155 mg.

1 cup all-purpose flour . . . 2 mg.

1 cup self-rising flour . 1565 mg.

1 beef frankfurter . . . . . 425 mg.

1 tablespoon Italian dressing 250 mg.

1 cup instant pudding. . 335 mg.

1 TV chicken dinner . . 1400 mg.

1 olive . . . . 165 mg.

1 cup baked beans . . . . 100 mg.

Fast Foods

1 Arby's Turkey
   Sandwich . . . . 1,060 mg.

3 pcs. Arthur Treacher's
   Fish . . . . 675 mg.

1 Burger King
   Whopper . . . . 990 mg.

1 Dairy Queen
   Hot Dog . . . . 830 mg.

Kentucky Fried Chicken:
   3 pieces chicken,
   mashed potatoes,
   gravy, cole slaw . . 2,285 mg.

1 McDonald's
   Big Mac . . . . 1,010 mg.

1 Taco Bell
   Enchirito. . . . . 1,175 mg.

N. Kaplan, M.D., *Clinical Diabetes,* Mar/Apr, 1984, American Diabetes Association

1. *Health Smart Gourmet Cooking* (A. Hackett, Hastings House Publishers) has many excellent low-fat recipes and useful preparation and cooking tips, similar to those in his public television cooking series.

2. Any of the Pritikin diet books (such as *The Pritikin Program for Diet and Exercise*). These books have good recipes for low-fat, low-cholesterol, high-fiber dishes. The full diet is very demanding for some to follow because of the low fat content.

3. *Bowes & Church's Food Values of Portions Commonly Used, 17th Edition* (J. A. T. Pennington and H. N. Church, Lippincott-Raven Publishers) is a handy reference giving grams of fat, carbohydrates, proteins, and other food values.

4. *The New American Diet System* (Sonja and William Connor, Simon and Schuster, 1992) and *Eater's Choice: A Food Lovers' Guide to Lower Cholesterol* (R. and N. Goor, Houghton Mifflin, 1995) are both innovative and useful guides to healthy eating (not specifically for people with diabetes).

5. *Fast Foods Facts* (M. J. Franz, 1997) and *Convenience Food Facts* (A. J. Monk and M. J. Franz, 1997) contain useful lists of food values from fast-food chains and name-brand processed foods. Available from Chronimed Publishing, P.O. Box 59032, Minneapolis, MN 55459-0032.

6. *Diabetes Forecast*, the monthly magazine of the American Diabetes Association, carries many helpful nutrition articles and recipes. The ADA offers several cookbooks for diabetes. The appendix at the end of the book gives addresses and telephone numbers for ordering *Forecast* and a catalog of ADA publications.

7. *The Restaurant Companion* (H. S. Warshaw, Surrey Books, Inc., Chicago, 1995) provides guidance and tips for restaurant dining in fourteen different cuisines.

8. *Eat More, Weigh Less* (Dean Ornish, M.D. 1993) and *Everyday Cooking with Dr. Dean Ornish* (Dean Ornish, M.D. 1996) both published by Harper Collins. Although these books are directed toward heart patients they are equally appropriate for those with diabetes. The recipes are totally vegetarian and the diet restricts fat intake to 10% of daily calo-

ries. This may seem overly stringent, but the recipes are good and its not a bad idea to head in that direction.

9. *Low Fat Living— Skillpower and Willpower* (Robert K. Cooper Ph.D. with Leslie L. Cooper, Rodale Press, 1996) shows how to get motivated and change lifestyles. They recommend between 20 and 25% total daily fat. Provided are 14 days of recipes for low-fat lunches and dinners, and much more.

10. *In the Kitchen With Rosie: Oprah's Favorite Recipes.* (Rosie Daley, Knopf, 1994) This book has the low-fat recipes created by Oprah's chef. The book shows ways to reduce the fat in many high fat foods such french fries, catfish, crabcakes, fried chicken, and sweet potato pie.

11. *Healthy Pleasures.* (Robert Ornstein PhD, David Sobel MD, Addison - Wesley) This book covers a lot more pleasures than food, but provides a perspective about the value of life's pleasures in enhancing health, with evidence to support it.

12. *Diabetes Interview.* (King Publishing, 3715 Balboa, San Francisco, CA 94121, 800-488-8468). This is a wonderful monthly publication that typically has one or two food-related columns and recipes, plus any news or research articles relating to food and meal planning. It also has news, research, and helpful articles about all aspects of diabetes. Gary is on their editorial advisory board.

13. *Calories and Carbohydrates.* (Barbara Kraus, Penguin, 10th ed, 1993). Includes tables for carbohydrate. *Carbohydrate Guide to Brand Names and Basic Foods* (Kraus, New American Library, 1992).

14. *Carbohydrate Gram Counter* (Corrine Netzer, Dell Publishing, 1994.) Includes tables for carbohydrate counting. *The Complete Book Of Food Counts* (Netzer, Dell/Bantam, 1994).

15. *The Tufts University Guide to Total Nutrition,* Stanley Gershoff, Ph.D. with Catherine Whitney. Harper Perennial, 1990.

16. *Total Nutrition.* Edited by Victor Herbert, M.D. from the Mt. Sinai School of Medicine. New York: St. Martins Press, 1995.

17. *The Wellness Encyclopedia of Food and Nutrition,* Sheldon Margen, M.D. and the editors of the University of California Wellness Letter. (Subscription Dept. P.O. Box 420422, Palm Coast, FL 32142).

18. *Jane Brody's Good Food Book,* Bantam, 1985.

19. *Low-Fat Living,* Robert K. Cooper with Leslie L. Cooper. Rodale Press, 1996.

20. *Carbohydrates, Calories, and Fat in Your Food: The Nutrition Guide,* Dr. Art Ulene, Avery Publishing Group, Garden City, NY, 1995.

21. *The American Dietetic Association's Complete Food & Nutrition Guide,* Roberta Duyff, 1996. Available from Chronimed Publishing, P.O. Box 59032, Minneapolis, MN 55459-0032.

Chapter Eleven

Living Actively
With Diabetes

"One of the good things about diabetes is that it
makes a virtue out of enjoying myself physically.
The little doctor in the back of my head smiles when
I go dancing or swimming, even when I make love.
My prescription includes having fun!"—Linda

In this chapter, we review the many ways that exercise improves diabetes
management and reduces the risk of complications. Included is an activity questionnaire that helps you assess your present exercise level and suggests ways to improve it. We conclude with guidelines to keep you
motivated so that you continue to stay active.

With so many people exercising, it may seem unnecessary to urge those
with diabetes to be active. Everybody knows the benefits of staying fit.
Exercise decreases the risk of heart disease, lowers high blood pressure,
improves physical fitness and general health, reduces anxiety and depression, and enhances your sense of well-being. As a person with diabetes,
you enjoy an extra bonus of being active: It helps you control blood sugar
and it lessens the risk of some complications.

How Physical Activity Helps You Manage Diabetes

1. Physical activity lowers your blood sugar by burning it as fuel.
   You can use exercise to return blood glucose levels to normal
   when tests are high (if test levels are not higher than about
   300 mg/dl [16 mmol/L]).
2. Steady exercise for more than twenty minutes enables your muscles
   to store glucose, further lowering blood sugar levels after you've
   stopped exercising. Your body utilizes this store when your blood
   sugar levels become too low. When you exercise regularly, your
   blood sugar levels will be more stable.

3. Consistent physical activity that is moderate or strenuous increases a cell's ability to use insulin. This lowers the necessary insulin dose.
4. Exercise builds physical fitness, strengthening the heart, circulatory system, lungs, and muscles. This reduces the risk of cardiovascular complications.
5. Exercise is a key to losing or controlling weight, and is as important as diet in doing so.
6. You can neutralize the effects of emotional stress with physical activity.
7. Exercising makes you feel good!

Regular physical activity is a key ingredient of your diabetes control regimen, especially if you want optimal control. Exercise reduces your body's overall insulin requirement, compensates for blood sugar highs, and gives you greater balance in blood sugar levels (once you have adapted to exercising). The cardiovascular benefits are especially important to you because, as a person with diabetes, you have a higher risk of heart and circulatory difficulties. So, in addition to improving your metabolic control, a consistent exercise program can help prevent a heart attack and improve your circulation.

The benefits of exercise also exist at an emotional level. The increased flow of blood and oxygen to the cells and the hormonal shifts that occur when we are physically active lift our spirits. A stressful day at work can be counteracted by a brisk walk or game of tennis. Mild depression may be lightened by an hour of working in the garden or riding a bicycle. When we are active, we have fewer mood swings and it is much easier to handle difficult problems.

How does all of this magic occur? As soon as we begin exercising, our muscles demand more energy. Blood flow to the muscles increases and more oxygen and glucose move into the muscle cells. Blood supply to the skin also increases, so the heat generated can be radiated out of the body. As an exercise session progresses, the liver releases additional glucose to fuel the muscles. Fats are also burned to provide further energy.

During physical work or play, insulin and counter-regulatory hormones such as adrenalin, growth hormone, and glucagon interact to ensure an adequate supply of glucose to the cells. Without insulin, this process breaks down in insulin-dependent diabetes. Despite the higher level of activity, blood sugar levels will rise considerably and excessive fat burning will produce ketones if insulin has been omitted. The effectiveness of insulin is increased by exercise because more insulin molecules connect to the cells, enabling glucose to pass through the cell walls.

After you stop exercising, the effects continue to accumulate if you have been playing or working at a moderate to strenuous level. The liver and muscles need to restore their supply of glucose, and they draw it from the bloodstream when you are resting. This process can go on for several hours following strenuous activity. This is why reactions sometimes occur long after you've stopped exercising.

Physical activity enables you to lose weight by burning fat and turning glucose into muscle, instead of more fat. Combining exercise with the proper meal plan allows a degree of weight control that cannot be obtained by diet alone. In fact, many weight-control programs now recommend at least one week of exercise before you begin dieting; the increase in activity level apparently makes appetite control easier.

The power of exercise to relieve stress symptoms is easy to explain: At the most basic level, the stress response is designed to prepare us to act physically. When stressed, we are ready for "fight or flight," so the most natural way to deal with stress is to move vigorously in order to use the hormones and glucose generated by it. This also enables us to release the physical tension that usually accompanies stress, assuming that the exercise includes a relaxed warm-up period.

Short-term benefits follow any period of increased physical activity. When you continue activity long enough to raise your pulse to the target range for your age, for fifteen to twenty minutes or more a day, you achieve what is called "the training effect" (discussed later in this chapter). If you do this regularly for a few weeks, you begin to enjoy the long-term benefits of exercise. A consistent program of physical training gives you greater sensitivity to insulin, usually allowing a significant decrease in insulin dosage or modification of your medication dosage if you have Type 2 diabetes. Your muscles store more glucose, which is readily available to balance low blood sugar. Reactions may become less severe as a result. Your body performs better, your lungs breathe deeper, your heart is stronger, and you feel better. You are living well.

Ernie's Dog Gets Him in Shape

Since completing the first edition of this book, I moved back to the city. I now live in a very steep section of the Oakland Hills. Our Siberian Husky needs at least three walks a day, so he's become my aerobic trainer. I've gone from a condition of gasping at the top of our first hill to being able to stride up a whole series of hills and hardly be winded. Not too long ago I climbed most of the way up the side of Yosemite Valley (on a trail, not the rock wall!) and was still enjoying myself. At age 62 I'm in better shape than I've been since my 30s.

Before we discuss beginning your program of physical activity, you may gain some insight into your present activity level by answering the following questions.

My Activity Profile

1. My typical day includes

_____ hours of sleep (7-8 hours recommended)

_____ hours of low activity (riding in or driving a car, reading, desk work, watching television, eating, talking while sitting or standing, etc.)

_____ hours of moderate activity (walking, gardening, mopping, light labor; sports such as golf or bowling, easy swimming, etc.)

_____ hours of vigorous activity (running, bicycling, tennis, basketball, etc.; moderate to heavy labor such as digging or carrying heavy objects)

2. At least _____ times a week I increase this to

_____ hours of moderate activity

_____ hours of vigorous activity

_____ This increase of activity happens only on weekends.

_____ This activity is distributed through the week.

_____ Although I am usually sedentary, I have occasional bursts of heavy physical activity.

3. I do some form of stretching or warm-up before physical activity.

_____

_____ I stretch to cool-down after exercise.

4. The physical activities I enjoy most are

_____

Activities I would like to learn are

_____

5. I have the following conditions, which need to be considered in designing my activity program:

_____ Difficulty recognizing the signs of low blood sugar
_____ Heart disease
_____ High blood pressure
_____ Poor circulation
_____ Retinopathy
_____ Neuropathy (especially if it involves decreased sensation in the feet)
_____ Fatigue
_____ Back pain (or other muscular or joint discomfort)
_____ Foot problems
_____ Other

(If you checked any of the above, discuss exercise with your physician. You may need tests to determine the level of activity advisable.)

6. I see the following obstacles to exercising:
_____ I don't feel I have enough time for it.
_____ I'm afraid I'll have too many reactions.
_____ I feel clumsy and uncomfortable with my body.
_____ I'm bored by physical activities; I prefer using my mind.
_____ I don't enjoy physical activity; it's a burden.
_____ I'd rather do other things.
_____ I don't have much energy.
_____ Other

7. I could overcome these obstacles to exercise by

_____

8. I would like to increase my level of activity by

_____

9. I would like to begin
_____ today
_____ this week
_____ this month

Beginning Your Activity Program

Without fail, wear a diabetes I.D. bracelet or necklace and inform any gym personnel, coaches, or fellow participants that you have diabetes and may need sugar in case of low blood sugar levels.

We advise you to begin any program of exercise gradually. You need to build strength, endurance, and flexibility so that you will be comfortable exercising. You also have to discover your particular balance between increased activity, insulin, and diet in order to avoid serious reactions. If you have diabetic complications or other physical conditions, you will need to proceed cautiously and with guidance from your doctor. If you are over 35, you should probably have a physical stress test to determine the level of exercise appropriate for you.

Choose activities that you enjoy. You should look forward to your exercise times as positive experiences, not as burdens or tasks. The following list contains several physical activities, ranked according to calories burned. If you have several favorite activities, you can choose among them to add variety and deal with changes in weather, mood, and physical state. Although you may prefer to have a partner when exercising, you should also have activities you can do by yourself. If your only physical activity tends to be your work, either on the job or at home, you will benefit more if you find new ways to enjoy it. Focus on your bodily movements as though they were a dance or a sport. Don't be so fixed on the end product that you ignore your body.

Let Me Count the Ways...

(The category of an activity depends on how energetically you do it. An asterisk indicates that an activity is good aerobic exercise.)

Light activity (50-200 calories burned per hour)

Stretching	T'ai chi chaun
Slow walking	Yoga
Light housekeeping	Slow social dancing

Moderate Activity (200-400 calories burned per hour)

Moderate to fast walking*	Gardening
Tennis (doubles)	Bowling
Stationary bicycle*	Swimming*
Ice skating	Ping pong and badminton
Making love	Jogging*
Volleyball	Jumping rope*
Bicycling	Golf
Calisthenics	Horseback riding
Canoeing and rowing	Square dance or folk dancing*
Fencing	Aerobic dancing*
Walking up stairs	Roller skating

Vigorous Activity (400-900 calories burned per hour)

Digging and shoveling	Running*
Hiking*	Chopping wood
Tennis (singles)	Waterskiing
Stair climbing*	Basketball
Bicycle racing	Football
Racquetball	Moving furniture
Ice skating	Hill climbing*
Squash and handball	Soccer
Skiing (downhill and cross country)*	

You should always warm up before vigorous activity. More importantly, you should cool down afterwards. Stretching and warming muscles for five minutes and beginning exercise at a moderate pace allows your pulse and blood pressure to increase gradually. Cooling down with five or more minutes of mild activity allows your body to return to normal in the same manner. Neglecting to warm up or cool down can cause risky, abrupt shifts in pulse and blood pressure.

Although any activity helps you become more fit, you will receive the greatest benefit from exercise that requires a fairly steady level of exertion and movement (such as jogging, dancing, or swimming). Stop-and-start activities (such as tennis and volleyball) and static straining (weight lifting) do not build the same level of fitness in your cardiovascular system. However, see strength training below!

Strength Training

Something has caught on recently—it's called strength training—and it isn't just for the young and already strong. It's exercise both young and old can enjoy. In order to be active we need muscle strength as well as the improved glucose control and vitality we get from aerobics. Strength training uses special machines or hand weights to provide resistance that strengthens and tones your muscles as you go through a series of exercises. There are people to help you get started at health clubs, adult education classes, and senior centers. Again, it's best to get information and some instruction before you begin.

▷ If you become faint, dizzy, or nauseated, if you experience severe shortness of breath or tightness or pain in your chest, or if you lose control of your muscles, stop immediately and contact your doctor.

▷ If your pulse or breathing rate does not return to normal within three minutes of stopping exercise, you are probably pushing yourself too hard and need to adjust your level of exercise.

▷ If you are fatigued by moderate activity, and especially if you continue to feel exhausted in the hours following, you are doing more than your current level of fitness will support. Cut back the duration or intensity of exercise until you feel stronger. (If this tiredness begins abruptly, it may indicate that you are coming down with a cold or the flu.)

▷ Be sure that you get enough water during exercise. You need to drink water every fifteen to twenty minutes during strenuous activity.

Exercise and Blood Sugar Levels

Home blood glucose testing and knowledge of your insulin regimen will help you avoid insulin reactions. If you test blood sugar before exercise, ten to fifteen minutes after you stop, and one hour after that, you will see how different types and amounts of activity affect you. (The ten- to fifteen-minute delay after exercising is necessary because sugar from the liver may temporarily raise blood sugar during vigorous activity.) You will have a rough idea of how much exercise it takes to lower high blood sugar levels and when you need extra food or reduced insulin.

If your blood sugar is under 120 mg/dl (6.6 mmol/L) before moderate to heavy activity, be sure to eat food that is absorbed quickly (fruit juice, dried fruit, etc.). By trial and error, you will discover how much you need to eat before a given amount of exercise to avoid reactions or high blood sugar levels. (See Chapter 5, Step 7a for suggestions on changing food and/or insulin to prepare for extra activity.) For insulin users, keep in mind when your insulin tends to peak—eat food if you are exercising at that time or match your activity to the times when insulin levels are not so high. The ideal time for exercise is about one hour after a meal; blood sugar is at a peak and reactions are less likely to occur. If you wait two hours or more, you should consider having a snack before physical activity, unless your blood sugar is high.

For insulin users, exercising the site where you injected the insulin (such as the thigh or the arm) causes the insulin to work faster. This can be an advantage if you need to bring down a high blood sugar level, or a disadvantage if you are at a normal level to begin with. If the level is normal, you should avoid legs as an injection site before a hike, or your racquet arm before a tennis match.

When you exercise strenuously or over a long period (over an hour), your blood sugar will continue to decrease after you stop. The muscles and liver are replenishing their stores. You may need a larger meal or extra snacks to avoid reactions in the hours following high levels or extended periods of exertion.

Keep in mind the overall interaction between insulin or pills, diet, and activity. You can vary any one or a combination of these factors to compensate for high blood sugar levels or changes in routine. This allows you a high degree of flexibility while maintaining good metabolic control.

However, if blood sugar is above 250 mg/dl (13.8 mmol/L), exercise has not been thought to be an effective way to lower it. When you exercise, your muscles need to burn glucose for energy. If your blood sugar is high, there is not enough insulin available to move the glucose into your muscle cells. Furthermore, exercise releases adrenalin, which also raises blood sugar. If ketones are present, they will also increase.

Still, a recent study has shown that in those subjects who started their exercise session with blood sugar levels greater than 240 mg/dl (13.3 mmol/L), in only 1% of those sessions did blood sugar rise. In all other sessions the average decrease was about 60 mg/dl (3.3 mmol/L) for people with Type 1 diabetes and 45 mg/dl (2.5 mmol/L) for Type 2.

We recommend using yourself as a research subject by testing your blood sugars before and after exercise. If your sugar is high before you start, see if it decreases or increases after exercise, and act accordingly. Extra insulin for those with Type 1 diabetes or less food for either Type 1 or Type 2 are the best ways to reduce high blood sugar levels.

If you are ill, you should avoid all but the mildest activities. Your body needs energy to deal with the stress of the illness. Exercise only adds to this physical stress and may worsen the condition.

The greatest benefits of exercise occur when you reach the training effect. This is achieved through sustained activity that raises your pulse to your target level for at least twenty minutes. If you do this at least three times a week (every other day), both your heart and metabolic system will function better, assuming you have no major diabetic complications.

However, recent studies have shown that even short periods of activity are beneficial, such as three short walks of 10 minutes each per day. Moderate walking at the rate of about one mile every 15 minutes is also helpful. Any activity is beneficial to your health, just as it is to lowering blood sugar levels.

You have a built-in meter right at your fingertips for measuring the effectiveness and safety of physical activity. Count the number of heartbeats you can feel in your wrist or neck (just above the collarbone toward the center of your throat) for fifteen seconds and multiply by 4. This is your pulse rate. Do this before, during, and immediately following exercise. The following table gives the meaning of different pulse rates, in terms of exercise intensity.

Listen To Your Heart

Pulse Rate (beats per minute)	Degree of Exertion You Feel	Comments
60-80	Very light	Of little value as exercise
80-100	Light	Useful if condition is very poor
100-120	Moderate	Intensity just right
120-140	Somewhat hard	
140-160	Very hard	Stop! unless you are an athlete in top condition

Those of you reluctant to stop and measure your pulse can use the degree of exertion that feels right to you as your guide. If you are unable to talk to a fellow exerciser, you might be overexerting yourself. If you work in the moderate to somewhat hard range, you will probably be at the level you need.

Another indicator of your level of physical condition is the time it takes your pulse to return to its resting rate after exertion. Measure your pulse after you have been resting for fifteen minutes. Move vigorously until your pulse is over 120, then rest and measure your pulse at one-minute intervals. If it takes more than three minutes to return to your resting rate, you are in poor physical condition and need to proceed cautiously with your exercise program. A more precise way of assessing your condition is to undergo an endurance or stress test at your doctor's office or at a local YMCA or YWCA.

If you have been fairly sedentary, you might find that even mild activity will bring your pulse up to a high level. Your body is at a low level of physical condition, and your heart has to work hard to handle any increase in activity. Your limits will gradually increase, so don't push yourself too hard. Twelve to twenty minutes a day at a pulse rate of 100 to 120 is a good beginning. (If you are over 60 and have not been very active, start with five minutes a day.) Stay at this level for a couple of weeks, and increase the duration and intensity of activity only when your endurance increases.

As you get in better condition, you will find that you are exerting yourself harder before you reach the same pulse rate as you did previously with less activity. The flight of stairs that left you breathless and your heart pounding a few weeks ago will be handled with ease. If you don't experience improved endurance, be sure to discuss this with your physician.

As you experience progress in endurance and performance, you will be able to gradually increase your level of activity. If your doctor approves, you can increase the duration and intensity of exercise every two or three weeks until you are at your peak. For a younger person without complications, peak performance will allow a pulse rate of 140 to 160 beats per minute for sessions of thirty to sixty minutes. It can take up to six months to reach this level of conditioning, depending on where you start. If you are older, a lower target pulse rate should be set, depending on age.

Pulse Rate by Age

Age	Recommended pulse	Pulse rate if you have history of heart disease, not to exceed:
20	130-170	150
30	124-162	143
40	117-153	137
45	114-149	134
50	111-145	131
55	107-140	128
60	104-136	120
65	101-132	113

How Often Do You Need to Exercise?

Three workout sessions a week can be enough to build conditioning. If you have diabetes, you also benefit from the blood sugar lowering effects. As we stated earlier, all activity appears to help. Ideally, you should include physical activity in your schedule every day. This regularity helps you maintain consistent blood sugar levels. You can't always meet this ideal, but you can use your skill at varying the ingredients of your regimen to deal with varying levels of activity. Diet or insulin dosage can be tailored to the kind of day you plan. A few more units of insulin or smaller meals will help maintain balance on inactive days.

What If You Have an Active Job?

Your work may be vigorous enough to keep you physically fit without further exercise. It depends upon the degree of exertion and the variety of movements you use. If your pulse stays in the range of 100 to 140 for extended periods during the day, you are working at a level that satisfies conditioning requirements. However, if your pulse is usually below 100 when on the job, you might need to exercise. If your job keeps you moving in repetitive patterns, you might need limbering exercises to avoid sore muscles and maintain flexibility.

Stretching

If you are already active in a sports program you know the value of stretching exercises. For the rest of us, it would be beneficial to begin stretching every day.

Muscles that aren't frequently used tend to shorten and tighten and become more prone to injury. To remain limber requires only 5 to 15 minutes of stretching each day. There are special aids available such as rubber bands and sticks that help you hold positions for the 15 seconds required to get the benefit of a stretch. You need to begin gradually if you haven't been working out or have limited mobility. This is supposed to feel good, so don't push yourself into pain.

Guidelines For Developing An Activity Program You Will Follow

1. Build on the physical activities you already enjoy doing. Your exercise program may take several hours a week for the rest of your life. Start with activities you enjoy, and then learn those you've always wished you could do. Avoid boredom by using several different forms of exercise.

2. If you feel short of time, do things simultaneously: socialize and exercise at the same time (friends don't always have to sit down!); use the exercise bicycle or stair climber while watching television, reading, or listening to music; hold business discussions as you walk.

3. Keep a balance between developing more endurance and staying comfortable. You need time to strengthen your heart and muscles and to learn how to adjust diet and/or insulin to your new level of exercise. If you go too fast, pain or low blood sugar might discourage you from continuing. This is especially important if you are over 35, if you have any signs of heart trouble, or if other complications have started to develop.

4. Use your knowledge of changing diet and insulin dosage to prepare for increased physical activity. It is better to have a few high blood sugar tests from eating more than it is to risk serious reactions. Feedback from your tests will tell you how much is enough. Exercise beginning thirty to sixty minutes after a meal is least likely to cause reactions. If activity comes two or more hours after eating, you should have a snack before you start, unless blood sugar is over 150 mg/dl (8.3 mmol/L).

5. If you have a distaste for exercise because you are an "intellectual" type, use the inner-sports approach. Techniques such a visualization, affirmation, and meditation help many people understand the strong relationship between mind and body and reinforce motivation to exercise. Another possibility is to keep an exercise log and monitor your progress.

Living Actively With Diabetes

6. If you are hesitant to exercise because of limiting physical conditions, ask your doctor for guidelines to ensure safety. You might consider joining a class specifically designed for people with physical limitations. Your YMCA, March of Dimes, ADA chapter, or adult-education school may have a program taught by someone trained to help you exercise safely and monitor your special condition. Organizations for the visually handicapped may also be of help.

7. If you are reluctant to exercise because you feel clumsy and awkward, begin by walking. It's hard to look clumsy while walking, and you can use walking to develop your coordination. The key is to pay attention to your body as you walk. Focus on your feet, legs, hips, arms, back, and shoulders. Let go of any tightness you notice. Later, you can apply this same awareness to any form of motion. You are likely to find any awkwardness decreasing as you learn to be conscious of your body and release its tensions.

8. If competitive activities make you anxious, avoid them. The stress they create for you will offset the benefits of the exercise. (Others may find the spirit of competition necessary to maintain motivation and avoid boredom.)

9. If you exercise outside, do it away from busy streets. Deeper breathing isn't so healthful when the air you breathe is full of carbon monoxide.

10. There is a great workbook available that may help you get motivated to develop an easy and specific plan for a walking program. It's oriented toward weight loss but is useful for anyone. It's the *Walking Off Weight Workbook* by Robert J. Sweetgall (Creative Walking Inc., P.O. Box 50296, Clayton, MO 63105, 1-800-762-9255). Call for a catalog and price list.

Chapter Twelve

Living Well
With Stress

In recent years, a lot of information has been gathered about the effects of stress on health. As people with diabetes, we have reasons to take special interest in the effects of stress:

▷ Simply having diabetes generates stress-inducing events.

▷ Physical and emotional stress can greatly affect our blood sugar levels.

▷ Chronic stress can contribute to the development of diabetic complications.

These three facts make an effective stress-management program a high priority for anyone with diabetes. If you follow such a program, you will be stabilizing your blood sugar levels by reducing the effects of stress on your metabolism. You will be lowering the risk of developing complications, and you will find it easier to live well with diabetes as you neutralize the stress of managing it.

Let's examine the three ways that stress affects diabetes.

Simply having diabetes generates stressful events.

How many simple events become stressful for us because we have diabetes? "Sorry, dinner's going to be a bit late." "I'm afraid your luggage got put on another plane." "Looks like that blister on your foot is infected." "No, there isn't a drugstore open here on Sunday." Our sense of security depends upon an amazing number of routines functioning smoothly. We are vulnerable to circumstances that may be trivial to others.

In almost every hour of the day, we must consider some aspect of our self-care and we may be confronted with a significant diabetes-related problem. Even our sleeping hours may be disturbed by the shaking cold sweat of a low blood sugar reaction (an event of great physical stress).

These day-to-day stresses of diabetes can create strong feelings of anxiety because they remind us of something greater: the fear of diabetic complications. This is true whether we have Type 1 or Type 2 diabetes. No matter how much we may try to forget the possibility of blindness, kidney failure, or heart disease, our mind remembers that we are at risk. Anything that suggests this risk becomes a source of further stress.

Now is an excellent time to practice stress management. Check to see how you responded to what you just read. What changes can you detect in your body? Do you feel edgy, tense, nervous, or suddenly tired? How is your mind responding? Do you want to stop reading to deny that you are at risk?

Close your eyes and say to yourself, "I am learning to take better care of myself. I am reducing the risks." Let the words relax you as you repeat them several times. If any other words try to deny what you are affirming, just hear them as static.

This illustrates one way of reducing stress: replacing the thoughts that trigger it with more reassuring thoughts.

Physical and emotional stress can greatly affect our blood sugar levels.

Diabetes gives us added sources of stress, and we are more vulnerable to its effects. Physiologically, the stress response creates a powerful shift in hormone levels. It can raise, and sometimes lower, blood sugar levels to two or three times their normal level. A botched and painful drawing of blood by an incompetent lab technician can result in an artificially high test result because of the emotional stress. Similarly, a scare while driving or a put-down from the boss can send blood sugar levels soaring. However, many brittle diabetics are people who simply don't know how to manage the stress in their lives.

Physical stresses such as infections, wounds, or burns are likely to have a powerful effect on metabolism, raising both blood sugar and ketone levels. These high levels, if uncontrolled, slow down healing and can result in medical emergencies and hospitalization. Blood glucose testing and adjusting insulin dosage (for Type 1) can be lifesavers when we suffer severe physical stress.

Chronic stress can contribute to the development of diabetic complications.

High blood sugar levels are thought to be the primary cause of complications, but there is growing evidence that stress also plays an important role. Heart disease, for instance, is strongly associated with poorly managed stress in the general population. With diabetes, high levels of stress hormones may contribute to such conditions as retinopathy. Stress is also a factor in hypertension (high blood pressure), which in turn contributes to the development of numerous complications. Clearly, effective stress management is an important component in any program to reduce the risk of complications.

Poorly managed stress has a major impact on the health of everyone—not just the health of those with diabetes. Many books, magazines, television shows, and classes have been addressing this issue and offering suggestions for handling stress. Stress is believed to contribute to heart disease, hypertension, and cancer. Although other factors play a role in these conditions, reducing your stress level is likely to increase your ability to live well.

Understanding The Stress Response

Stress is an inherent part of living. When changes occur in our environment, our bodies react. There are similarities to these reactions no matter what the external stimulus (called the stressors) may be: a threat of physical attack, an emotional blow, a joyous event, a burst of energetic activity, or an actual injury or illness. The stress response is our body's attempt to maintain or restore healthful conditions to itself.

You can appreciate the stress response by remembering the last time you had a very low blood sugar level (if you have Type 2 diabetes, this is usually only experienced if you are using insulin as well as medication). You probably felt shaky and nervous, your pulse sped up, your blood pressure increased, and you may have become sweaty and emotional. These were responses to the physical emergency of low blood sugar. The adrenal hormones released as a result of this physical stress caused the symptoms you experienced. (They also signaled the liver to release glucose and glucagon into your blood stream in an attempt to correct the low blood sugar.) The same hormones also neutralize the effects of insulin so it will not lower blood sugar any further.

If you had become unconscious, this response might have been enough to bring you around, if you were lucky. The body treats this situation as an emergency because the brain needs a certain level of glucose to function effectively and may be damaged if blood sugar levels fall too greatly.

If the stressor is the threat of a mugging, negative criticism from a fellow worker, or a bad fall, you will probably experience the same response. Hormones are released, blood sugar levels rise, insulin becomes less effective, and you are ready for "fight or flight." Your energy is mobilized for an all-out effort.

This mobilization has a negative effect on metabolic control, unless it is in preparation of a major physical event. Your pancreas is unable to produce enough insulin to burn the extra blood sugar stimulated by the stress. If this occurs, your next test will be high, and if you don't know about the effects of stress, you might shake your head in puzzlement, saying, "But I didn't eat any more than usual!" You may not even be aware of the source of distress, and the symptoms of the stress response can be subtle enough to go unnoticed, though blood sugar levels still rise.

Ernest's Traffic with Stress

I'm generally very polite and restrained, even earnest, but in traffic I used to express myself rather emphatically when other drivers treated me unkindly... until the last and absolutely final time I ever made an obscene gesture on the freeway. I was chased down Interstate 5 through Seattle, onto city streets and back to the freeway for seven miles before I finally ditched my offended pursuer. I did my best to meditate while weaving in and out of traffic, but I still ended up with blood sugar at 500 mg/dl (27.7 mmol/L) by the time I got home.

The threat doesn't have to be so real, though, to raise my blood sugar. A number of times I have found that my emotional participation in a movie I'm watching has been enough to produce similar increases. On the other hand, there have been times when blood sugar has gone down to a reaction level after I got angry and expressed it strongly.

One other aspect of the stress response has a special importance for people with diabetes. Both physical and emotional stress can have a powerful effect on blood ketone levels. In some adolescents, ketones have increased tenfold during family arguments.

The effects of stress do not stop with those directly related to diabetes. Your muscles become tense. When you are unable to relieve this tension, headaches, back pain, and other muscular disorders can occur. Your digestive system becomes involved, with changes in the secretion of stomach acids, digestive hormones, and the muscle tone of the alimentary canal. Blood fat and cholesterol levels increase to provide energy for action. Pulse and blood pressure increase. The whole body participates in the stress response. If the cycle is not completed by action, the tension, hormones, glucose, fats, and other stress products stay at unnaturally high levels. If the stress is chronic and poorly managed, your health suffers.

From the point of view of its stress-producing activity, it is immaterial whether the agent or situation we face is pleasant or unpleasant; all that counts is the intensity of the demand for readjustment or adaptation...[We need] to distinguish between distress, which is always unpleasant, and the general concept of stress, which also includes the pleasant experiences of joy, fulfillment, and self-expression. —Hans Selye in *Stress Without Distress*

Dr. Bruce Lipton, a cellular biologist, views our stress response as one of two systems of protection or defense, our immune system being the other. Our external adrenal stress-related system is designed to protect us on the outside, while our immune system protects us on the inside. They share a common budget that is divided between them. If we live in fear of external threats, we devote less energy to our internal environment and steroids released by the adrenals suppress the immune system. When there are fewer threats from the outside, we become more at peace with ourselves, and our immune system activates to help our physical machine run more smoothly. The larger the proportion of our budget we allocate to our internal environment, the happier and healthier we will be, advises Lipton.

Based on existing studies, it is difficult to predict whether stress is likely to raise or lower blood sugar levels in people with diabetes. The gap in our understanding is partly due to the difficulty of doing reliable stress research. (One study in the late 1940s would probably be rejected today by research review committees on the grounds of cruelty. In it, the doctor tested his subjects' blood sugar level and then berated them for being weak and spineless for controlling their diabetes so poorly. Then he tested again and found higher blood sugar. He apologized.)

Although scientists are not certain about the relationship between stress and diabetes, you do not have to wait for their conclusions. Armed with your blood glucose test kit, urine ketone test strips, and logs, you can do the research that is most important: Determine how stress affects you as an individual. (Apparently the impact of stress is highly individual.)

Note distressing or exciting events and periods; study your test results in relation to these events. See if there is a difference in blood sugar levels during a week when you are depressed and a week when you are happier than usual. What happens after a quarrel or a frightening episode? The following questions can help you determine how stress affects your diabetes.

1. Does stress seem to have much effect on your blood sugar levels? If so, do your blood sugar levels increase or decrease?
2. Does the type of emotion aroused influence the direction or amount of change in blood sugar?
3. What difference do you see between short, intense moments of distress and long, drawn-out episodes? What impact do you find from stress that extends for days or weeks at a time?
4. Are the effects on blood sugar levels different when you express feelings rather than hold them in? (One study found blood sugar in one woman unaffected after she became angry and hit her mother-in-law over the head. We hope that more modest forms of expression prove adequate!)
5. Do you have positive tests for ketones in your urine after stressful incidents? If so, when?
6. How do attempts to cope with stress through self-gratification (such as overeating, drinking, and not exercising) disrupt control?
7. What overall patterns do you see in the ways you respond to stress?

As you understand more about how stress affects your control of diabetes, you will be better equipped to handle it. You will know that you need to check your blood sugar level after certain experiences to see whether you need extra insulin. You will know whether you need to modify your insulin dose during times of increased or decreased stress (only for those with Type 1). And you will know which stressful experiences you need to manage more effectively.

Recognizing the signs and symptoms of stress

Acute signs and symptoms

Pounding heart, rapid pulse	Sweating
Trembling, shaky	Easily startled
Dry throat and mouth	Diarrhea or frequent urination
Difficulty concentrating	Indigestion
Change in blood sugar level	Compulsive eating
Emotional and physical tension	Tension headache

Chronic signs and symptoms

General irritability	Nervousness
Easily fatigued	Migraines

Depression	Nightmares
Loss of appetite	Missed menstrual periods
Anxiety	Stuttering
Insomnia	Chronic muscular pains
More accidents and mistakes than usual	

—adapted from *The Stress of Life* by Hans Selye (McGraw-Hill, 1976)

Some of us are more aware of feelings and physical sensations and have no difficulty recognizing the signs of stress. If you have trouble recognizing its symptoms, you need to develop more awareness of the stress. Ignoring the effects of stress does not decrease its impact. And if you know when stress is building, you are better able to deal with it. With more awareness of your body, you are also better able to detect the onset of low blood sugar.

At times, you may mistake a low sugar reaction for a stress response, or vice versa, because the symptoms overlap. You may have signs of low blood sugar such as blurred or double vision, tingling or metallic taste on the tongue, and confused thinking. If in doubt (and if you cannot test your blood at the time), eat something sweet and see if the symptoms decrease.

Doing Something About Stress

There are four main styles of managing stress:
1. Reduce the frequency of stressful incidents by
   a. Making changes in your family, social, or work situation.
   b. Changing beliefs and emotional reactions that trigger stress for you.
   c. Gaining skills that allow you to function more effectively.
   d. Preparing for events likely to be distressing.
2. Reduce the intensity of your stress response by
   a. Learning to relax
   b. Meditating
   c. Praying
   d. Using biofeedback or receiving acupuncture treatments
3. Putting the stress response to work by becoming physically active.
4. Decrease your consumption of stimulants.

As with other aspects of diabetes regimens, coping with stress is a highly individual matter. Vulnerability to stress, the level of arousal, and the effectiveness of particular coping techniques vary from person to person. Fortunately, there are many different approaches to stress management, so you can find at least one that works for you.

The only requirement is this: Whatever you do should decrease your stress level. Find an approach that suits you.

1. Reduce the frequency of stressful incidents

a. Make changes in your family, social, or work situation. You may find it easiest to act on your environment, demanding or requesting changes in the people and conditions that produce stress for you. For the less assertive, you may be able to withdraw from whatever it is that distresses you. For instance, you might have a doctor who doesn't listen to you or who tries to motivate you with fear. Explain how that approach affects you, and ask for changes. If your physician doesn't respond, or if you choose to avoid the confrontation, change doctors.

b. Change beliefs and emotional patterns that trigger stress for you. You may prefer to focus on yourself, using the source of stress to determine the areas of your personality that need change. With the same insensitive doctor, you might discover that the cause of your stress is a belief such as "No one thinks anything I say is important." By eliminating this belief, you will reduce your stress and find it easier to speak with more confidence.

Similarly, you can work with feelings of stifled anger triggered when an authority figure ignores you. By detaching yourself from such responses, you learn to utilize the energy they release. (See Chapter 15 for more on working with beliefs and feelings.)

c. Gain skills that allow you to function more effectively. Often the source of distress is a sense of inadequacy that can be corrected by performing tasks that are important to us. This might involve learning, working, relating, or simply enjoying life. For example, you might overcome your physician's resistance to listen by taking a workshop in assertiveness training or communication skills (assuming this is not the only relationship in which you have difficulty getting your point across).

d. Prepare for events likely to be distressing. We often do this negatively by imagining everything that can possibly go wrong, sometimes in great detail. This skill of visualization can be turned into a positive resource by relaxing and imagining the potentially stressful event. Imagine yourself performing with strength and clarity. This visualization/rehearsal technique is routinely performed by world-class athletes prior to competition. Go through the experience in detail several times, especially if you see yourself faltering. Visualize yourself performing successfully, but don't try to use the visualization as a map when you get to the actual event. Real life calls for spontaneous, not rehearsed, action.

2. Reduce the intensity of your stress response by learning to relax

Your body knows how to relax, but sometimes your mind forgets to use this essential skill. When you practice it during a distressing incident, you can lessen the physical impact of the event. Even if you forget to relax until afterward, you still benefit from releasing the tension that developed under stress. A relaxed body deals with stress more effectively and provides the best conditions for creative problem solving. Some studies indicate that people with diabetes who regularly practice relaxation improve their metabolic control. It also just feels better to be relaxed!

Relaxation techniques include visualization, massage, music, autogenics, meditation, acupuncture, prayer, and biofeedback. If you learn several ways to relax, you will have one to use no matter what situation you face. This chapter contains several examples of relaxation techniques.

Whatever relaxation techniques you choose, practice them while sitting, standing, or moving, as well as while lying down. It is important to learn to relieve tension in any position, especially since it is more likely to strike when you're up and about.

Visualization can involve all of the senses to produce relaxation. Examples are imagining warm water flowing gently across tense muscles; imagining each breath carrying tension out of your body; or imagining a fragrant garden filled with the sounds of birds singing. Your body releases tension in response to this visualization process.

Autogenics uses words to instruct the body to relax. By telling yourself that your arms and legs are becoming heavier, and then warmer, you are suggesting that the results of relaxation are beginning to take effect. As you repeat the phrases, your body responds by relaxing further. Physicians in Europe have reported decreased insulin requirements by those who regularly practice autogenics.

Massage can relax tense muscles, as well as lead to a sense of well-being. Self-massage of temples, neck, shoulders, feet and calves can relieve tightness and pain. Learning specific acupressure points increases the effectiveness of massage.

Acupuncture, while not something you would typically do to yourself, can be very relaxing. Many people go to an acupuncturist for regular "tune-ups" that are reported to last several weeks to months. Five-Element acupuncturists, who focus on the spirit, are perhaps most suited for these tune-ups, although all acupuncturists deal with stress.

Quiet and peaceful music can be used to create a relaxing environment. (In fact, relaxing music might help you work with this book.) Our bodies respond to excess noise with tension, but they often relax when the sounds around us are tranquil. (The resource list at the end of this chapter lists records and tapes that can be used.)

Meditation is a centuries-old means of contacting inner sources of strength and calmness. The physical effects of meditation have been shown to quiet the ravages of stress in our bodies.

Prayer may be seen as a meditation of words directing awareness to a sense of unity and connectedness. Some envision their words being received by a deity; others imagine them joining the wholeness of the universe.

3. You put the stress response to work by becoming more active physically

Since the stress response prepares us for physical activity, exercise is an ideal way to utilize the physical changes produced by stress. Try running up and down stairs after you learn you will not get that hoped-for-promotion. Jog or dance after a quarrel with your lover. Thirty to sixty minutes of moderate to brisk physical activity will use the adrenalin and begin lowering blood sugar levels. (If you have very high blood sugar because of stress, you may need extra insulin.)

4. Decrease your consumption of stimulants

Caffeine and nicotine, along with their other negative effects, can add to stress. Though they are advertised as calming, they are stimulants.

Any one of these techniques for managing stress will benefit your health. If you have a stressful life, you may need to combine several of them to cope with the demands on you. Find the right combination for you, and be gentle in its application. Don't make stress management one more source of stress in your life.

Relaxation Exercises

Remember to practice relaxation in a variety of situations—while sitting, standing, and moving, as well as lying down. You can relax anytime, not just while flat on your back. However, you may want to start learning to relax when lying down, with your eyes closed.

Utilize time spent waiting. No matter where you are, you can use those in-between times to let go of tension. As long as you don't start snoring, no one will care what you are doing.

Breathe Away Tension

Begin by observing your breathing. What part of your torso are you using? How deep or shallow is your breathing? How fast? Are you holding your breath unconsciously?

Next, focus on the air moving through your nostrils. Follow the air into your lungs, feeling your chest and stomach expanding and contracting with each breath.

Focus now on each exhalation, imagining that the air is carrying tension out of your body. If you are alone, sigh or hum gently with each breath.

Finally, focus on each inhalation, imagining new energy coming into your body with the air.

Visualize With Any or All of the Senses

Imagine yourself immersed in a sensory bath of fragrant, warm breezes, tropical showers, glowing light, and gentle, natural sounds. Picture warm water and breezes flowing over your body, and through the muscles, opening and relaxing them.

Another method is to let your mind return to a specific time when you felt happy and deeply relaxed. Relive the event in as much detail as you can.

Talk Your Body into Relaxing

When our minds talk, our bodies listen. Doctors in Europe have created a discipline of relaxation called autogenic training based on this simple truth. This method uses repeated phrases to suggest that the body is experiencing relaxation. Repeat each phrase slowly (and silently) five or six times:

"My right arm is becoming heavier."
"My left arm is becoming heavier."
"My right leg is becoming heavier."
"My left leg is becoming heavier."
"My right arm is becoming warmer."
(and so on through the other limbs).

Meditate

Among the numerous approaches to meditation, one of the easiest to learn is called mindfulness. With this, you step back from the constant flow of thoughts and sensations and simply watch the parade.

Find a posture you can maintain comfortably for ten to twenty minutes without moving. Balance your body so you are not leaning forward, backward, or to the side. (Or lie down if you can stay awake.)

Begin with awareness of the breath passing through your nostrils, and focus on this sensation. Let each breath remind you to observe the flow of thoughts, feelings, perceptions, and body sensations. Just watch, without commenting on or judging what you see.

Naturally you forget to "just watch" and you become immersed in the process of thinking and feeling. You forget even the simple task of sensing each breath. Then your breathing reminds you to detach and step back again.

You move between watching and marching along in the parade of your mind. Gradually, the periods of watching become longer and the mind grows quieter.

Resources for Stress Management

Books on Relaxation

New England Deaconess Hospital and Harvard Medical School Mind-Body Institute, *The Wellness Book,* 1993

Patricia Carrington, *Freedom in Meditation,* Anchor Books, 1978

Daniel Girdano and George Everly, *Controlling Stress and Tension,* Prentice-Hall, 1979

Joseph Levine, *A Gradual Awakening,* Doubleday, 1984

Hans Selye, *Stress Without Distress,* Signet, 1975

Jenny Sutcliffe, *The Complete Book of Relaxation Techniques,* People's Medical Society, 1994

Music to Help You Relax

Gregorian Chant and other early church music (before Baroque)

William Ackerman, *Passages,* Windham Hill Records

Brian Eno, *Music for Airports* or *Plateaux of Mirrors,* ECM

Steve Halprin, *Spectrum Suite,* SRI Records

Georgia Kelly, *Seapeace,* Global Pacific

Environments (natural sounding records—waves, bird song, country streams, and the like) Cyntonic Research, 175 5th Ave., New York, NY

Guided-Relaxation Tapes

Emmett Miller, *Letting Go of Stress and Health and Wellness*

Classes on Stress Management

Your local chapter of the American Diabetes Association may offer or know of a stress-management class especially designed for people with diabetes. Or you can call their national information line, 1-800-DIA-BETES.

YMCA and high school or college adult-education programs usually have general stress-management classes.

Section Four
Support for Living Well

Chapter Thirteen

Living Well
With Your Medical Team

Of all chronic medical conditions, diabetes probably has the most sophisticated, well-developed team of health professionals dedicated to helping you learn about and manage the disease. There is even an American Association of Diabetes Educators (AADE) with over 10,000 members. Membership includes a wide variety of professionals interested and involved in working with diabetes.

Diabetes Health Professionals

Physicians

Most likely, your primary care giver is either a family physician or an internist. Your physician may have special interest or expertise in diabetes. There are also subspecialists—endocrinologists and diabetologists—who have special training in diabetes. Any of these physicians can help you live well with your diabetes. You have the right to choose a physician with whom you have a mutually rewarding relationship. You may find one who is more responsive to your individual needs, more knowledgeable about the options available and more willing to work with you. These qualities are more related to the physician's personality than to training. Don't feel guilty if you decide to change doctors because you want a better relationship.

If complications develop, your physician may refer you to a specialist in the area of your complication such as a dermatologist for skin problems, a neurologist for nerve problems, a cardiologist for heart and circulation problems, a nephrologist for kidney problems, a gastroenterologist or neurologist (since these problems in a person with diabetes are usually due to neuropathy) for digestive or bowel problems, or an ophthalmologist for eye problems. We recommend that you see an ophthalmologist at least once a year for preventive purposes.

Podiatrists and Dentists

Diabetes can affect you from head to toe. It is wise to have regular (yearly, and more often, if recommended) preventive maintenance on your teeth and gums and your feet. You should be sure that your dentist and podiatrist are aware that you have diabetes. It will affect the signs and symptoms they look for and the kind of treatment they may give you.

Diabetes Educators

In this category, we include nurses, nurse educators, nurse practitioners, dietitians, nutritionists, patient educators, and exercise specialists. Other health professionals named in this chapter can also be considered diabetes educators if they consider diabetes education a part of their professional responsibility. The knowledge, skills, and attitudes involved in living well with diabetes require someone who is well trained to help the patient learn them. A nurse or patient educator can teach most areas of diabetes education and may refer you to a specialist if you need detailed information in specific areas. For example, an exercise specialist can help design a program of exercise suited to your interests and level of fitness, or a dietitian can create a program of food, nutrition, and weight management.

Several years ago, a national program of certification for diabetes educators was begun. Those who pass a comprehensive exam become Certified Diabetes Educators and are entitled to put the initials CDE after their names. A CDE is likely to be well informed about the latest methods of diabetes management. However, keep in mind that many excellent diabetes educators are not certified.

Psychologists, Psychiatrists, Counselors, Behavioral and Mental Health Specialists, and Other Psychotherapists

These professionals are available to help you with crises or difficult changes that you wish to make in your life. They can help you overcome resistance to following the diabetes regimen you choose, if you need more than the techniques presented in this book. They can also help you deal with the emotional and problem-solving aspects of crises such as the onset of complications. To find someone who specializes in diabetes or other chronic illness counseling, contact your local chapter of the American Diabetes Association or call 1-800-TEAM-UP-4. (See Chapter 14 for more on professional psychological support, as well as lay support.)

Pharmacists

Pharmacists are extremely helpful in providing information on medications and how they affect diabetes. They can also inform you about insulin and the selection and use of a wide variety of diabetes products. Pharmacists are the fastest growing group among diabetes educators.

Working With The Team

The idea of a team implies the coordination of roles and responsibilities to accomplish a mutually shared goal. You are the focus, and the team's goal is to help you live well with diabetes.

It is your responsibility to convey your needs, concerns, questions, and problems to individuals on the team. We urge you to speak up

▷ when you do not understand something you are told.

▷ when too much is being said at once.

▷ when you think you will have difficulty carrying out a recommendation.

▷ when you do not agree with something you are told.

▷ when you want to know if there are alternatives to the recommended plan.

Most health professionals prefer that you voice lack of understanding or disagreement from the beginning rather than say nothing because you feel awkward or embarrassed. You make the ultimate decisions about your care, and they want you to understand their recommendations and be willing to follow them.

It is your health professional's responsibility to communicate the care options available to you. They should use words you understand, speak slowly enough for you to follow, and write down or provide printed information about their recommendations. They should outline the risks and benefits of alternative courses of action and explain any side effects of recommended tests, medications, procedures, or treatments.

We have reproduced here a sample diabetes health record developed by the Diabetes Coalition of California, in collaboration with the American Diabetes Association California Affiliate and the Juvenile Diabetes Foundation International. It is intended to help you monitor the care your physician and diabetes team provides. Discuss your targets with them.

Health Record

Evaluations	Date of Visit			
Review daily blood glucose (BG) records (every visit)	——	——	——	——
My target (pre-meals): ____				
Blood Pressure (every visit)	——	——	——	——
Target: ____				
Weight (every visit)	——	——	——	——
Target: ____				
Foot Exam (every diabetes care visit)	——	——	——	——
Dilated Eye Exam (every year)				
HbA1c (every 3 months)	——	——	——	——
Target: ____				
Microalbuminuria (every year)	——	——	——	——
Target: ____				
Triglycerides (every year)	——	——	——	——
Target: ____				
HDL/LDL (every year)	——	——	——	——
Target: ____				
Flu Shots (every year)	——	——	——	——
Pneumonia Vaccine (generally once)	——	——	——	——

Discuss these issues regularly with your health care provider to improve your diabetes management skills:

▷ Smoking Counseling   ▷ Hypoglycemia (low BG)
▷ Medications   ▷ Hyperglycemia (high BG)
▷ Nutrition Therapy   ▷ Sick Day Rules
▷ Physical Activity   ▷ Psychosocial Issues
▷ Weight Management   ▷ Pre-pregnancy Counseling
▷ Complications   ▷ Pregnancy Management

We have also reproduced the Basic Guidelines for Diabetes Care and the accompanying Explanatory Notes, developed by the Diabetes Coalition, upon which the previous Health Record is based. You can share a copy with your physician and use it to become more informed about your care. It is consistent with the ADA Standards of Care.

Basic Guidelines for Diabetes Care

Physical Assessment	Blood Pressure, Weight (for Children, add Height; plot on Growth Chart) Every visit. Blood Pressure target goal <130/85 mm Hg (children: <90 pctl age standard). Children: normal weight for height (see standard growth charts).
	Foot Exam (for adults) Thorough visual inspection every "diabetes visit"; pedal pulses, neurological exam annually.
	Dilated eye exams Type 1 (Insulin-Dependent Diabetes Mellitus): 5 years post diagnosis, then every year by a trained expert. Type 2 (Noninsulin-Dependent Diabetes Mellitus): shortly after diagnosis, then every year by a trained expert.
Lab Exam	HbA1c Quarterly, if treatment changes or is not meeting goals; 1-2 times/year if stable. Target goal 7.0% or 1 percentage point above lab norms; children, modify if necessary to prevent significant hypoglycemia.
	Microalbuminuria Type 1: 5 years post diagnosis, then every year. Type 2: begin at diagnosis, then every year.
	Blood Lipids (for adults) On initial visit, then annually for adults. Target goals: Cholesterol, Triglycerides (mg/dL) <200; LDL <130 unless CHD, then <100; HDL >35.

<table>
<tr>
<td rowspan="1">Self-Management Training</td>
<td>

Management Principles and Complications

Understanding diabetes, medications, glucose self-monitoring, hypo/hyperglycemia, chronic complications, psycho-social assessment (special attention needed for adolescents); initially and in follow-up visits. Children: appropriate for developmental stage.

Self Glucose Monitoring

Type 1: typically test 4 times a day; others as needed to meet treatment goals.

Medical Nutrition Therapy

Initial: assess condition/needs, assist patient in setting nutrition goals. Follow-up: assess progress toward goals, identify problem areas; by a trained expert.

Physical Activity—Assess patient initially; prescribe physical activity based on patient's needs/conditions, initially and in follow-up visits.

Weight Management—Must be individualized for patient; initially and in follow-up visits.

</td>
</tr>
<tr>
<td>Interventions</td>
<td>

Preconception Counseling and Management

Consult with high risk perinatal programs where available (e.g., "Sweet Success" Regional Perinatal Programs of California). Adolescents: special counseling advisable, beginning with puberty.

Pregnancy Management

Consult with high risk perinatal programs where available.

Smoking Cessation

Screen, advise, and assist; initially, then annually.

Vaccinations

Influenza and Pneumococcal, per CDC recommendations.

</td>
</tr>
</table>

Adopted by the Diabetes Coalition of California 1995 & 1997. These guidelines should be used in conjunction with the following Explanatory Notes. These guidelines are consistent with ADA Clinical Practice Recommendations.

Explanatory Notes to Basic Guidelines for Diabetes Care.

1. These guidelines are intended for use by primary care professionals.

2. The guidelines are meant to be basic guidelines, not enforceable standards. (Where an internal quality assurance program has demonstrated that less frequent testing does not jeopardize patient care, less frequent testing may be acceptable; e.g., dilated eye exams every two years vs. every year.)

3. One or more of the following criteria were used for inclusion of an item in the guidelines:

   a. Published evidence demonstrated either the efficacy or the effectiveness of the item.

   b. Published studies on cost-identification, cost-effectiveness, or cost-benefit analysis of the item demonstrated favorable economic results.

   c. A preponderance of expert opinion held that the item is considered to be essential to the care of persons with diabetes.

4. It is assumed that the following are routinely occurring in the medical setting:

   a. A history and physical appropriate for a person with diabetes are performed. Visits are sufficiently frequent to meet the patient's needs and treatment goals.

   b. Abnormal physical or laboratory findings result in appropriate interventions which are individualized for each patient.

   c. Self-Management Training is provided by allied health professionals who are experts in the provision of this training. For children/adolescents and their families, training from a diabetes team or team member with experience in child and adolescent diabetes is strongly recommended to begin at diagnosis.

   d. Physicians consult current references for normal values and for appropriate treatment goal values, both for children and adults.

   e. Specialists should be consulted when patients are unable to achieve treatment goals in a reasonable time frame, when complications arise, or whenever the primary care physician deems it appropriate. Under similar circumstances, children/adolescents should be referred to specialists who have expertise in managing children and adolescents with diabetes.

5. Additional comments on specific items included in the guidelines:

   Children/Adolescents—For specific diabetes care, see references.

   HbA1c/Self Blood Glucose Monitoring—HbA1c target goals should be achieved gradually over time. Targets goals should be less stringent for children, the elderly and other fragile patients. Clinicians have found that making the patient aware of his/her HbA1c values and their significance helps motivate the patient toward improved glucose management. This principle also applies to self blood glucose monitoring. Target goals should be individualized for each patient.

   Blood Lipids—Abnormal blood lipids are often under-treated. An active, progressive treatment and monitoring plan should be instituted.

   Microalbuminuria—Need not test for microalbuminuria if albumin has previously been found in the urine.

6. A list of general and specific references is available (Diabetes Coalition of California).

As you work with members of your diabetes team, you may wish to bring this book with you. Go over parts of the book that are relevant to you with your health professional and ask questions about anything that is not clear to you. You may wish to show them the special note in the Preface to this book.

The most important tool of your diabetes care team is communication. We hope this book encourages communication between you and the members of your team.

Chapter Fourteen

Living Well
With Others
With Diabetes

"I always felt lonely and a little weird, like I was the only diabetic in the world who lied to her doctor or ate lemon meringue pie. The only thing worse than my guilt was my depression over feeling so out of control. I didn't think anyone could understand what I was up against, until I went—unwillingly— to a diabetes support group. For the first time I got to talk to people who were struggling with the same issues that had me down. They taught me I could do something to get myself under control."—Jean

Creating A Diabetic Support Network

Diabetes is a demanding companion that isolates us from others. Our friends and relatives often have little understanding of the frustrations and challenges we face. Often we feel that we would only bore them with the countless details of regimen we stay aware of every day. We need support from those who have a knowledge of diabetes to help us cope with our feelings, answer our questions, and enable us to follow our complex and challenging regimen.

Contact with others who are attempting to live well with diabetes is a vital component to our self-care program.

Support from other people with diabetes is especially important when you decide to improve your level of management. The experiences, knowledge, and understanding of others who have gone through this process make the path much easier. They can help you see when you are trying to move too fast or when you are forgetting important aspects of regimen. They can also offer encouragement and practical tips. This level of help is an excellent complement to your medical team's support.

Support is especially important when diabetes is first diagnosed or when complications first appear. These are times of crises when we are filled with emotions and countless questions. Others with diabetes can help us deal with these challenges and learn the lessons of living well.

Those who are close to us need support as well. Being the mate or parent of someone with diabetes has its own unique demands. Just ask a person who has found a loved one unconscious or who watches one of us consistently overeating. They can learn from and be encouraged by others with diabetes and their families.

Anyone with diabetes may encounter problems that require professional mental health assistance. Our support system may be weak, or the particular challenges we meet may require the aid of someone with professional training. Some of the signs of needing to see a psychotherapist (including psychologists and psychiatrists), counselor, behavioral specialist, or social worker include

1. Chronic depression.
2. Repeated self-destructive behavior such as "forgetting" insulin, going on frequent eating binges, and not learning to handle insulin reactions.
3. A sense of helplessness that blocks learning and action.
4. Unwillingness to ask for help from an informal support system.
5. Participation in negative family or social situations that detract from self-care.

If you feel you need more support than your network or group can give, take this as a sign of healthful perception, not as evidence that something else is wrong with you.

Setting Up Your Support Network

There is an abundance of diabetes support resources. Local American Diabetes Association chapters, hospitals, clinics, diabetes centers, or individual physicians may sponsor continuing support groups that you can attend. Your local ADA office should know if anything is available in your area (or call the ADA information line 1-800-DIABETES). You may find that there are only general educational meetings in your area. Although not specifically devoted to emotional support, these events are good places to meet other people with diabetes and begin building your diabetes network.

Using the diabetes network is an effective way to develop your support system. You can find people who function as diabetes networkers; they are often storehouses of information on people, resources, and meetings. "You're trying to get control of your eating? Talk to Joe Dodds. He's winning that battle and can really help you." "You're afraid of laser treatment and keep putting it off? Joan Mason can tell you how she overcame her fear." Don't feel that it is an imposition to ask for help. Most people enjoy an opportunity to help someone, especially when they share a common interest in diabetes. Networkers are special people who love the process of making connections. As you gather your own information, you might find that you want to serve this function as well.

Talk to your friends, relatives, doctor, pharmacist, clinics or hospitals with diabetes education programs, and the nearest ADA chapter. Indicate that you want to contact people with diabetes who have positive attitudes and can encourage you. If you need support, it doesn't help to begin networking with people who will make you feel worse.

You may run into obstacles as you begin, so be prepared to persevere in building your network. Some doctors are protective of their patients and will discourage them from learning from others with diabetes. And some people with diabetes avoid others completely. You may have to make a number of calls before you start getting positive responses, or you may find support from the beginning.

Soon you will have several people you can call when you need support or information. Perhaps there will be a person who shares a compulsive eating pattern with you, and you agree to call each other when the urge strikes. If you have a complication developing, you might know someone who has dealt with the same problem. Or you may just want a sympathetic ear when it all feels like too much.

Perhaps occasional telephone contact or conversation over a diet soda or cup of coffee will satisfy your need for support. You'll go through a sorting process, dropping out of contact with people who just complain and turn away from encouragement. You may have friends of friends calling you because they have heard you are interested in mutual support.

You will soon be giving support to others, offering resources you know about such as a new development in diabetes care you have just read about, a drugstore that sells insulin at a discount, or a doctor who works well with patients. When you encourage another, you encourage yourself. A principle of mutual support is that giving and receiving are the same.

Living Well With Others With Diabetes

Often, you will be able to offer guidance or information well suited to someone else's needs. However, there will be times when there is little you can do. Don't feel that you must always have an answer. Your responsibility is to listen, show that you care, and share what you know. Sometimes "You'd better talk to your doctor about that" is the most useful thing you can tell someone. As your network grows, you will be able to suggest others who can help with particular problems.

Developing A Support Group

Informal networking can provide very effective support, especially for people who are uncomfortable in groups. A group, however, offers certain bonuses. You can obtain feedback from a variety of points of view, and you have a larger body of experience to draw upon. A group can bring in guest speakers or even set up a training program dealing with aspects of diabetes management. Also, a group is usually more effective than individuals in handling a crisis such as the development of complications.

A support group is most effective when it is part of an ongoing network. If members feel free to contact one another between meetings, support is always available. Members maintain contact even when they are not able to attend every meeting. The meetings themselves are more relaxed, since they are only one of several times of sharing.

If you find no existing diabetes support group to join, you can start one by following the networking steps just described. Ask the people you contact if they are interested in creating a group. Find out what they are willing to do, what they want out of the meetings, and how often they would like to meet. You will find some who enjoy organizing and leading meetings, and others with practical skills such as typing or access to copying machines. Share the work load so that you do not have to carry the entire burden. Be clear about the tasks people are assigned and specify when they need to be completed. "You're willing to call Sarah, Phil, Joan, and Larry? The meeting is on the tenth, so can you do that by the second?"

You may want to proceed informally, or you may prefer to set up a coordinating committee from the beginning. Two or three other members are enough to work with you to organize the group, planning meetings, and develop other activities. It will become clear which decisions need to be made by the whole group, and which by the committee. Some groups want to share the organizational tasks and decisions, and others prefer to use most of their meeting time for support and learning. In your initial conversations with potential members, you will get a sense of how they feel about this question. It can be explored at length in the first meeting.

The First Meeting

Establish a positive tone at the first meeting, without doing so there might not be a second meeting. The details of this first meeting depend upon the wants and needs of the group. We will describe three ways of conducting this session, though there are countless others.

Shared Leadership Everyone shares in the creation of the group. At the beginning, the facilitator or discussion leaders ask the group to work together to develop guidelines, structure, and topics. Everyone in the group should answer the following questions:

▷ What do you want out of the group?

▷ What do you want to avoid?

▷ How do you want the group to operate—no leader, rotating leaders, professional facilitators?

▷ What guidelines for discussion are important to you?

▷ What are you willing to do to help the group function?

The leader encourages everyone present to describe their preferences. After discussing each question, an agreement may be reached, a vote may be taken, or further discussion may uncover solutions that satisfy conflicting views.

The strength of this approach is that it encourages a high level of participation and responsibility. It reflects the level of individual responsibility demanded by diabetes. However, if some group members are dealing with major problems, they could find it difficult to give their attention to organizational questions. If you have someone in crisis, find out how they feel about beginning the group this way.

There should be a limit set for the organizational discussion; at least half of the meeting should be devoted to discussing living well with diabetes.

Committee Leadership A coordinating committee is responsible for defining initial guidelines and structure of leadership. This method is appropriate if you sense those coming to the first meeting are shy. The discussion leader briefly describes the proposed structure and asks for approval or recommendations for change. It is then possible to begin the support work. With good topics for initiating discussion, group members can quickly experience the value of being in a support group. However, it may take more effort to involve them in keeping the group going.

Outside Leadership If you or the other members lack confidence in a self-directed group, a counselor or social worker might be hired to lead the first few meetings. Look for someone experienced at facilitating groups and willing to build the group's capacity to function on its own. A local college, hospital, or public health department can help you find such a person, who might even be willing to volunteer their time. If not, the group will have to be willing to pay fifty to one hundred fifty dollars for each meeting.

Any of these structures can be effective. Choose the one that seems most appropriate to the people in your group. For more information on conducting this first support meeting, read the general comments on meetings that follow, especially the sections on guidelines, stress level, and evaluation.

Conducting Successful Support Meetings

Clearly stated guidelines help instruct new members, and remind old members, of the group's basic values and meeting format. Print the list and read it at the beginning of the first few meetings. This helps to keep the discussion within bounds and avoids pitfalls of discussing individual regimens in a group setting. Your group can create its own guidelines or use the following as a model.

Guidelines for a Diabetes Support Group

1. We are here to support one another in facing the challenge of living well with diabetes. By helping one another, we help ourselves. We intend to maintain a positive climate for discussing our experiences, feelings, problems, and solutions.
2. We will feel free to share any information about ourselves within the groups, but we will not disclose anything we hear to people outside the group.
3. We will respect one another's right to remain silent as much as his or her right to speak. And we will be sure to create opportunities for the silent to speak.
4. The proper care of diabetes differs from person to person. We will remember that regimen is individual and not try to advise someone else on the basis of our own practice.

5. If we hear something that suggests possible changes in our own regimen of physical care, we agree to discuss such changes with our physician before acting.

6. If we feel anyone is passing on misinformation, we will not be afraid to challenge the information. When there is a difference of opinion or doubt, we will determine the facts with a health professional.

7. One of our functions is to share feelings. When we do this, we will give support but avoid interpretation and analysis. If any of us opens to deep emotions during the meeting, we will allow room for this. At the end of the meeting, one of us will check with the person to be sure they are OK.

8. We will feel free to express anger but not to direct it at other group members.

9. Many of the topics we discuss at an informational level may arouse strong feelings and stress reactions. When any of us senses stress or tension, we will feel free to ask for a moment of silence to calm our emotions. When the group stress level is high, we will take time for guided relaxation or another stress-reduction technique.

10. When one person is discussing a problem, we will encourage that person to find their own answers before offering ours. When we make suggestions, we will do it gently, without pushing.

11. If any of us is an alcoholic or drug user, we agree to come to meetings only when we are sober or straight.

12. If any of us decides to stop coming because we can't handle the issues the group discusses or the way the group functions, we will discuss our reasons in the meetings or contact someone in the group and give feedback on what is causing the difficulty.

13. Having diabetes challenges us to learn the lessons of life we are faced with. We are together to support this learning.

Leading Effective Meetings

These guidelines imply that many of the leadership functions in a group can be shared by all members. If each person takes responsibility for maintaining discussion, awareness of stress levels, respect for feelings, and other questions of process, the meetings will practically run themselves. When there is an understanding of the group's guidelines, it is possible to function without a discussion leader.

Living Well With Others With Diabetes

It can also be effective to designate one person discussion leader for each meeting, with the role rotating to another member each time the group meets. This is especially true if new people come regularly.

The facilitator will do the following:

1. Read the group's guidelines at the beginning of each meeting.
2. Mention any departures from the guidelines if they occur.
3. Lead introductions and note the subjects people wish to bring up.
4. Direct the discussion, quieting side conversations and opening new subjects when the last has been completed.
5. Stay attentive to stress levels and call for relaxation when the level is high.
6. Reserve space for discussing group business, such as a change in meeting place.
7. Conclude each meeting with a time of evaluation and appreciations.

When a different member handles this job at each meeting, the whole group becomes experienced leaders. It becomes natural for everyone to share the leader's tasks. If the evening's facilitator fails to notice the high level of stress, it can be corrected by any member of the group.

Introductions Members can introduce themselves by describing their relationship with diabetes and sharing something about their life outside diabetes. They can also mention subjects they would like to discuss during the meeting. The facilitator should list subjects on a chalkboard or large pad of paper. Also, knowing who has Type 1 or Type 2 diabetes and who is a parent or partner of a person with diabetes, helps keep information relevant. The information about one's life outside diabetes helps group members see one another as complete persons, not just as people who have diabetes.

Starting Discussion Reviewing the subjects people mention during introductions may be all that is needed to begin a discussion that lasts all evening.

The facilitator can read the list and ask the group which topic to discuss first. Another way of beginning is to assign a subject that establishes a positive mood: "The most useful thing I've learned about living with diabetes is…" or "How has diabetes improved my life?" It is surprising how willingly most people talk when such simple questions are presented.

Guiding Discussion Sometimes meetings flow spontaneously, with little need for guidance from the facilitator. However, there are times when some direction is needed. One person may be cut off prematurely; a quiet "I'm not sure Francis was finished speaking" will return the floor to the speaker.

There may be shy members in the group who will say little or nothing during the meetings. You can open space for them by saying, "Do any of those who have not said much want to speak?" Allow them time to speak up, but do not pressure them. They may prefer to just listen for a while, and learn from other's experiences.

Setting a Positive Tone A support group is more attractive if members emphasize abilities rather than disabilities, and solutions rather than problems.

Members need room to describe the difficulties they experience, but they should be encouraged to overcome these difficulties rather than be a victim to them. Ask questions in such a way that they elicit positive responses, such as "How do you deal with your feelings about diabetes?" rather than "What psychological problems does diabetes cause?"

Awareness of Stress and Feelings Many of the issues discussed at a support group can raise stress levels. Feelings of vulnerability will be aroused by even the most boring and technical description of laser treatment: "My doctor shot this blue beam through a thick contact lens. The flashes were really bright. He said he did 800 zaps the first session." When the group is discussing subjects such as complications, it is important that the facilitator and group members watch for signs of stress. Some of these signs include a tendency to quickly change subjects or give in to nervous laughter.

It is always appropriate for a group member to ask, "Is anyone else feeling anxious?" and call for a stress check in which people sense how they are reacting to the discussion. If enough of the group shares a discomfort, the facilitator can lead a relaxation exercise. By doing this, members learn to be aware of and manage stress as it occurs. This also makes participation in the group a more positive experience. A diabetes support group should reduce, not increase, stress levels.

Avoiding Misinformation Members must feel free to challenge information they believe to be inaccurate or incomplete. Keeping the facts straight is important. A self-led group may want to enlist a physician or nurse practitioner who can answer questions between meetings.

Living Well With Others With Diabetes

Handling "Difficult" Members You may lack the necessary assertiveness to confront the person who dominates the discussion, drains the group with complaints and discouragement, or sarcastically criticizes others. As facilitator, one thing you can do is refer the difficulty to the group: "Jim seems to have a lot to say tonight. Does anyone else want to say anything?" Or suggest doing something that will change the tone: "Betty has pointed out a few things she doesn't like about doctors. I'd like to hear if any of you have anything good to say about your doctor." Or just say what you are feeling: "I'm frustrated. It sounds like everyone's doing everything wrong, according to Cliff."

Evaluation At the end of the meeting, each member describes what they most appreciated about the evening's discussion and mentions any changes that would improve the sessions. This feedback keeps the group on task.

Meeting Format

Support group meetings can follow a variety of formats. Each facilitates a different type of discussion, so it is good to vary the format occasionally. Some of the possibilities include the following:

1. General discussion of questions and concerns members bring up at the beginning of the meeting.
2. Sessions organized around a specific topic. The coordinating committee can choose the topic in advance, or the group can decide the topic at the beginning of the meeting.
3. Discussion in subgroups, such as insulin dependent and noninsulin dependent, diabetic and nondiabetic family members, or married and single people. With this format, people are able to spend more time on questions unique to being the spouse, or a single person with diabetes, and so on.
4. Discussion in pairs. The group can break up into pairs to discuss topics or just get better acquainted. This is important for people who are more comfortable talking one-on-one than in groups. When the group reassembles, members can summarize their learning from the more intimate conversation.
5. Question-and-answer or instructional periods with a guest speaker. A nurse practitioner or psychologist can give instruction in stress management for diabetes. You might ask a physician to answer questions such as "How can we most effectively use of our office

visits?" A dietitian might be asked to describe new research affecting nutrition and diabetes. (Guest speakers can be effective early in the development of a group to enlist new members.)

6. Films related to diabetes as a way to focus discussion. *Diabetes— Focus on Feelings,* for instance, is effective for exploring feelings about living with diabetes.

7. Social events, such as parties, picnics, and potlucks to share favorite recipes.

Some Topics for Discussion

▷ How has diabetes been my teacher, helping me learn about living?

▷ What attitudes, beliefs, or skills have helped me cope with diabetes?

▷ What do I wish I had known about living with diabetes at the beginning?

▷ What benefits do I receive from diabetes?

▷ What are three things I like most about myself? How do they (or how could they) help me deal with diabetes?

▷ What attitudes and skills do I need to learn to deal with diabetes better? How can I learn them?

▷ How does diabetes affect my relationships, both intimate and casual?

▷ How did I feel when I first learned I had diabetes?

▷ What can I do to create a more effective relationship with my doctor and health care team?

▷ Given my need to respect the demands of diabetes, what can I do to improve the quality of my life?

▷ How can we cut the costs of managing diabetes?

The elements selected for a diabetes support group should be determined by its members. There is no universal formula for support groups, just as there is no universal regimen for diabetes care. Feel free to experiment until you find a combination that works for everyone.

The following is a description of how one group met in Seattle.

A Meeting Of A Diabetes Support Group

Five of the regulars are present at the agreed-upon meeting time, so they begin with a relaxation exercise and introduce the topics for the evening. Three more people, one of them new, come in during the introductions. The newcomer says she wants to find out about blood glucose testing, so this is discussed first. The three members who are doing blood glucose testing talk about how it has improved their control. They recommend that the newcomer attend a class at a diabetes clinic. Later in the evening, the hostess brings out a blood test strip and a lancet, and the woman tests her blood.

A man with Type 1 diabetes and his wife arrive late because the man had a serious insulin reaction just before dinner. As he describes what happened, it becomes evident that he is on a metabolic roller coaster. Group members emphasize the importance of working closely with one's doctor to get regulated. They also suggest specific actions that would help such as making his schedule more regular, keeping detailed records, handling stress more effectively, and sharpening his awareness of reaction symptoms. A young woman who has had diabetes most of her life says with conviction, "It is possible to learn to control diabetes."

The man's wife describes her distress over the difficulties she goes through with her husband. Others acknowledge that it can be as difficult to live with someone who has diabetes as it is to be a diabetic. Another spouse offers to meet the woman for coffee and share some of the things that have helped her live with her husband's diabetes.

One member notes that the stress level seems high after talking about personal relationships. She asks if others would enjoy a relaxation break. Many people nod, and the facilitator reads a relaxation exercise, going through the steps of the relaxation as she reads.

A 32-year-old woman who works in an office says she has been using the relaxation technique she learned at the previous meeting. She says she does it several times a day at her office, and believes that her blood sugar control has improved. She suggests relaxation to the man who had the reaction.

The facilitator notes that only thirty minutes of the meeting are left, and she asks how the group wants to end the meeting. The man who had been delayed by the reaction says he wonders if his difficulty with control has something to do with his beliefs. He asks the group to talk about the beliefs that help them maintain control. A thoughtful discussion follows in which people describe the beliefs that help them. Those who feel they have very little control speculate on the beliefs they think might help them.

A coordinating committee member asks about the possibility of shifting the meeting to another night because of conflicts in several members' schedules. Another evening is found. Everyone agrees to meet on a different night next time. She also asks for a volunteer to type up a new membership list.

The meeting ends with the facilitator and other members expressing appreciation to individuals and to the group as a whole.

"Housekeeping" Issues For A Support Group

Several practical aspects of an ongoing support group need to be handled. The members of the coordinating committee can work with the group on these matters.

Information System Coordinating committee members can be those who talk to potential members and whose phone numbers are listed on printed announcements. A membership list can be the basis of a phone chain that allows group members to communicate between meetings. Each committee member calls two people, who each call two people, and so on through the list. The phone list indicates who calls whom.

If the group wishes to grow larger, information can be distributed by networking through doctors, nurses, pharmacists, dietitians, friends, and relatives, as well as the local ADA chapter. If these channels fail to bring new members, you can send press releases to local newspapers and make spot announcements on radio and television stations.

Group Size This depends on available space and flexibility of meeting times. Large groups (more than ten members) can work effectively if they use subgroups and pairs to give everyone a chance to participate. Small groups function well because of their intimate nature.

Meeting Frequency Every other week is probably the best schedule for the meetings. A weekly meeting may feel burdensome; gathering once a month may not allow the group to develop momentum.

Meeting Place Private homes, schools, churches, community centers, and bank conference rooms are potential meeting places. Some support groups meet in hospitals or public health buildings, but the association with illness can discourage some people from coming. Using homes creates a more comfortable atmosphere; as long as the site is changed every month, meeting in homes does not become a burden on any one member.

Attendance Some members will come regularly; others will come only when they feel a special need. If a group is viewed as only one aspect of a diabetes network, irregular attendance becomes less frustrating to those people organizing the meetings. They can stay in touch by phone, and those who do not appear regularly will know they can get support by calling or visiting another member.

Screening and Referring Occasionally, someone who needs professional physical or psychological assistance will come to a support group. This might be someone who does not have a physician, is dangerously out of control metabolically, or has serious mental problems. Only those who seriously disrupt meetings should be screened out. However, the group should not try to solve problems that require skilled help. Members should indicate that professional guidance is needed and, if necessary, help the person find a physician or mental health professional.

Other Activities Of The Support Network

Support activities can be initiated by your diabetes network. Your network may or may not be affiliated with the local chapter of the American Diabetes Association, and you might find that an independent organization is more creative than working through an official group. If your local ADA already has a good level of participation, any of the following activities might be easily accepted.

Training for Support Giving

People with diabetes and family members can learn communication skills, stress management, problem-solving techniques, and guidelines of peer support. Such a training program can be developed with mental health professionals from a local college or clinic. (Crisis centers often have volunteer training workshops that could be adapted to diabetes.)

Support for the Newly Diagnosed or Those in Crisis

Beginning with hospital or home visits, network members can provide encouragement and practical information to newly diagnosed patients and their families. They can also visit people after a major emergency such as diabetic coma, insulin reaction, or treatment for complications. This is a time when motivation to improve self-care is high. Contact with someone who has dealt with and learned from similar crises can be inspiring.

Study Groups

Those interested in learning about a particular subject might form a study group. For instance, three or four people who want to learn the intensive regimen could work together, helping one another master the information they need to attain optimal control. This would make the learning process easier and ensure the emotional support needed to make lifestyle changes. Or people with retinopathy could work together, collecting and sharing information on the condition and its treatment.

Residential Houses

A live-in treatment center for adolescents with diabetes was operated in Gainesville, Florida. This was available for children who had serious difficulties managing diabetes. The program included individual and family psychotherapy and intensive instruction in diabetes care. When families were willing to participate in the center activities, the children showed a significant improvement in management. A diabetes network could take the lead in developing professional and community support for the creation of such a center.

Summary

Support is available from the community of people who have diabetes—those who best understand the meaning of living with diabetes. We can work together to deal with feelings, share information, and learn the skills needed for diabetic management. This can happen through personal networking, or in support groups that meet regularly. Both methods of giving and receiving support are effective. If diabetes networks or groups do not exist in your area, you can create them using the information in this chapter.

Chapter Fifteen

Living Well
With Yourself

You are the best available source of support for living well with diabetes. You are always there and you know yourself well; no one else can take care of you as well as you can.

Having diabetes can affect how you feel about yourself, which affects your willingness to live healthfully. The goal of this chapter is to help you become aware of your strengths and resources, and learn to neutralize patterns that weaken your ability to care for yourself well.

You are resourceful. You are stronger, more creative, and more able than you may realize. Some of these strengths can be hidden, or used in only one area of your life, others can be expressed in negative ways. Your strength can be redirected to increase your ability to live well with diabetes.

For example, the teenager who refuses to test or follow a diet and schedule shows great strength of character. Although this strength is focused on rebellion and denial, it is a valuable resource. This teen can learn to turn "won't power" into "will power" and improve his or her self-care.

After months of receiving support, a man acts as a victim of diabetic complications. He is overwhelmed, helpless, and depressed. Where is his strength now? Perhaps he is strong in the tenacity with which he holds onto his role as victim, refusing to adapt to his situation. Continuously feeling sorry for oneself takes a great amount of energy. A negative self-image can be changed to create the flexibility needed to live well with the changes being experienced. Negative feelings can be redirected into positive action. This redefinition can reveal surprising resources that can be applied in a healthy way.

We often develop skills in one area that we never apply to the rest of our life. Photographers learn about tests, processes, measurements, precision, and combining a complex series of actions to achieve a given result. They have the skills necessary to learn a diabetic regimen. Salespeople are skilled at communication and persuasion. Perhaps they could use these strengths to sell themselves an improved regimen.

Let's explore the resources you can use to live well with diabetes.

Going Into Your Storehouse

Do this exercise in a quiet place where you won't be disturbed. At each step, close your eyes and allow both words and images to help you find answers. Make notes before you go to the next step.

1. Think of three areas of your life, large or small, in which you are successful. See yourself in action. What strengths do you demonstrate here?
2. Think of three activities you enjoy. See yourself enjoying them. What personal qualities do you have that allow you to enjoy these activities?
3. What do you believe about yourself that enables you to act with success? With enjoyment?
4. Remember one of the best times in your life. Tell yourself the story of that time or recall scenes from it. Which of your qualities made this such a good time?
5. What strengths do you utilize in your work (or schoolwork, if you are a student)?
6. What strengths do you express in your relationships with friends?
7. What special qualities do you experience only when you are alone?
8. If you were to fulfill your true potential, what hidden qualities would you feel free to express?
9. What qualities would you like to develop?
10. What are some of your most negative traits or limitations?
11. Can you find a strength that each of these limitations contains? Can you think of a way to make them serve you?
12. Now, review your answers and examine how these qualities can:
  ▷ Help you deal with diabetes.
  ▷ Enable you to improve your self-care.
  ▷ Help you feel better about having diabetes.
  ▷ Assist when you are fearful or unwilling to do what you know you should do.
  ▷ Allow you to resolve problems in relationships with others.
  Write down your thoughts or discuss them with a friend.

After you do this exercise, observe your life with these questions in mind. See what traits could help you live well with diabetes. Explore how the qualities you have just identified can improve your self-care.

Recognizing your resources will help you deal with diabetes creatively. You can reinforce this positive step by learning to overcome the negative self-image, limiting beliefs, self-judgments, emotional reactions, and behavioral patterns you experience because of diabetes.

A Case Of Mistaken Identity

Beliefs, feelings, and actions create your sense of who you are. You often become closely identified with this sense, forgetting that it is only learned behavior. Many of your limitations seem so real that you can't imagine exceeding them. You forget that you learned to see yourself as inadequate, helpless, rebellious, or sick.

This mistaken identity becomes self-perpetuating. When you believe you are weak and unable to follow a regimen, you act weak and unable. You may feel depressed and eat a pint of ice cream, thus making your sugar-clogged body feel uncomfortable. The evidence grows. Beliefs, feelings, and actions reinforce one another and strengthen your negative self-image.

Responses to the threat of diabetic complications illustrate the way false identity functions as a system of beliefs, feelings, and actions.

If you believe that diabetic complications and an early death are inevitable, you are likely to feel anxious, fearful, and depressed. You might bury your feelings and live for the moment, ignoring the measures that improve your odds. The idea creates the feeling; together they lead to action. When you believe nothing will help, you will do nothing to manage diabetes. However, some manage so compulsively that their stress levels decrease the benefits of a tighter regimen.

On the other hand, if you can reduce the risk of complications and early death, you become more hopeful. Anxiety may still affect you, but you learn to handle it and maintain a positive attitude. When you do, it is much easier to follow a regimen and do the things that reduce your risks. Following your regimen encourages positive feelings, and the immediate benefits make a difference.

Beliefs and feelings affect actions, and in turn actions affect beliefs and feelings. Neither pattern is an inevitable response to having diabetes; either way, you choose the way you respond. You can become aware of your beliefs, feelings, and actions relating to diabetes and change them when they lead to negative results. This is an incredibly powerful concept: You can change how you feel about an event or a situation. Once you identify its origin ("I am feeling upset because my blood sugar test was high and I thought I had taken the right amount of insulin"), you can tell yourself to put it behind you, that feeling upset is not going to help or change anything, and that you may as well feel neutral and go on to something else.

Change comes from seeking a deeper identity and detaching from seeing ourselves as our limitations. Not, "I am weak, sick, and unable," but, rather "I am the person who can see these negative patterns without judgments. I am the person who chooses the life I live. I am the person who learns, grows, and changes. With this image of myself, I find it easier to use the information I have learned."

With a positive self-image as a foundation, you can work for specific change at the level of belief, feeling, or behavior. Or you may move from one level to another, integrating changes in beliefs, emotions, and actions.

Changing Beliefs

A belief is a statement about yourself or the world that shapes your life. It may be conscious or unconscious. Some beliefs give you power; some make you feel weak.

I am capable of learning to manage diabetes; or
I just can't manage; it's all too complex.

Diabetes is a teacher, challenging me to be my best; or
Having diabetes is a punishment.

People accept me as I am; or
People judge me for having diabetes and think I'm a bother.

Some beliefs restrict your ability to act, and produce feelings of helplessness. Others are enabling, empowering, and encourage positive feelings. Limiting beliefs are often so deeply ingrained that you believe them to be true. They are reinforced by the feelings and actions that result from them.

If you believe you cannot control the amount you eat, your actions will prove you correct. You will feel depressed and eat even more to bury your feelings. The cycle can be broken by recognizing that beliefs such as these are not truths, but rather learned habits of thinking. When you view them as habits rather than facts, you reduce the power they have over you.

Many of your beliefs will be related to facts such as that people with diabetes have a higher risk of kidney failure than the general population. However, it is a mistake to believe "I will have kidney failure." A more appropriate belief is "I can act to reduce my risk of kidney failure." This belief is empowering and has a factual basis, because most people with diabetes do not develop kidney disease.

Uncovering Your Beliefs About You And Diabetes

Watch for hidden beliefs as you work on diabetes learning, especially at times when you feel stuck. Catalog the beliefs that empower you, and those that limit you, in your life with diabetes.

Some techniques for uncovering beliefs are as follows:

1. Ask yourself a repeating question: "What do I believe about (diabetes, home blood testing, complications, my diabetic regimen, how diabetes affects my relationships, my doctor, my age, etc.)?"

   Another way of doing this is to alternate between "What do I believe about?" and "What should I believe about?"

   Repeat the question for each topic a dozen or so times, writing down whatever beliefs come to mind.

   Example: What do I believe about myself as a diabetic individual?

   Sample—Beliefs: I am more vulnerable than other people. I should get special consideration. I will probably die in my sixties. My problems are a bother to others. I am unwilling to follow a strict regimen; this is a sign of weakness. Others should take care of me. I really want to be fully responsible for myself. I have learned to live better because of diabetes. I value my life because I know how vulnerable I am.

2. In a concrete situation—especially at a time of distress, frustration, or failure—ask "What beliefs have created this problem?

   Example: I have forgotten to take my morning dose of insulin or pills and don't notice the signs of high blood sugar until late afternoon. (I am scheduled for a job interview that day.)

   Sample—Beliefs: If I'm sick, I won't be held responsible for anything. Diabetes isn't really serious. I'm invulnerable. Hurting my body is better than facing difficult challenges. I'm weak and deserve to be hurt. I want someone to take care of me.

3. Choose an enabling belief you would like to adopt. Repeat it, holding out one hand as though it were speaking the belief. Let the other

hand state the limiting beliefs that oppose it. Keep repeating until you understand the conflicting beliefs and begin to resolve the conflict.

Right hand: A blood sugar test is free of judgments.

Left hand: It shows I've eaten like a pig.

Right: A blood sugar test is free of judgments.

Left: Big Brother is watching me.

Right: A blood sugar test is free of judgments.

Left: It makes me worry to see how high the test will be.

Right: A blood sugar test is free of judgments.

Left: Can I ever learn to control myself?

Right: A blood sugar test is free of judgments.

Left: I'd like to stop worrying so much.

Right: A blood sugar test is free of judgments.

Left: I really want to know the truth.

4. Write or speak a fantasy in which you are easily doing something that now seems difficult or impossible. Write down all the reasons the fantasy could not come true. Then write down the beliefs that would enable you to make the fantasy real.

After completing any of these exercises, underline the beliefs that seem most powerful, indicating those that limit you and those that free you. Then choose the limiting beliefs you would like to change.

Identifying limiting beliefs is the first step toward changing them. Awareness is often enough to dissolve the power a belief has over your feelings or behavior. However, you may have to take further steps to replace a belief with one that enables you to live as you wish.

There are many techniques for changing beliefs. Some are developed by behavioral psychologists, others by people in the human potential movement. (Techniques 3 and 4 in the preceding section are good for changing, as well as uncovering, beliefs.) Some techniques for changing beliefs are as follows:

1. Create a positive phrase that clearly states the belief you want to adopt. Use your own words. Find ways to remind yourself that this new belief is entering your life (for example, put signs around the houses and repeat the phrase every day).

    Example: To replace the phrase "I am unable to follow a diabetic regimen" try "I am improving my regimen step by step. I will continue until I have excellent control." The new belief is encouraging but not overwhelming.

2. Imagine yourself doing the things that would indicate you are living according to the new belief. Create a scene in your mind where you see yourself acting as you wish.

Example: With "I am improving my regimen..." I see myself testing blood, keeping records, exercising, and doing other things that mean improvement for me.

3. Recall a scene from your life in which a limiting belief was active. Recreate the scene in detail, noting how the belief was expressed in your feelings and actions. Imagine how you would have lived the scene if you held the new belief at that time.

Example: My old belief is "I must keep my diabetes a secret. I'll be rejected if people know."

I'm embarrassed at lunch because a friend keeps insisting I eat her cake and I don't want to tell her I have diabetes. I'm afraid she won't go out with me if she knows. I get angry and uptight, and she is hurt.

I want to adopt the new belief "I am open about having diabetes. Anyone who rejects me isn't worth having around anyway."

I see myself at lunch, smiling when my friend presses me to eat the cake. I say, "I've got a little secret I'm going to let you in on. I'd love to eat the cake but I really can't unless I take more insulin. I have diabetes." I sigh as she responds with surprise and caring. I answer her questions and feel relieved to have torn down that wall between us.

4. Trace the roots of beliefs and cut them. You learn beliefs from your parents or other people who have had a great influence on you. When you have trouble weakening a particular belief, determine who you learned it from. Visualize yourself giving it back to the source, or cutting the connection. With a belief specific to diabetes, you might have to look for an underlying belief.

Example: I have a set of related beliefs: "I am more vulnerable than other people. I should get special consideration. I will probably die in my sixties." These beliefs are from my father, who had rheumatic fever as a child. He was sure he had cancer years before it finally developed. He was 67 when he died.

I would rather believe: "I am both vulnerable and strong. I will give myself special consideration by living well. I will die when I die, and I can't predict when that will be."

I see myself telling my father why I won't follow his example anymore. I give him a box containing his beliefs and he throws it into the fire. He smiles at me and says, "Go ahead. You are free to outlive me."

Beliefs are closely related to emotions. Working at changing beliefs can help relieve negative feelings. It helps to have tools for working directly at the emotional level.

Dealing With Feelings

Living with a complex, life-threatening condition such as diabetes adds many emotional triggers to our lives. The threat of long-term complications creates an underlying anxiety for many of us. A delayed meal, cut foot, or having no sweets available when blood sugar drops too low can become major emergencies. Diabetes even affects our relationships with others.

Our feelings affect diabetic control through the stress response and our willingness to follow regimen.

Throughout this book, we have examined a number of emotional issues specific to diabetes. We focus here on ways to gain awareness of and handle your feelings as they relate to your self-care.

The following exercises will sharpen your emotional awareness and ability to work more effectively with your feelings.

In this work, you may find strong emotions coming to the surface (particularly if you are dealing with a tough situation). If you do not usually feel things very deeply, this can be an alarming experience. You may want the aid of a friend, support group, or professional.

What Am I Feeling?

1. Breathe. A very simple way of finding out what you are feeling is to sit quietly and breathe more deeply than usual. Feel your stomach, chest, throat, and face. Relax and breathe and allow the feelings to emerge.

2. Imagine. Visualize what you are feeling. Create scenes in your mind that act out your feelings.

3. Move. Let your body tell you what you're feeling by moving or dancing. Allow the movements to come spontaneously, without worrying about appearing graceful.

4. Descend. Often there are layers of feeling below the emotion you're conscious of. The experience of being caught in an emotion may stem from underlying feelings. Breathing, relaxing, and visualizing are ways to expose these deeper layers. After you've experienced each level, ask yourself, "What feeling is below this one?" Continue exposing layers to learn more about what you are feeling.

(The exercises for getting in touch with beliefs in the previous section are also likely to bring feelings to the surface.)

Just getting in touch with an emotion is often all you need to do about it. You may feel it for a time, express it, and go on with life. Other times, a feeling may seem eternal and inescapable. Perhaps you've just seen a relative with diabetes who has recently become blind, and you feel depressed. Or you've been on a food binge for two days and are filled with guilt and anger. You can probably supply your own examples all too well.

What You Can Do About Feelings

1. Accept what you are feeling. Don't compound the problem by chastising yourself for feeling the way you do. You have every right to feel whatever you are feeling. Use the techniques described above to explore this experience with a sense of curiosity.

2. Express the feeling and communicate your emotions. Draw, paint, write poems, speak to a friend (or into a recorder), sing, or dance. Communication often enables you to let go of a feeling that seems endless.

3. Detach from the feeling. Detachment is not suppression of emotion; it is a refocusing of awareness to achieve a broader sense of yourself. The emotion is present, along with your bodily sensations and perceptions of the world around you, as well as a self-awareness that observes the emotions, senses, and perceptions you experience.

   Example: I am feeling hopeless and depressed. I can't escape this feeling. I feel the texture of the rug beneath my feet. My breath is shallow; My nose is dry as I breathe. I want to escape and go to sleep. I've never felt such deep despair. I see wind blowing trees outside the window; I hear the wind in the leaves. My stomach is tight. I smell the rose across the room. I hear music from downstairs; it's a song I like. My chest relaxes when I think of the words. Depression seems like a ball inside of me, instead of me locked inside it. The ball is dissolving. My breath is deep now. I have tears in my eyes. I'm alive again.

"It should recompense us well to study the qualities of our emotional spectrum, studying them not as a pathologist dissects but as an artist cares for his materials. Or perhaps as one who loves. For the quality of our emotions belongs to ourselves perhaps more than any other aspect of being. To love ourselves, then, means to love these pure qualities. In a strange way purely expressed emotions engender a degree of empathy and love as part of our interrelations. 'Seeing' them as they are eases the burden and boundary that separates man from man."—Dr. Manfred Clynes

Changing Behavior

The discussion of our actions extends throughout this book. How we act is an important aspect of living well with diabetes. The introduction and Chapter 1, in particular, explore the techniques and attitudes that support changing our behavior. Rather than repeating any of these themes we ask you to review those sections.

Telling The Story Of Yourself

Earlier in this chapter, we emphasized the interaction between three levels of diabetes self-care: beliefs, feelings, and behavior. Now we would like to explore the integration of the three. Work at any of these levels produces change, and at some point you will want to bring them all together. This may happen after you've gained greater clarity, or when you are caught and don't know what to do.

An effective way of integrating levels is to tell your story. See your whole situation by telling yourself what is happening. Move between what you are feeling, the beliefs and images that surround your feeling, and the things you are doing. Observe how the different levels reinforce each other. Identify the limiting beliefs that are preventing you from moving forward. Recognize how your actions reinforce beliefs.

You can write this narrative or say it aloud to a friend or into a tape recorder. Use the most direct language possible.

Example:

I'm frustrated, angry, and guilty. I've been on a binge for two days and can't stop; I have no self-control. I'm probably taking years off my life when I do this. I must hate myself. I began eating Tuesday morning, just after Dr. Blast told me my tests were lousy and that I had to take better care of myself or I'd be in trouble. I've been trying hard and it doesn't seem to do any good. Nothing I do works out right. Why can't she understand how hard I've been trying?

Now I'm poisoning myself with candy and pastries. My blood sugar must be 500! Every time I eat something I feel worse. I'm angry at how weak I am. I'm afraid of what this is doing to me, and that I'll never learn how to take care of myself.

There was a blind woman at the newsstand in the lobby of Dr. Blast's building last Tuesday. I never even noticed her before then. I forgot about her right away, but now I can see her face so clearly. I'm terrified I'll go blind like her. I don't believe there's anything I can do; I can't do anything right.

No wonder I'm in such a mess. I must be stronger than I think if I can keep myself feeling this bad and acting so stupid for so long. My eyes are still fine and there's a lot I can do to keep them that way. Dr. Blast was worried and doesn't know how to be gentle. I can be gentle; gentle and strong.

This example focuses on a specific situation. You can also gain insight by telling your story in a more expansive manner. Describing your life with diabetes through the years can give you extraordinary perspective, and understanding. You might do this with a friend who has diabetes or another medical condition, sharing stories at length.

When you have reached a level of achievement, exploring how you got there both rewards and reinforces the changes you have made. Don't be bashful about giving yourself credit for the work of living well with diabetes.

Living well with yourself is a matter of balancing the needs of diabetes with the other demands in your life. It is also a balance between acceptance and reaching for something better. As this sense of equilibrium grows, you will find that it is a deep source of support, even in times of distress.

Living Well With Diabetic Complications

Chapter Sixteen

Neutralizing The Threat Of Complications

"Complications?! I don't want to hear about them.
That's too depressing."

If this is how you feel when you turn to this section, we can sympathize. After living with diabetes for over forty years each, your authors have experienced all the fears and uncertainties you might feel. Ernest has experienced a major complication—temporary loss of vision in one eye, and when that cleared, a temporary loss of vision in the other. Treatment was successful, and his vision is still clear fifteen years later. So we know there is hope to counterbalance the threat of complications.

If you learn the information in the next three chapters, you will have the ability to improve your odds for avoiding complications. You can limit, postpone, or altogether avoid the effects of diabetic complications on your future health. You will know how to increase your chances of preventing them and what their early symptoms are so you can seek treatment before it's too late. If you are already dealing with their unwelcome arrival, you will be able prevent them from dominating your life, no matter what disabilities they bring.

The DCCT (see chapters 1 and 4) proved that complications are not an inevitable result of diabetes. How we live with diabetes can slow, prevent, and even reverse the development of its side effects. So learn these chapters—today, tomorrow, next week, or whenever you're ready, but do it soon!

Roget's Thesaurus captures the emotional quality of the word complication when it lists entanglement, snag, snarl, and difficulty as synonyms. Diabetes by itself is a relatively friendly condition. But when we consider its potential complications, it becomes threatening.

An essential part of the diabetes self-care program is staying open to new information about complications. Face the fears they present, but also learn the facts. This doesn't mean studying every last detail of what can go wrong, but you do need to know the following:

▷ Changes in regimen and lifestyle that will reduce your risk.

▷ Early warning signs that enable you to seek treatment if a complication begins to develop (both laboratory test results and symptoms you can recognize yourself).

▷ Treatments now available and under research for each complication.

▷ Ways of reducing anxiety over the possibility of developing diabetic complications, or dealing with feelings that come up if they do begin.

When you know these things, you have the power to turn the odds in your favor. You may be able to avoid complications altogether, or if they do develop, escape their more serious consequences.

In this and the next two chapters:

▷ We examine recent developments in diabetes care that can reduce the risk of complications.

▷ We offer techniques for dealing with the anxiety, fear, and uncertainty caused by the threat of major complications.

▷ We explore the physical and emotional needs of a person experiencing a major complication of diabetes.

▷ We discuss the specific long-term complications of diabetes, and the steps you can take to possibly avoid them.

Taking It Easy

No other aspect of diabetes education is as promising—or as threatening—as the subject of diabetic complications. We want you to live well while you work with these chapters. That means taking it easy, and using techniques for reducing stress, and remembering that reducing stress is likely to lower your risk of developing complications. Our purpose is to inform you of the many ways to minimize the risk, not to overwhelm you with the risk itself.

Special care must be taken in discussing complications with diabetic children.

Neutralizing The Threat

We are at risk for serious disabilities and early death, yet we can choose to live well with the risks and the anxiety they evoke. What could better express the concept of this book? We can reduce both the risk and the anxiety. Even if we are disabled by one or more complications, we can still go on living well.

We have said many times that diabetes is a teacher. Here the lessons are challenging: living peacefully with physical and emotional risk; accepting vulnerability while living a full life; coming to terms with aging and mortality; identifying with inner healthfulness, no matter what the state of the body. When you deal with the questions raised by complications, you grow as a human being.

A medical dictionary defines complication as a disease process that may or may not accompany a primary disease. You may have had a doctor who warned you of your higher risk of stroke and heart attack. Or you may know someone who has become blind, lost a foot, or whose kidneys have failed. You may have read of the diabetic nerve disorders that can result in pain, loss of feeling, or impotence.

The possibility of developing complications is the most serious consequence of diabetes, so serious that many of us avoid the subject. (Avoidance has been reinforced by parents and doctors who use the threat of complications as a motivation-through-fear device.)

"I ignored my fear of complications, I felt good so I didn't give it any thought. I knew that complications existed for other people—but not for me. Then all of a sudden I realized I was lazier and more lethargic. I felt drained. It gradually got worse, to the point of my kidneys failing." —Jim

We believe that hope is a better motivator than fear. You have a basis for hope—you can limit or avoid the effects of complications. To do this you need to be informed, and you need to act on what you learn.

1. Complications are not inevitable. You have a risk, but there is no guarantee that you will develop major complications of diabetes.
2. You can reduce your level of risk by improving your diabetes self-care program. Maintain better control of blood sugar and blood pressure, practice stress management, eat healthfully and lose weight if necessary, and live an active lifestyle.
3. Treatment for most complications is becoming more effective. In many cases, negative results can be reversed or reduced, especially when detected early.

These three ideas provide an essential context for considering diabetic complications, so we will examine them here in detail.

Complications are not inevitable. When you read statistical reports on diabetic complications, you may believe you cannot avoid them. "Blindness is 25 times more common in individuals with Type 1 diabetes" is a typical statement. Those are dramatic odds, but actually, less than 1 percent of us will lose our vision. The majority of people with diabetes do not become blind. Even without taking special precautions, you have a good chance of avoiding a major handicap.

Statistics are misleading—if not terrifying—for a very fundamental reason: They are based on an earlier era of diabetes care when the medical knowledge and tools we now have were not available. It was also a time when individuals were much less interested in a healthy lifestyle. But the DCCT results have shown that the statistics for the present generation of those with diabetes can be improved.

Michael and Cousin Melvin

Ernest began counseling a 13-year-old boy named Michael who had recently developed diabetes. Michael's doctor had asked him to test his blood sugar, but he seldom did so. "It reminds me of being in the hospital at the beginning. They were testing me all the time," Michael complained. Ernest asked what the tests had meant to Michael. "They remind me I'm diabetic. I want to forget it. I don't care." Michael talked more about being in the hospital. "I kept hearing about my uncles and how they died of diabetes when they were in their forties."

"Michael, I think it's time you heard about my cousin Melvin. He became diabetic the year after they first used insulin with people. He's almost 80 now and he's still going strong without any complications. What happened to your uncles doesn't happen to all of us!"

Ernest asked Michael if he'd like to adopt a cousin. Melvin agreed to this, and the next week Michael told everyone about his new cousin Melvin. Michael wanted everyone to know he had a chance.

You can reduce your risk by improving your management of diabetes. You can increase your odds by the way you live. Older studies of people maintaining a moderate level of control showed they were less likely to develop major complications. Now that a near-normal level of control is possible, you can reduce your risk even more. The risk is still there, but it is much smaller. Good nutrition, an active lifestyle, blood pressure control, and stress management also make complications less likely to occur.

(The development of complications is determined by a number of factors other than metabolic control. Genetics, stress, and other lifestyle matters may also play significant roles in particular individuals. It is possible to be well controlled and still experience a serious impairment.)

Treatment for most complications is becoming more effective. If a complication develops, you are more likely to find a treatment that will reverse or limit its advance. This is especially true if you are aware of its symptoms and seek treatment early. Thousands of people with diabetes avoid disability thanks to laser treatment, kidney transplantation, early treatment of foot disorders, and other new developments.

But There Are No Guarantees

Despite these advances, risks are still present for you. There are many variables: how long you have had diabetes, at what age it began, the kind of lifestyle you live, your genetic makeup, and other factors still poorly understood. You can do everything possible to reduce your risks of developing complications, and they can still occur.

Diabetes makes a clear demand: Learn to do your best, and live well with uncertainty. Learn to cope with anxiety and maintain hope, no matter what happens. This is not altogether different from the demand the world at large makes upon us all.

You and Diabetic Complications

This exercise will help you see how you relate to the possibility of diabetic complications developing. Answer spontaneously, even though the feeling or belief that comes may seem "wrong".

1. What did you feel as you read the beginning of this chapter?

_____

_____

2. Which of the following statements describe(s) the way you have dealt with complications in the past?

_____ I don't want to think about the possibility of complications.

_____ I worry about them quite a lot.

_____ It makes me angry that diabetes could do that to me.

_____ I do everything I can to reduce the risk.

_____ I can do more to reduce the risk.

_____ I just do everything I want to, since I don't know how long I'll last.

_____ I probably spend too much time taking care of my diabetes.

_____ I feel depressed quite a bit.

_____ I feel guilty because I have not taken good care of myself.

3. I believe I will probably live to the age of _____

4. The complication I fear the most is_____

5. I believe

_____ I will escape major complications.

_____ I am very encouraged by the findings of the DCCT.

_____ I will certainly develop a major complication.

_____ There is nothing I can do to change what will happen.

_____ If one complication develops, others will follow.

_____ If I become (or am) disabled in any way, my life will be damaged beyond repair.

_____ I will be able to learn to live well with the disability.

_____ I will be a burden to others.

Other beliefs I hold about complications include

_____

_____

Positive beliefs that neutralize any negative beliefs listed above include

_____

_____

6. Is there anyone close to you who keeps reminding you of what can go wrong? Who uses threats to motivate you? Have any of your doctors done this?

7. My present level of control is _____. My level of regimen is _____ (See your questionnaire results in Chapter 4.)

8. I intend to make the following improvements in self-care in the next months

_____

_____

9. I can get support for my feelings about complications and for making changes from

_____

_____

10. I do not intend to make any changes in self-care at this time because
    _____ I am already doing everything possible.
    _____ I do not believe it will do any good.
    _____ I do not feel I have the time and energy needed.
    _____ I feel the changes would reduce my freedom or pleasure.
    _____ I feel overwhelmed by the demands of diabetes.
    _____ Other

If someone you loved gave the reason(s) checked above for not improving their diabetes self-care, what would you say to that person?

Make an appointment with yourself to re-ask this question in a few months. Mark it on your calendar.

Reflect on your answers to these questions. Look for changes in beliefs or behavior that will help you lessen the threat of complications. For example, if you do not have the time needed to improve your self-care program, ask yourself what changes in your life would give you that time.

Dealing With Anxiety About Complications

The best way to deal with anxiety about diabetic complications is to reduce your risk of developing them. A complete diabetic regimen makes complications less likely and handles your day-to-day need for metabolic control. The following list indicates the things you can do.

Ways You Can Reduce Your Risks

1. Improve your metabolic control, and continue improving it to the highest level you are comfortable with, ideally with a HbA1c less than 7%.
2. Learn to handle stress well.
3. Follow a healthy meal plan that is low in fat and high in fiber. Limit sweets and rapidly absorbed carbohydrates.
4. Engage in regular physical activity.
5. If you are overweight, lose weight.
6. Act to prevent high blood pressure by controlling stress and weight. Seek treatment for hypertension if your blood pressure is high (above 130/85).
7. If you smoke, quit.
8. Get the amount of sleep and rest you need.
9. Know the warning signs for each complication.
10. Consider taking a multivitamin pill with emphasis on the anti-oxidants.

Except for item 1, this is the same prescription for good health that doctors give those without diabetes. It is especially important for you because each item will improve your odds of avoiding other disease as well as diabetic complications (or of limiting them if they have already started).

You may have already adopted some of the measures and need to make only a few changes. Or you may need to alter your life in every area. Begin where you feel most willing to change. If your sense of urgency is great, begin with metabolic (blood sugar) control, the most fundamental way of reducing risk. Give yourself the best chance for a long and healthful life by following the complete preventive program. At least give yourself the benefit of stress reduction and self-acceptance if you choose nothing else from this list. Only you can determine the ingredients of a lifestyle that will work for you.

Even if you are doing everything on the preceding list, or are in the process of learning to, you can still experience anxiety. A useful skill to develop is the art of living well with uncertainty. For all the talk of risks and odds and possibilities, you simply cannot know whether you will end up with one or more diabetic complications. You can do your best to avoid them, but a degree of uncertainty is inevitable. Face the possibility that you will become disabled as a consequence of diabetes, but also realize the possibility that you will remain free of major complications. Decide to live well with yourself, no matter which path is given to you, and return to the task of living well right now.

Learning about complications should be a process in which you use stress-reduction techniques such as relaxation, meditation, prayer, and whatever else is effective for you. Learn the information in small parts, and give yourself breaks that allow you to focus on positive aspects of life. Participation in a diabetes support group or conversations with others who have diabetes can help you deal with the feelings that come up. Some will find counseling sessions helpful while they are dealing with this threatening subject.

Another way of dealing with your feelings is to explore the beliefs and attitudes you have about the possible consequences of diabetes. Neutralizing negative beliefs and adopting a positive attitude can help relieve the anxiety, depression, or anger you may experience. For instance, a typical belief is, "I've been so out of control that I can't possibly avoid complications." This is a belief, not a fact. A more helpful belief is, "If I improve control now, I may still escape major complications."

If You Decide Not To Act Now To Reduce The Risks Of Complications

You may feel unwilling at this time to make the changes in your life that will lessen the risk of complications. If so, it is important that you make this a conscious decision. Look at the reasons you give for maintaining your present level of self-care. Discuss them with someone you trust and explore them within yourself through writing, inner dialogue, prayer, meditation, or whatever method works for you.

Find a point of view that allows you to begin making the necessary changes, while dealing with your reasons for not changing. For example, if lack of time is your reason for not changing, find changes that do not require additional time, or learn to use your time more effectively.

Neutralizing The Threat Of Complications

If you decide not to change, accept your decision and any anxiety that goes with it. You are increasing risks in your life, but you are not guaranteeing the development of complications. We all make risk/benefit decisions about our lives each day. Self-acceptance is healthful for body and mind, and it gives you a positive foundation for making future decisions.

We suggest you make a date with yourself in a few months to re-ask the question of what you are willing to do to reduce the risk of complications. Your life may change enough to make other choices.

Chapter Seventeen

If Complications Develop

"How long can you mope and pine after disaster? You've got to ultimately pick up your life and sing."
—Rev. Karl Baehr (*Diabetes Forecast*, Nov./Dec. 1983)

"When my kidneys started to go, it stimulated me to educate myself. I put time and energy into finding out what I could do to help myself. It was a great deal of motivation. It scared me a lot. I knew how sick I could become. That terrified me—what my body could do with me having no control over it. I also realized there was something I could do to gain control. —James

The Early Signs

Diabetic complications usually show early signs of development. They often appear in laboratory tests; however, you may notice the signs yourself, or your doctor may notice them during a routine exam. Your ophthalmologist may tell you that you have background retinopathy, a condition found in the majority of people who have had diabetes for ten years or longer. Or your physician may tell you the beginning signs of kidney disease are present, shown by protein in your urine.

You may shrug off the diagnosis, or you may find the news very disturbing. But this "bad news" can provide the motivation to improve your self-care regimen. Taking action will enable you to delay or halt the progress of the disorder, and perhaps even reverse it. (The early signs of each complication are described in the next chapter. If you know these warning signals, you will be able to begin preventive treatment early.)

Handling The Crisis

The onset of a major diabetic complication can be a crisis, no matter how well you handle it. It reminds you of your vulnerability. The beginning of one disorder may suggest that others will follow. You can feel angry and frustrated if excellent self-care has not prevented complications. At the same time such feelings arise, you might have to make serious decisions about treatment and lifestyle changes.

All of this creates a major challenge that demands your time, energy, and the support of others. You will live well through this crisis if you deal with the many practical, emotional, and social needs it generates.

At first, you might react to the crisis in a way that allows you to deal with the shock of diagnosis. Some people go through a stage of denial, ignoring both the doctor's recommendations and their own feelings. Others enter a period of withdrawal while they absorb the impact of the news. Still others become convinced that the worst will happen to them. Some feel guilty and go on a food binge, believing that nothing will help them.

Understand what your pattern of response to the diagnosis of a complication has been. If your response is negative, do not fault yourself for reacting this way. You've had to deal with a stressful piece of news. But recognize the limitations of this initial reaction and allow yourself to move on to a more functional response.

Treatment and Self-Care

You will have to absorb new information, learn new skills, make important decisions, and change aspects of your life at this time. These changes may feel overwhelming, especially when you are dealing with your emotions. You can regain control of the situation if you define the tasks facing you. Break them down into manageable steps. Establish how much time is needed, what resources and support you will need, and what information you must acquire. By organizing the demands, you are better able to deal with them. (The questionnaire at the end of this chapter will guide you through this process.)

You will probably be faced with decisions about treatment and regimen. In some cases, specialists will describe complicated procedures that can be difficult to follow. If you do not understand what is being recommended, ask for an explanation in language you do understand. If you still don't understand, ask your internist, family practitioner, or diabetes educator to help you. Ask if there are written materials or audiovisual aids describing the treatment. You need to understand what you are being asked to undergo.

You should know the risks of the recommended treatment. What are the odds for success? For a negative outcome? What will happen if you do nothing? Are there alternative treatments available? If you have any doubt about the treatment your doctor suggests, seek a second opinion from another physician with equivalent expertise. (Do not go to a general practitioner or an internist for a second opinion about eye treatment. You need an ophthalmologist, preferably one who specializes in retinal diseases or diabetic retinopathy.) If your doctor does not have much experience working with diabetes, you should probably find someone who does to guide the treatment of complications. Always ask your doctors how experienced they are in a treatment or procedure. (For example, ask how many procedures were done in the last week or month.)

In addition to prescribing a specific treatment, your doctor may suggest that you improve your self-care regimen at this time. Improvement in blood sugar control may help you handle the condition that has developed. It will also make other complications less likely to occur. You will need to proceed cautiously in tightening metabolic control if you have advanced retinopathy or kidney disease. In a number of studies of those with Type 1 diabetes, these complications worsened (at least initially) when a high level of control was achieved too quickly. When retinopathy or kidney disease is clinically evident, blood sugar levels must be lowered gradually, over a period of three or six months. This is true whether control is improved through multiple insulin injections or the insulin pump. Although we're not aware of studies of Type 2 diabetes, it makes sense that control should be improved gradually here as well, particularly if insulin is initiated.

You will need to be cautious in your exercise and physical activity at this time, depending upon the specific complication you have. This is especially true if you are beginning an exercise program after a period of inactivity. Discuss exercise and physical activity with your doctor. You may want to enroll in a medically supervised exercise program that monitors your physical condition.

This is also a good time to improve your diet. Begin by eating more fresh vegetables and fruits, and cut down on animal and saturated fats. Also, add more beans, pasta, and other high-fiber foods to your meals.

Having diabetic complications is stressful, so this is an especially important time to manage stress well. Stress interferes with blood sugar control, and it plays a role in the development of diabetic complications. Do your best to limit stress in your life, and learn to relax under anxiety.

The emotional impact of the changes in your body is a highly individual matter. You may feel overwhelmed, frightened, depressed, or angry. You may do your best to feel nothing at all. If a major body function is involved, such as loss of vision, amputation, or kidney failure, it is natural to go through a grieving process. You will find yourself going through a series of emotional reactions, rather than experiencing just one. Allow yourself to feel what you are feeling, if you are unable to function, ask for help.

Family and friends are often able to help. However, a support group, or professional counseling may be necessary. This is a time when most people need support. Immediate family members usually experience their own stress about what is happening to you, so it is best not to rely solely on them. (In some cases, their input may be so negative that it is better to seek support elsewhere.) Others who have dealt with complications will know what you are going through. They can help you sort things out at a practical level, and offer encouragement at the same time. If informal support is not enough, you might want to see a psychologist or psychiatrist or a social worker who specializes in medical counseling. A diabetes educator who is trained in dealing with complications is also a good resource. (The American Association of Diabetes Educators provides a toll-free number for referrals, 1-800-TEAM-UP-4.)

The onset of a diabetic complication is a time when you gain a new appreciation of your internal resources for coping. Such a crisis often puts you in touch with your personal strength and spirituality. You may also gain encouragement from remembering those who helped you in the past. Chapter 15 describes many techniques to help you handle your emotional responses.

If Complications Develop

The diagnosis of a diabetic complication is a major challenge. This questionnaire will help you clarify what is happening, how you are responding, and what you need to do.

1. What diabetic complication(s) has your doctor diagnosed?

_____

_____

2. At what stage of development is the complication?

_____

_____

3. What treatment does your doctor recommend?

_____

_____

4. What risks are involved with this treatment?

_____

_____

5. What are the odds for a successful outcome?

_____

_____

6. What does your doctor think will happen if you do nothing?

_____

_____

7. What changes in regimen or lifestyle does your doctor suggest?

_____

_____

_____

_____

8. Do you think you will have trouble making these changes? (If so, see Chapter 3.)

_____

9. Outline the steps needed to make these changes. Also include any decisions you need to make about treatment, or things you have to do to undergo treatment.

_____

_____

_____

10. How are you coping with the diagnosis of the complication so far?
_____ I am trying to ignore what the doctor told me.
_____ I am ignoring my feelings.
_____ I am paying attention to my feelings.
_____ I am reading everything I can find about the complication.
_____ I am talking with people who have been through this.
_____ I am feeling withdrawn. I don't want to talk to anyone.
_____ I am worrying a lot and dwelling on the worst possible outcome.
_____ I am blaming myself and feeling guilty.
_____ I am living it up. I'll enjoy myself while I can.
_____ I am doing everything possible to take care of myself.
_____ I am becoming too dependent on my family and friends.
_____ I feel completely overwhelmed.
_____ Other

11. How would you like to change your reaction?

_____

_____

12. How are you feeling about the diagnosis?
_____ Angry
_____ Frightened or anxious
_____ Guilty
_____ Depressed
_____ Hopeless
_____ Hopeful
_____ Grief-stricken
_____ Calm
_____ Other

13. What support can you count on? (Name the people.)
   _____ Family
   _____ Friends
   _____ Diabetes network
   _____ Other support network
   _____ Professional and religious counselors
   _____ Other

14. If you do not have enough support, what steps can you take to find the help you need?

_____

_____

For Your Family Or Friends...

Someone close to you is going through a crisis that, most likely, is affecting you as well. Give them support and encouragement, and seek the same from others for yourself. This is a time when you will all need support from one another

If you find you or your loved one reacting negatively, understand that something shocking has occurred. If the negative reaction from your loved one persists, suggest some appropriate responses. If your own reactions remain negative, seek outside help and find others who can provide support to your loved one until you can.

Find a balance in the assistance you give; issues of dependency can arise. Your friend may feel that they are being a burden, or may attempt to be overly independent. Define where help is needed, but don't reinforce feelings of inadequacy by doing things they are able to take care of. Also, be realistic about any physical limits imposed by the disorder.

Chapter Eighteen

Complications Simplified

"I want to know the risks I'm facing as a diabetic. Why stick my head in the sand and pretend I'm not worried? I tried that and it didn't work worth a damn. I kept hearing horror stories, anyway. I finally pushed through my fears and read about all the things that could happen to me. Glad I did. I found out what I could do to improve my odds for avoiding them."

—Marybeth, 50 years old,
Forty years with diabetes
with only minor complications

In this chapter we review background information on the causes of diabetic complications and the likelihood of reversing or preventing them. We also offer a comprehensive program for reducing your risks of developing complications. We review in detail the nature of the major disorders of diabetes, specific preventive measures, and the options for treatment. As we've discussed earlier, the DCCT (Diabetes Control and Complications Trial) proved that in Type 1 diabetes, the better your blood sugar control, the greater the likelihood of preventing or minimizing complications affecting the eyes, kidneys, and nerves. Data from a smaller Japanese study show that this applies to Type 2 diabetes as well.

If you feel tempted to skip this chapter, we suggest you read at least the sections describing what you can do to avoid the various complications. This is the most important reading you can do. Then, later, return to read the rest of the chapter.

Why Do Diabetic Complications Develop?

Although medical library shelves bulge with studies trying to answer this question, it still is not fully resolved. Still, the broad outlines of an answer do exist.

One major explanation centers on the many abnormalities found in the system of a person with poorly controlled diabetes. The basic inner ecology is profoundly out of balance, especially in the circulatory and hormonal systems. When blood sugar is chronically high, excess sugar disrupts the structure and biochemical processes within the body's cells, particularly those of blood vessels, nerves, kidneys, and eyes. These repeated imbalances create the building blocks for diabetic complications. There is increasing evidence that some of these building blocks are the result of excess glucose reacting with protein in the body, creating AGEs (advanced glycosylation end products). For example, one study showed that AGEs accumulate faster in the arteries and circulatory system in people with diabetes than those without. The increase was positively related to the severity of diabetic kidney disease in these patients.

One imbalance caused by high blood sugar is hormonal. When combined with the biological disruption of emotional or physical stress, the damage from this is compounded. This means that stress management can play a vital role in reducing your risk of complications.

One crucial result of circulatory changes is a tendency for those with diabetes (both Type 1 and 2) to develop high blood pressure. Though hypertension has no symptoms of its own, it contributes strongly to the development or worsening of retinopathy, kidney disease, and cardiovascular disease. If hypertension is present, control of it may be as important in preventing complications as keeping blood sugar levels down. (The lifestyle factors associated with high blood pressure include obesity, high intake of salt, smoking, stress, and lack of exercise.)

Finally, recent studies show increasing evidence of the importance of genetic factors in complications. We inherit tendencies toward or resistances to some of the disorders related to diabetes.

So, in each individual, the onset of a diabetic complication will be determined by a unique combination of past blood sugar imbalances, hormonal imbalances, hypertension, environmental influences, and genetic tendencies.

Can Complications Be Prevented Or Reversed?

This question has been resolved since the last edition of this book! As we've stated several places earlier, the DCCT has given clear answers that blood sugar control matters—the closer blood sugar is to normal, the better the chances of preventing or slowing the development of complications. And every little improvement helps!

Still, major questions remain unanswered: how early must one maintain this level of control in the course of diabetes? How do the different factors that cause complications interact? How do other aspects of self-care influence the risks? Are there levels of blood sugar above which complications are more likely to develop—the threshold effect? (It may be around an HbA1c of 8.0 to 8.1%.)

Diabetes research examines relationships among a limited number of factors—control of blood sugar levels and development of complications studied statistically in a group of people. But each of us as individuals are influenced by a whole life system generally outside the researcher's capacity for study. Diabetic control must be seen as one of a variety of factors determining our future—diet, exercise and activity level, patterns of managing stress, emotional life, immunological responses, heredity, and other influences yet to be discovered.

If we look at the question of preventing complications in this broader frame of reference, improving blood sugar control becomes one important part of a healthy, balanced lifestyle that is of immediate and long-term benefit to people with diabetes. Despite researchers' specific uncertainties, the total benefits of improving diabetes control are well worth the costs. The degree of control you maintain, though, must be determined by your other life demands. That is why we describe three levels of control to help in your decision making. Our goal is to help you be realistic in your choices and not fool yourself about what you are and are not willing to do to control your diabetes.

Reducing Your Risk Of Developing Complications

Do you believe the hoped-for cure for diabetes or breakthroughs in treatments of complications will allow you to ignore preventive measures? Don't fall for this illusion. Diabetes' side effects accumulate over time, cause deterioration of basic body systems, and, in many cases, are not reversible. If you just wait for a cure, it may not work for you because too much damage may have already occurred. Preventive measures, started as early as possible, are much more effective than later treatment.

The following information on reducing your risk of complications expands on the list of actions that appears in Chapter 16. Yes, "Reducing the risk" does not necessarily mean "avoiding complications." But by following these preventive measures, you will improve your odds. And, if complications do develop, they are likely to appear later, progress more slowly, and be more treatable, perhaps with methods not yet perfected or discovered. It is also likely that you will have to deal with fewer complications.

Ways to Reduce Your Risk

1. Improve your metabolic control and continue improving it until you achieve the best level with which you can live well. While other factors play important roles, blood sugar control is clearly central to reducing your risk for diabetic complications.

   Improvements in your level of control will make complications less likely to develop or delay their onset and severity. As we have said before, there is no guarantee, simply improved odds.

2. Learn to handle stress well. In the short run, poorly managed stress interferes with blood sugar control, causing either high tests or swings between high and low. In the long run, excessive levels of stress hormones are probably a major contributor to many diabetes complications.

3. Follow a diet low in fat, high in fiber, and with controlled salt consumption, as well as moderation of sweets and rapidly absorbed carbohydrates. Low salt consumption helps control high blood pressure. Restrictions of cholesterol and total fat, especially animal fat (and other saturated fats like coconut and palm oils) help maintain a healthy circulatory system. In addition to having a beneficial effect on blood sugar, high-fiber diets have been associated with a lower incidence of colon diseases, including cancer.

4. Live an active lifestyle and/or exercise regularly. Physical activity provides a foundation for good metabolic control as well as helping control weight and stress. It also has significant benefits for cardio-respiratory fitness.

5. If you are overweight, try seriously to lose weight. In addition to contributing to metabolic control, weight loss will decrease your risk for cardiovascular disease and hypertension.

6. Act to prevent high blood pressure by controlling stress and weight. Seek treatment if your blood pressure is high (the American Diabetes Association recommends treatment if blood pressure exceeds 130/85).

   High blood pressure dramatically increases the risk of kidney failure and visual loss from retinopathy. As in people who do not have diabetes, it increases the risk of heart and circulatory illness. A program of prevention and treatment can be found in the section on hypertension later in this chapter. Following this program is one of the most important preventive actions you can take.

7. If you smoke, quit. Smoking usually increases the risk of vascular disorders and heart disease, risks already heightened in diabetes. Smoking has a negative effect on arteries, small blood vessels, blood pressure, and circulation, thus contributing to arteriosclerosis, hypertension, and coronary artery disease.

8. Get the amount of sleep and rest that you need. Adequate sleep and rest minimize stress and contribute to good metabolic control.

9. Consider taking a daily multivitamin. Scientific evidence supporting the preventive role of vitamin and mineral supplementation in diabetes is still sketchy. Many claims for substances such as vitamins E and C, bioflavonoids, and brewer's yeast are made in health magazines, yet few reliable studies consistently support these claims. There may be definite benefits in moderate vitamin and mineral supplementation. The medical community is more actively studying these substances in general, as well as for their particular use in people with diabetes (for example, the value of the antioxidant properties of certain vitamins, and the possible benefits of magnesium or chromium supplements in certain people with diabetes).

   Large doses of vitamins C (thousands of units per day) and E (over 250 units per day) should be avoided if advanced retinal disorders (proliferative retinopathy) or kidney disease (nephropathy) have developed. Such megavitamin self-treatment may have a damaging impact on these conditions, increasing capillary fragility.

This is not an all-or-nothing program. Each item on the list improves your chances. If you want to do more than you are now doing but are having difficulty making all of the changes suggested, review the information on learning and change in Chapter 1.

The Major Complications Of Diabetes

The rest of this chapter describes the conditions specific to diabetes or that take a special form in people with diabetes. We have not covered the cardiovascular complications whose course is similar in those with and without diabetes. You can find good sources of information on heart disease at the end of the chapter.

As you read this section of the book, be aware of the stress it is likely to trigger. Don't just plow through it, ignoring the feelings that naturally arise as you study such threatening material. Pause often, relax, and reassure yourself. Talk about your feelings with someone close to you, or write them down. Live well, even with this very difficult information about diabetes.

Complications of the Eyes

Diabetic Retinopathy

What Goes Wrong? Abnormalities in blood sugar level, blood chemistry, and hormone levels produce an oxygen or circulatory shortage in the eye's retina and blockages of small blood vessels. At first, this results in background retinopathy—minor changes in blood vessels of the retina. When the process intensifies, new blood vessels form in the retina in an attempt to increase the supply of blood and oxygen. These vessels are weak and prone to leak blood and fluid into the retinal tissue or the vitreous liquid (the jelly-like substance between the retina and the lens) of the eye. Together with other blood vessel abnormalities in the retina, these hemorrhages can lead to decreased or total loss of vision. These changes also create a risk of retinal detachment or macular edema (excess fluid in the portion of the retina used for sharp vision).

Signs and Stages of Development Background retinopathy begins to develop after five to twenty years of diabetes. It is a mild condition characterized by small, scattered changes in the retina. Vision is not affected, and the disorder is no cause for alarm. The condition can be detected only through an ophthalmological examination by a doctor trained to recognize it.

Proliferative retinopathy may develop after fifteen years of diabetes, or sooner. New fragile blood vessels and fibrous scarring are found on the retina. Unless there is retinal detachment or hemorrhages interfering with vision, it can only be discovered through an eye examination. (Possible visual cues of this condition include the presence of flashing lights, floaters, and blurred vision.) Photos of your retinas may be taken, with and without a fluorescein dye, to indicate points of leakage.

If proliferative retinopathy continues to develop, vision-blocking hemorrhages or retinal detachment may occur.

Macular edema is a thickening of the retina or the collection of fluid around the central part of the retina used for fine vision (the macula). This thickening results in blurring or fuzziness of vision.

The Risk More than 90 percent of people with Type 1 diabetes have mild or background retinopathy after 15 years of diabetes. By 20 years, up to 50 percent have developed some degree of proliferative retinopathy. Before laser treatment was introduced, many people with diabetes experienced severe visual loss or blindness from advanced retinopathy. This risk has been dramatically reduced by the laser. Relatively few now become blind from this condition. For people with Type 2 diabetes, proliferative retinopathy is less common—after 20 years only about 20 percent of insulin-users and 10 percent of non-users develop proliferative retinopathy.

Prevention

1. Have an ophthalmologist examine your eyes each year after you have had diabetes for five years. Even if your vision is normal, you may have changes that can benefit from laser treatment.
2. Check your own vision in each eye weekly (or even daily), looking for any changes: increased blurriness, floaters, fuzzy areas. (Good vision in one eye may mask worsening vision in the other, so make sure you close each eye to check the sight in the other.)
3. Report any changes in vision to your doctor immediately.
4. Keep blood sugar as close to normal as possible.
5. Maintain normal blood pressure. (Practice preventive measures for high blood pressure.) Adhere to treatment for hypertension, if prescribed.
6. Maintain your target weight.
7. Avoid smoking.

Treatment Your internist or family physician is trained to examine your eyes for retinopathy, but if you have Type 1 diabetes, you should start having a yearly examination by an ophthalmologist five years after diagnosis. If you have Type 2 diabetes, yearly exams should start when you are diagnosed. This is recommended because those with Type 2 may have diabetes for several years before diagnosis and retinopathy may have already begun. All treatments for retinopathy are performed by ophthalmologists. If the first stages of proliferative retinopathy are diagnosed, you may need examinations every three or four months.

Laser photocoagulation is the recommended treatment for retinopathy once a certain level of new vessel formation or macular edema is reached. This is an office procedure in which an ophthalmologist uses a laser to make hundreds of microscopic scars along the retina. Local anesthesia can be used, but usually the process causes only moderate discomfort. The treatment increases the oxygen available to the central area of the retina and promotes healing of the new vessel growth. This decreases the risk of blindness by 50 to 60 percent.

Risks of treatment, occurring very rarely, include further bleeding and inadvertent scarring of the central area of the retina. Possible side effects include a moderate restriction of peripheral (side) vision, a slight decrease in sharpness of vision, and decreased night vision.

A large, multi-center national study (the Early Treatment Diabetic Retinopathy Study, ETDRS) has shown that "focal" laser treatment decreased visual loss by about 50 percent in those patients with clinically significant macular edema. This is defined very precisely for the ophthalmologist and requires a special, painless exam. You may have clinically significant macular edema that would benefit from treatment, but you may not know it because your eyesight is still normal. It is essential that you have your eyes checked even if your sight appears unaffected.

Vitrectomy is a surgical procedure used when retinopathy is too advanced to be treated by laser (because extensive hemorrhages fill the vitreous fluid in the eye, blocking the retina). The fluid is removed and replaced with a clear saline solution. The operation may also remove scar tissue and fibers that can cause retinal detachment. This process is riskier than laser treatment, so ophthalmologists usually prefer to wait six to twelve months to see if blood in the vitreous will clear without treatment.

Cautions If proliferative retinopathy has developed, you should avoid activities that cause a sudden rise in blood pressure or a sudden flow of blood to the head: straining with bowel movements, bending over quickly, high diving, scuba diving, lifting heavy weights, head stands, and so on. Hemorrhages in the eye can result from these activities as well as from blows to the head. Discuss the general level of physical activity appropriate for you with your ophthalmologist.

At the proliferative stage, you should not tighten your diabetes control quickly. Control should be improved gradually, over several months. A sudden change to tight control can cause retinopathy to worsen (usually only temporarily) at the proliferative stage.

It is important to cope with the emotional stress accompanying this threat to your vision. High levels of stress may cause periods of high blood pressure and add to the threat.

Chronic high blood pressure should be controlled with medication.

High doses of vitamin C (over 500 mg per day), used by some to treat colds, should be avoided. This vitamin in large doses affects blood clotting and thickness.

Diabetic Cataract

What goes wrong? The lens of the eye becomes cloudy as an indirect result of high blood sugar. The immediate cause is excess sorbitol, the alcohol of glucose, in the lens. This changes the chemical balance of the lens because it tends to accumulate in the cells. (People with diabetes may also be more likely to develop the more common age-related form of cataract.)

Signs and stages of development How cataracts affect vision depends on the pattern of cloudiness that develops in the lens. Opacity may occur at the center, around the sides, or diffusely throughout the lens. The initial stage of development may be detectable only through ophthalmological examination. In the mature phase, a milkiness can be seen from the outside, and vision decreases, with fogginess and halos around lights.

Prevention

1. Maintain excellent blood sugar control.
2. Some biochemical research indicates that taking 1,000 mg of bioflavonoids daily may help. This food supplement may reduce sorbitol in body tissues.
3. Research continues on aldose reductase inhibitors, drugs such as sorbinil, which counter the action of the enzyme that converts sugars into the sorbitol causing cataracts. Early results have been mixed. However, if successful, a drug may be available to prevent diabetic cataracts.

Treatment Cataract surgery involves the removal of the cloudy lens, replacing it with a plastic lens. This process is usually done under local anesthesia. It restores vision in 90 to 95 percent of patients. Surgery is really recommended only when the disruption of vision interferes with your daily life.

Risks This procedure carries the usual surgical risks of infection and bleeding that can further compromise vision. The risk is low.

Take a break

Especially if you are reading straight through this chapter, you need one. Relax, check your feelings, and give yourself some warm love and friendship. Taking in all this information is a difficult task. Do not think that you can just absorb it without emotional impact. After working with these hard facts for years, your authors still feel them deeply.

Kidney Disease (Diabetic Nephropathy)

What goes wrong? Normally, the kidney filters blood, clearing out waste products and recirculating blood chemicals and proteins that are then reused. This is done by networks of capillaries (called the glomeruli); however, these fine blood vessels can become severely damaged by years of high blood sugar. A layer of the capillary—the basement membrane—becomes thickened.

With this thickening, kidney function is progressively altered. The selective filtering by the kidney is impaired. First, protein (albumin) that should be retained in the bloodstream is passed through the kidney into urine (a condition called microalbuminuria and albuminuria or proteinuria). Then, toxic waste products that should be filtered out of the blood remain in circulation (azotemia). Serum creatinine and blood urea nitrogen (BUN) levels become abnormally increased. (Creatinine and BUN are chemicals normally found in the blood and passed into the urine. Their levels rise if the kidney is not working well. Temporary increases may occur occasionally from causes such as eating a large amount of meat or heavy exercise.)

This stage eventually leads to a condition known as uremia: an excess of urea and other nitrogen wastes in the blood that produces symptoms of kidney failure, such as fatigue, decreased appetite, nausea, and vomiting.

The good news is that for people who have had diabetes for more than forty years and have not developed proteinuria, it is unlikely that nephropathy will develop. Moreover, it appears that 60 to 70 percent of people with insulin-dependent diabetes and 60 to 90 percent with Type 2 diabetes will never develop clinical kidney disease. Those with Type 2 diabetes are less likely than people with Type 1 diabetes to develop end stage kidney disease, but because there are so many more people with Type 2 diabetes, about the same number of each develop kidney failure.

Signs and stages of development The early stages of kidney disease are revealed only by urine and blood tests. Here we provide technical information on these signs to help you understand the results of tests your physician may report. The early signs of kidney disease can be strong motivators for preventive action on your part.

Stage 1 Changes in the kidneys begin to develop slowly over many years, with no obvious clinical signs or symptoms. The normal kidney excretes a small amount of protein (albumin) in the urine (less than 30 mg in a 24-hour period). With new, more sensitive tests, it is now possible to measure such small amounts clinically (rather than in a research lab). A urine protein level between 30 and 300 mg per day is called microalbuminuria.

Substantial evidence now indicates that persistent microalbuminuria predicts the later development of diabetic kidney disease (particularly in people with insulin-dependent diabetes). So urine protein in the range of 30 to 300 mg per day—along with the typically increased blood flow and filtration rate through the kidneys—can now be considered Stage 1. If nephropathy is going to develop, this stage may last an average of fifteen to seventeen years and has traditionally been considered the silent period of nephropathy.

Stage 2 The next development may occur after fifteen to seventeen years of diabetes on average. Standard urine tests may show abnormally increased albumin excretion, greater than 250 to 300 mg per day. At this stage, the kidney is leaking out protein, but BUN and creatinine—other indicators of disease detected through blood tests—have not yet started to rise. If Stage 2 is reached, development of further disease is highly likely. Proteinuria may be present in urine for several years without other evidence of kidney disease. (Remember, there is great individual variation for these statistics, and many will never develop kidney disease.)

Stage 3 In this stage, BUN and serum creatinine levels slowly rise. Once an individual's creatinine exceeds 2 mg/dl (milligrams per deciliter), it is possible to estimate roughly the time progression of disease and the percentage of kidney function remaining. Simply divide the creatinine level into 1 and multiply by 100 to get the percentage remaining. For example, a creatinine level of 4 gives approximately 25 percent remaining function. (Most people don't have symptoms until function drops to 5 to 15 percent.) Your physician can give you a rough estimate of the rate of progress of kidney disease.

Stage 4 At this point, the kidneys are failing. BUN and creatinine levels are high enough to cause symptoms of kidney failure. These symptoms include poor appetite, vomiting, ankle swelling or other signs of fluid accumulation, weakness, lethargy, drowsiness, fatigue, and nausea. Weight gain, mostly from excess fluid accumulation, is continuing to occur. Do not scare yourself if you have any of these symptoms. Individually they are signs of a large variety of low-threat disorders. Urine and blood tests done in the laboratory and interpreted by your physician are the only way to determine the presence of kidney disease.

In Stage 4 kidney disease, dialysis or kidney transplant is necessary to preserve life.

Monitoring and Prevention Although no evidence suggests that improved blood glucose control will affect the progression of kidney disease once Stage 2 has begun, there is evidence that action in Stage 1 may benefit you. Researchers recommend that you generally strive for control as good as possible when your tests show microalbuminuria (30 to 300 mg/dl). In addition, there is some evidence that keeping your HbA1c below 8.1% may substantially decrease your risk of developing nephropathy (a "threshold effect"). Furthermore, if microalbuminuria begins, there is convincing evidence that taking an ACE inhibitor, a drug commonly used to treat high blood pressure, may slow or prevent further development of kidney disease. The following guidelines for monitoring kidney function are one approach:

For the first five years after your diabetes diagnosis (Type 1 or Type 2), you should have a routine check for protein in the urine each time you visit your physician for your diabetes and a test for microalbuminuria at least yearly. BUN and creatinine should be measured at least yearly if proteinuria is present, and creatinine clearance every two years. The urine test for microalbuminuria is a very effective screening test—a recent study of people with Type 2 diabetes showed that not only is increased microalbuminuria associated with greater risk of kidney disease, but also heart disease and nerve disease. (This also has been shown to be true for people with Type 1 diabetes.) It is believed that microalbuminuria may be a signal of general damage to the blood vessels throughout the body, not just in the kidneys.

After five years or in the person who is past puberty, in addition to the above, you should have a 24-hour urine test yearly to measure total daily protein.

Once overt (dipstick) proteinuria or elevated serum creatinine or BUN is detected, you should have your kidney function monitored at least two or three times a year. Make sure you see a nephrologist (kidney specialist) to work out a long-term therapeutic strategy and to discuss the possibility and implications of renal failure.

Additional preventive measures in kidney disease

1. Maintain the best possible metabolic control.
2. Avoid ketoacidosis (diabetic coma) by carefully managing infections and stress.
3. Avoid high blood pressure by controlling your weight and limiting your intake of salt or sodium (for instance, do not add salt to foods). Take any hypertension medication prescribed. (Hypertension promotes the development of diabetic kidney disease.) For hypertension, drugs like ACE inhibitors or certain calcium-channel blockers are especially useful for people with diabetes.
4. Use relaxation techniques as a further way of lowering blood pressure.
5. Avoid urinary tract infections. (Know the symptoms: burning or pain or urination and cloudy urine.) Seek treatment promptly if they occur. Such infections can contribute to kidney damage.
6. To minimize the risk of infection, you should not be catheterized unless it is absolutely necessary.
7. Use of dye-contrast agents in X-ray or other radiological studies should be avoided unless absolutely necessary. (They tend to be toxic to the kidney.)

Treatment In the first stage, your internist or family practitioner is equipped to watch for signs of advancing kidney disease. By Stage 2, a kidney specialist (nephrologist) should be consulted to monitor your condition. Treatment in Stages 3 and 4 is by a nephrologist, preferably one experienced in diabetic kidney disease.

Stage 1 Strictly following the preventive measures described above is likely to allow you to avoid or postpone diabetic kidney disease. The fact that you have an early warning sign in the microalbuminuria test gives you a valuable gift of motivation. The best possible self-care can keep your kidneys intact.

Stage 2 With excellent self-care—including all the preventive measures just described—you can probably extend the life of your kidneys by many years. The key is controlling your blood sugar and weight, using ACE inhibitors as prescribed, and getting any additional needed treatment for high blood pressure and urinary tract infections. Care at this stage is designed to extend kidney function by controlling hypertension and avoiding urinary tract infection and drugs toxic to the kidney (such as those used in some radiographic studies).

Stage 3 At this stage, your kidney function has deteriorated and toxic products are building up in the bloodstream. Blood sugar control may help other body systems but it cannot reverse kidney disease at this stage. Restricting protein in your diet may be recommended, although this is still controversial. More specialists are recommending high protein intake (especially animal protein) even in Stages 1 or 2. Diuretic pills to help you lose any accumulated fluid may be prescribed.

Stage 4 Once kidney failure occurs, the two choices for treatment are dialysis or a kidney transplant.

Dialysis is a demanding procedure in which a machine performs the blood-filtering function of the kidneys. You are attached to the machine, using blood vessels in your arm, typically for four hours, three times a week. The experience is taxing, but it can add years to your life. Peritoneal dialysis uses the peritoneum (the lining of the abdominal cavity) to filter toxins out of the blood. It is possible to do this procedure at home or at work, and it may provide a motivated person with more flexibility.

Kidney transplants allow a more normal life than dialysis. The technique has advanced rapidly, increasing the organ acceptance rate and long-term survival rate. Successful transplantation no longer depends on receiving a kidney from a relative, because matching of cadaver kidneys has improved significantly. Five-year success rates range from 70 to 90 percent, depending on the source of the kidney donated.

Cautions Avoid ketoacidosis (diabetic coma), urinary tract infections, use of dye contrast agents in X-ray studies, and catheterization; follow treatment for high blood pressure.

Time for another break

Even if your kidneys are still completely healthy, what you have just read may be frightening and depressing. If you do have signs of kidney disease developing, you will probably need to deal with strong emotional reactions. Chapters 3, 12, and 15 can help you handle these reactions. Don't be afraid to seek outside aid in a diabetes or kidney disease support group or from professionals.

Nerve Disorders (Diabetic Neuropathies)

What goes wrong? Several families of nerve disorders may develop as complications of diabetes, producing pain, lack of sensation, digestive and urinary difficulties, and impotence. Fortunately, many of the disorders usually disappear after a few months to a year. Others are successfully treated with a variety of drugs. Good metabolic control probably reduces your risk of developing a neuropathy.

The reasons why diabetic neuropathies develop are still not completely understood, but clearly the overall cause is higher-than-normal blood sugar. The ability of nerves to carry messages, and the nature of the messages themselves, may be altered by several chemical effects of poor control. The insulation of the nerves (the myelin sheath) is damaged. Sorbitol (a glucose-related alcohol) and fructose accumulate in nerve cells. The speed at which messages travel is slowed. Myoinositol content of nerve tissues is reduced. (This deficiency may be corrected by drugs.) Glucose attaches to protein cells. The net result: a nerve disorder.

Neuropathies are caused by elevated blood sugar, but the DCCT showed that good metabolic control will allow you to minimize the risk of developing these complications and slow their progression if they do develop. The Kumamoto study in Japan showed similar results for those with Type 2 diabetes.

The various forms of neuropathy are rare among children with diabetes. Neuropathies usually do not develop before fifteen years of having diabetes. Generally, if the symptoms are mild in the first few years of neuropathy, they are unlikely to develop to an extreme degree.

Prevention Maintain good metabolic control. Be aware that chemical toxins or alcoholic beverages may accelerate the development or progression of neuropathy.

Peripheral neuropathy

In this disorder, impairment occurs in those nerves extending down the legs and arms—the peripheral nervous system. Two main forms of disorders occur: those that develop gradually, usually without pain, and those with rapid onset and significant pain.

Gradual peripheral neuropathy is marked by numbness, tingling, itching, burning, a decreased sense of touch, a decrease in deep tendon reflexes, or any combination of these. These symptoms are usually found on both sides of the body and occur more frequently in the feet and legs than in the hands and arms. (Your doctor checks for this disorder when testing your reflexes and when using a tuning fork, sharp devices, and a monofilament to test your sensations. The monofilament is a quick and easy way for your doctor to test the feeling in your foot and predict whether your foot is at risk for sores or ulcers.) Another possible symptom is the loss of the sense of orientation (proprioception) in the feet and legs—not knowing by feel which way a foot is turned, for instance. While not painful, peripheral neuropathy can lead to serious foot problems.

Treatment seems to be limited to improving control of diabetes. Myoinositol and sorbinil may prove to be effective against this form of neuropathy.

Peripheral neuropathy that has come on rapidly and with pain is a temporary complication, but the pain can be intense. It develops within a matter of days or weeks and generally lasts from six to eighteen months. The chief symptom, a burning pain like a "toothache" in the feet or legs, is usually worse at night.

Treatment focuses on reducing the pain, first with aspirin or acetaminophen or the nonsteroidal anti-inflammatory drugs (NSAIDs) such as ibuprofen, Advil, etc. Narcotics such as codeine, or drugs such as imipramine, Elavil, or Prolixin, may provide relief. The anticonvulsant drugs, phenytoin or carbamazepine, although not substantiated in controlled clinical trials, may be worth a therapeutic trial. Some larger medical centers now have pain clinics offering a wide choice of treatments beyond drugs. Recently, capsaicin cream has helped nerve pain from contact that typically doesn't cause pain (like light touch, bedding, or clothes).

Autonomic neuropathy

This disorder affects the nerves that control internal organs, genitals, small blood vessels and sweat glands of the skin, bladder muscles, and the gastrointestinal tract. Some of the conditions that can result include impotence, difficulty urinating or sensing when the bladder is full (which can lead to bladder infection), diarrhea, stomach upset due to retention of food, dizziness after standing up, loss of the normal sweating response, and weakening or disappearance of the symptoms of an insulin reaction.

The symptoms of autonomic neuropathy are usually not temporary, as with some other forms of neuropathy. However, effective forms of treatment are available for most of the specific disabilities. Impotence from neuropathy, for instance, can be effectively overcome by a surgical implant that allows full sexual functioning. Several nonsurgical approaches, including external vacuum aids and drug injections, are also available, as is alprostadil (MUSE), a microsuppository that is inserted relatively painlessly into the end of the penis, which has just come on the market. An oral drug is also being investigated. Tests are often given to distinguish clearly between neuropathic impotence, impotence due to blood vessel problems, and impotence caused by psychological factors, tests essential to avoiding unnecessary treatments.

We do not know to what extent metabolic control can reverse any of these conditions caused by autonomic neuropathy. Evidence so far indicates that stricter control can reverse the other form of neuropathy: peripheral.

Complications of the Feet and Legs

What goes wrong? Two diabetic complications join forces to threaten the feet and legs : peripheral neuropathy and peripheral vascular disease. With proper self-care and regular foot examinations, you can neutralize this threat and reduce or eliminate the risk of losing a limb.

When peripheral neuropathy (described above) causes numbness and lack of feeling, injuries to the feet may go unnoticed, leading to infection and amputation. Pressure sores and ulcerations can develop on the feet and not be discovered until severe infection has set in.

This risk is compounded by the presence of peripheral vascular disease, a common disorder that takes a unique form with diabetes (described in this chapter under "Complications of the Heart and Circulatory System"). This disorder causes decreased blood flow in the legs and feet. This, in turn, means a decreased flow of the oxygen, white blood cells, and nutrients needed to fight infection. Either of the peripheral disorders can lead to limb loss. Together, the two multiply the risk.

One other foot problem can develop from lack of sensation. If any bone or joint disorders begin, symptoms may not be evident until they reach an advanced stage (neuroarthropathy). You are able to go on walking and standing without pain on feet and ankles that need immediate attention. This is not a common condition, but it is one more argument for excellent daily foot care.

Prevention of complications of the feet and legs
1. Maintain the best possible blood sugar control.
2. Do everything possible to prevent peripheral neuropathy, peripheral vascular disease, and hypertension.
3. Wash and inspect your feet daily. (If you can't see clearly or get close enough, have someone else do it for you.)
4. Check for blisters, bruises, cracks, cuts, and scratches. A sore, scratch, or red area that could be ignored by someone without diabetes should be watched very carefully by someone with diabetes. Use mild antiseptic and antibacterial salve on minor injuries. See your doctor for any sore that does not improve or heal within a few days. If the sore becomes infected or swollen, or if white or yellow pus appears, take no chances. See your doctor. You need to avoid serious infection, which can lead to gangrene and loss of a toe or foot.
5. Athlete's foot and fungal infections of the toenails should also be caught early and treated aggressively. Long-term care using antifungal cream or ointment or the new oral antifungal drugs (such as terbenafine) may be necessary.
6. Massage your feet with anhydrous lanolin (available from your pharmacy) or polysorb. Do not rub lotion between the toes. (Massage helps maintain good circulation. Foot cream prevents dry, cracked skin.)

7. Do not cut or use patent medicines on corns or calluses. File calluses gently with an emery board. See your physician or a podiatrist for any large or painful lumps on your feet or for any changes in the shape of toes, toenails, or other parts of the foot.

8. When trimming toenails, gently round them to follow the shape of the toe. Avoid creating sharp points that dig into the next toe or sharp angles that cause ingrown toenails. Over-the-counter medicines for ingrown nails should also be avoided, as they may cause unwanted effects.

9. Select shoes that fit well and feel good. Break them in gradually. Always wear soft, seamless socks with shoes. Avoid sandals with straps between the toes.

10. Inspect shoes daily for rocks, nail points, or damage.

11. Avoid very hot or very cold water. Do not use heating pads or hot water bottles on your feet. Wear socks to bed if your feet are cold.

12. Do foot and ankle exercises to stimulate circulation. (Two good exercises: rotating your feet at the ankle with your leg raised when you first wake up; standing with the front one-third of your feet on the edge of a step and raising and lowering your body a dozen times.)

13. Do not smoke. Nicotine is very damaging to the circulatory system.

Treatment Early treatment of any foot disorder is essential, because infections can advance rapidly when circulation is poor. The primary guideline is to be alert and call or see your doctor for what may appear to be minor blisters, cuts, or sores. The earlier these can be treated, the less likely they are to become serious.

Other Skin and Joint Complications

We want to mention briefly the thickening of the skin and possibly the connective tissue that may affect up to one-third or more people with Type 1 diabetes, and probably those with Type 2 as well. It is usually painless and causes little if any disability. However, it can restrict joint movement, particularly in the wrists, hands, and fingers, and may be the cause of otherwise unexplained musculoskeletal problems. It can also affect the shoulder and neck. Because it is believed to result from glucose attaching itself to tissue proteins (AGEs), it may represent an early warning of other complications such as retinopathy, neuropathy, and nephropathy. Aldose reductase inhibitors may relieve some of this limited joint mobility (LJM).

Less well known among medical professionals is the increased prevalence of frozen shoulder (adhesive capsulitis) among those with diabetes. In one large study, 11 percent of 800 study participants with diabetes had frozen shoulder compared with 2.3 percent of 600 without diabetes. If you notice any pain or limitation in the range of motion of your arm or shoulder, see your doctor. It is much easier to treat in the early stages (with stretching exercises or other physical therapy) than after it progresses.

Complications of the Heart and Circulatory System

In most cases, the characteristics of the following disorders are not unique to diabetes. We differ from those without diabetes only in having a higher risk for these problems, a risk that begins earlier in life (about 10 years earlier). This risk can be reduced significantly by excellent self-care. In fact, just like most of the population without diabetes, we are most likely to die from these cardiovascular diseases, rather than anything specific to diabetes.

These are diseases primarily of the larger blood vessels (macrovascular) in contrast to the microvascular complications of retinopathy, nephropathy, and neuropathy.

The primary risk factors for cardiovascular diseases (heart attack, stroke, arteriosclerosis, and peripheral vascular disease) are

▷ Smoking

▷ High fat and cholesterol levels in the blood

▷ Obesity

▷ Lack of exercise

▷ Family history of heart and circulatory disease

▷ High blood pressure

High levels of insulin circulating in the blood is also believed to be a contributing risk factor. Most of those with Type 2 diabetes have high blood insulin levels for some time during the course of their disease, because their pancreas works extra hard to bring down the blood sugar. (The association of many of the above risk factors with high insulin levels has been called Syndrome X or the Reaven Syndrome.)

Prevention of cardiovascular disorders

A general preventive program for your heart and circulatory system includes many of the basic elements of the full diabetic regimen. Most of these are fundamental to a healthy lifestyle for anyone. They include the following:

1. Maintain normal body weight. If you are overweight, lose weight.
2. Limit sodium consumption to 2,000 to 4,000 milligrams per day if you have high blood pressure.
3. Avoid foods high in saturated fat and cholesterol.
4. Learn and use effective techniques of relaxation and stress reduction.
5. Live an active lifestyle, with aerobic activities if your condition allows.
6. If you smoke, stop smoking.

Because information on stroke and heart attack is widely available, we will discuss only high blood pressure and peripheral vascular disease. These conditions have unique significance in diabetes.

High Blood Pressure

Prevention of chronically high blood pressure ranks close to blood sugar control as a means of avoiding diabetic complications. It also plays a major role in treating complications; lower blood pressure helps to slow or reverse the progress of eye, kidney, and circulatory problems. So here is a keystone of living well with diabetes: Act to maintain normal blood pressure before it starts to climb, and begin treatment promptly if it does go up.

What goes wrong? Hypertension is more common among those with diabetes, and it tends to begin at an earlier age. It has no noticeable symptoms, so it can be diagnosed only through a series of blood pressure readings (consistent readings above 130/85, according to the American Diabetes Association which recently lowered this target level from 140/90, emphasizing the importance of good blood pressure control). The causes of high blood pressure are not completely known. Contributing factors include obesity, stress, smoking, inactivity, and genetic tendency.

Hypertension occurs more often in people with diabetes because high blood sugar and fats contribute to its development. Once narrowing of arteries due to fat deposits (atherosclerosis) or kidney disease start, these disorders further heighten blood pressure.

Although you feel no immediate symptoms, hypertension has very serious consequences for those with or without diabetes. In any person, hypertension:

> ▷ Intensifies the buildup of fatty deposits, narrowing the blood vessels in a condition known as atherosclerosis, which increases all of the risks below.
> ▷ Causes your heart to work harder, enlarging it, and adding to your risk for heart attack.
> ▷ Increases your chances of developing peripheral vascular disease.
> ▷ Makes strokes more likely.

Those with diabetes have a higher risk for all of these disorders, a risk made even higher by hypertension. But there are further effects specific to diabetes. High blood pressure also contributes to the development and progress of kidney disease and hastens the development of retinopathy.

Hypertension is called the silent disease, because its effects are not experienced directly. But it speaks loudly in its impact on our health.

Prevention General preventive measures for circulatory disease are given at the beginning of this section. Following the recommendations is one of the greatest gifts you can give yourself, hundreds of times more valuable than the relatively small sacrifices involved.

Treatment For both Type 1 and Type 2 diabetes, when blood pressure consistently goes above 130/85, it is time to start treatment for hypertension. Fortunately, the first stage of treatment is to do the very things recommended for prevention, if you are not already doing them. You may not need medication, assuming that your blood pressure is only mildly elevated and that other complications do not require it. You might want to buy a blood pressure cuff (sphygmomanometer), the device for measuring your blood pressure, so you can monitor your pressure at home between medical appointments.

If an antihypertensive drug is prescribed at the first sign of high blood pressure (and if you are willing to follow the recommendations above), ask your physician if there is any special reason to go directly to medication. If there is not, you both can consider a six-month trial to determine whether relaxation, sodium restriction, weight reduction, and other steps will bring your blood pressure down. Most people with high blood pressure need antihypertensive drugs, but if you can control blood pressure without them, you avoid the potential side effects of the drugs. However, if there is any sign of kidney disease, it is probably wise to begin taking an ACE inhibitor (see below).

Great care must be taken in choosing an antihypertensive medication, because many have side effects potentially harmful to people with diabetes. Don't be afraid to ask your physician to choose the drug with the fewest possible side effects for you and your diabetes. It will be a matter of finding a medication least likely to raise your blood sugar or undesirable lipid (fat) levels in the blood.

There are more than twenty-five different drugs available to lower blood pressure, including many particularly useful for people with diabetes, such as ACE inhibitors. Some (propranolol and other beta blockers), however, eliminate the warning signs of an insulin reaction and block the release of the hormone that helps us recover from hypoglycemia. One of the most popular diuretics used for hypertension, hydrochlorothiazide, tends to increase both blood sugar and blood fat levels. Others reinforce the difficulties with impotence some men with diabetes have. Adrenergic inhibitors are the worst offenders. These include reserpine, clonidine, and methyldopa.

You may feel uncomfortable raising the choice of drugs with your physician. We suggest that you say something like: "I've read that some of the common blood pressure drugs are not as good for people with diabetes as others. Can we discuss this? Which one(s) are you going to prescribe for me?" Most likely, your physician will respond with an explanation indicating an awareness of a considered choice and that more monitoring of blood sugar or potassium may be needed. Possible major side effects to watch for should be discussed.

If kidney disease has started, treatment for hypertension becomes more complex and even more important. High blood pressure hastens deterioration of kidney function. Kidney impairment further increases blood pressure. This vicious cycle can be slowed and possibly halted if medication and nondrug therapy are started early enough. Antihypertensive treatment (including ACE inhibitors) and perhaps restriction of animal protein in your diet are the only ways believed to slow the advance of existing kidney disease. Under your physician's care, you should begin all of the general measures listed earlier to prevent circulatory disease. But you will need stricter control of salt in your diet (no more than 1 gram per day). The selection of drugs at this point is crucial and should be made by a physician familiar with diabetic kidney disorders.

What goes wrong? Poor circulation develops in the legs and feet of people with diabetes, mostly through atherosclerosis. The decreased blood flow prevents adequate supplies of oxygen and nutrients to reach cells in the feet. This is one of the major causes of the difficulties described under "Complications of the Feet and Legs." Disorders of this type can result in serious infection, gangrene, and amputation. For this reason, foot care is one of the most vital aspects of your regimen.

Symptoms Aching, cramping, or pain sometimes occurs in the legs while walking. This pain usually subsides in a few minutes when you rest. (Its technical name is intermittent claudication.) Other symptoms are

▷ Cold feet.

▷ Aching in the legs or feet when lying down.

▷ Feet that become red or purplish when your legs hang down.

▷ Pulses in the feet that become weaker, particularly after a brisk walk.

▷ Feet that become pale when raised above your body.

▷ Reduced blood pressure at the ankles.

Prevention The basic measures to prevent cardiovascular disease, described earlier, all apply here. You should also review and follow the foot care recommendations given under "Complications of the Feet and Legs."

Treatment Treatment of peripheral vascular disease seeks to avoid the consequences of poor circulation. Pentoxifylline may help to relieve symptoms. Surgery to bypass the diseased blood vessels, or angioplasty to open them up, may be necessary to relieve severe persistent pain.

Summary

Complications are the most disturbing aspect of having diabetes. We face serious risks, yet we can defy this uncertainty and face the consequences of diabetes bravely, even if we do develop a complication. We are free to reduce the risks and improve our odds.

We are, after all, individuals, each with our own unique history. Some of us will live long without major complications. Others will delay the onset and lessen the severity of the disorders that result from diabetes. Ever-improving treatment will enable us to limit their consequences in our lives. By learning to follow the balanced and healthy lifestyle this book presents, we will be able to live well with diabetes, even if its complications develop.

Resources for Diseases of the Heart and Blood Vessels

There is no single book that covers the entire field of heart disease adequately. Look for these or other books in your local library or bookstore.

Dr. Dean Ornish's Program for Reversing Heart Disease, Ivy Books, New York (1996).

Heartcare, rev. ed. American Medical Association. Random House, New York (1984).

Your Heart: Questions You Have... Answers You Need, Peoples Medical Society, Allentown, Penn. (1996).

Heart to Heart: Cleveland Clinic Guide to Understanding Heart Disease and Open Heart Surgery. N. V. Richards. Atheneum, New York (1987).

Mayo Clinic Heart Book, K. Michael D McGoon, ed., William Morrow, New York (1993).

Women and Children Living Well

Chapter Nineteen

Living Well As A Diabetic Woman

This chapter was written by Cathy Feste for the first edition. We have edited it minimally and brought it up to date. Cathy is a nationally recognized health motivation specialist, president of her own wellness consulting business, and the author of the best-selling book *The Physician Within*.

As a woman who has lived with diabetes for 40 years, I know that it carries with it some special challenges. I have seen my blood sugars swoop when a period is approaching. I saw my insulin requirements nearly quadruple during my pregnancy. As I nursed my baby, I faced the additional challenges of low blood sugar as my body burned extra calories.

Those are physical issues. But there's another side to life with diabetes. Being unwilling to miss out on the fun and fulfillment of life has required extra creativity. As a teenager, I found that cheerleading and marching band worked out fine if I hid LifeSavers in my uniform. Girl Scout canoe trips were not a problem if I kept insulin, syringes, testing strips, and carbohydrates in airtight plastic containers that would float. These early successes gave me the confidence as an adult to ski in the Rocky Mountains.

Living well as a diabetic woman requires adapting to certain physical requirements without sacrificing the quality of life. It's a constant balancing act. This chapter discusses the major physical issues unique to women with diabetes. It also explores some emotional and spiritual concerns associated with the disease.

Physical Issues

Diabetes presents women with special challenges during pregnancy, menstruation, and menopause. The interactions between blood sugar and hormone levels during these times affect our blood glucose regulation. Control, in turn, has a profound effect on pregnancy. Awareness of these effects will help you to manage both your diabetes and these aspects of your womanhood.

Menstruation

Interviews with both diabetic women and doctors reveal that, although hormones affect blood glucose levels, the effect is not uniform in all women. Even more frustrating is the fact that the effect can vary in the same woman; some months the blood sugars may rise dramatically, and some months they fall. Living well with the hormonal challenge requires a team effort. It is important for you to have medical advisors on your team who are knowledgeable and experienced in diabetes as well as female issues. They will best understand the general effect of hormones on blood sugars. Your job as a member of the team will be to record blood glucose levels accurately before, during, and after your menstrual periods. If you find a definite pattern, then together you can determine an appropriate course of action. If, for example, your blood sugar levels are consistently high the week before your period begins, then you may be able to successfully anticipate the increased need for insulin. However, it may not be that easy if your needs cannot be anticipated. The hormonal impact may vary or your periods may be inconsistent.

There is an individualized and changeable hormonal impact on blood sugar levels. Your choices are as follows.

1. With the help of your medical advisors, make a monthly plan of action designed to anticipate and meet your needs.
2. Do nothing anticipatory, but deal with the fluctuating blood sugars with the same strategies you use to cope with any stress-related, unpredictable blood sugars.

In addition, remember the strategy used by every woman in dealing with a period: When you can't exactly predict when it's coming, you start carrying some form of protection with you toward the end of the month so that you're prepared when it starts. We get frustrated and angry about periods when we are not prepared for them. The same is true of diabetes. Insulin reactions or high sugar levels are far more frustrating to us when we are ill prepared to handle them. When we handle them well, we increase our entire sense of well-being.

Birth Control

Since blood glucose should be under control before a woman becomes pregnant, it is important that a woman with diabetes practice birth control as soon as she becomes sexually active. Various methods are available. The method of choice will be determined through careful consideration of its effect on the woman's health as well as her personal preference.

In her book *The Diabetic Woman,* Dr. Lois Jovanovic recommends that if a woman does not have high blood pressure, she may use low-dose birth control pills. Their impact on insulin doses is minimal. Dr. Jovanovic writes that research shows that birth control pills do not increase the risk of blood clots. (Women with diabetic retinopathy should seek the advice of a specialist in diabetic retinopathy.) Dr. Jovanovic further points out that some women will require higher-dose pills that do affect glucose and insulin requirements.

If birth control pills are not chosen, women can use barrier methods such as the diaphragm, condom, or cervical sponge. Talk this over with a trusted medical advisor.

Pregnancy

The outcome of diabetic pregnancies has improved dramatically. Many years ago, women with diabetes had miscarriages at an alarmingly higher rate than did their nondiabetic counterparts. Today, a healthy woman with diabetes can expect an outcome similar to that of the general population if

1. She is seen and closely followed by a knowledgeable medical team experienced in diabetic pregnancies. Teams vary from center to center, but they usually include specialists in endocrinology, diabetology, obstetrics, dietetics, nursing, psychology, and social work or family counseling.

2. She is educated about caring for diabetes and is motivated to act on what she learns.
3. Her diabetes is under control before she becomes pregnant.
4. She keeps blood glucose levels within normal limits throughout the pregnancy. Research indicates that babies in utero tolerate low blood sugars much better than they tolerate high blood sugars.

The mother's health should be assessed before she conceives. If she has existing complications, especially of the kidney and eye, she must be informed about what effects the pregnancy might have on her health and the health of her baby. After an evaluation by a doctor extensively educated and experienced in both diabetes and pregnancy, the potential mother can make an informed choice about whether or not to attempt a pregnancy.

Ask your physician how many diabetic pregnancies he or she has managed. Also ask for a description of how your physician manages diabetic pregnancies. You need to have an obstetrician and a diabetes care specialist who are knowledgeable and experienced with diabetic pregnancies. If you know of no such physicians, ask your local American Diabetes Association chapter for a referral.

"When I decided to get married, my physician said to me: 'I think it's fine if you get married. But don't ever have children. Don't spread your genes around.' Because I am an educator, I believe that people ought to be given information and then make their own decisions. I felt that this doctor was giving me his personal opinion rather than information upon which to make a very important decision. So, my husband and I saw a genetic counselor who gave us not only information, but also a great deal of encouragement about the genetic issues involved. Appropriately informed about genetic issues and my good health, my husband and I chose to have a baby."

Another essential element of a successful pregnancy is good health insurance. Even an uncomplicated diabetic pregnancy includes extra tests and visits to the medical team. A complicated pregnancy could include a lengthy hospitalization as well as intensive neonatal care for the baby. Make sure you have good health insurance before you become pregnant.

Throughout pregnancy, you should keep your blood sugars as nearly normal as possible. Chapter 5 of this book provides detailed information for learning the intensive regimen needed for this level of control. Your doctor will adapt this regimen to your individual needs. Besides the impact on the overall successful outcome of a pregnancy, it is important to keep blood sugars in normal range for the sake of the baby's size. The pregnant mother's blood sugar crosses the placenta. When the sugars are high, the baby's pancreas produces insulin to normalize them. In the process of using the mother's blood sugar, the baby gains weight. The baby's weight is one of the factors that determines the method through which the baby is delivered. Babies of normal weight can be delivered vaginally if the health of both the mother and the baby is otherwise good. Large babies must be delivered by Caesarean section.

Close blood sugar control presents numerous challenges. Ironically, close control increases the risk of severe insulin reactions (hypoglycemia). Fortunately, this is not a great problem for the baby, because babies can tolerate low blood sugar much better than high blood sugar. The risk of low blood sugar is to the mother and her diabetes management. One undesirable result of low blood sugar is a swing to high blood sugar (hyperglycemia) and a bouncing effect that can upset one's control for a day or longer. Testing blood sugars more frequently is an excellent strategy for avoiding hypoglycemia.

One reason blood sugars rise too high following a low-blood-sugar episode is that people sometimes eat more than they need to counteract the lower sugar level.

"While I was pregnant, I forced myself to drink four ounces of juice and then wait a full fifteen minutes before taking anything more if the symptoms had not subsided. To help me wait, I pretended that it was a middle-of-the-night feeding for the baby. I viewed this strategy of treating low blood sugar as good practice for motherhood."

With self blood glucose monitoring, we now have tools to tell us the impact of the food we eat. This is especially helpful when we need to assess the impact on low blood sugar. After you have eaten, you should wait fifteen minutes before rechecking blood sugar. After fifteen minutes, if the reading is still low and has not moved toward normal levels, drink another glass of juice or milk and retest in another fifteen minutes.

Doing periodic 3:00 a.m. blood tests can help to prevent problems with very low blood sugars. Report middle-of-the-night low blood sugars to your doctor. A change in your insulin dosage may be required. You may already be doing 3:00 a.m. blood tests on days when you are unusually active and are more inclined to an ongoing blood sugar-lowering effect. Knowing your body and your unique responses to activity, food, and stress is extremely helpful.

Close control of blood sugars will mean that your lifestyle during pregnancy will be closely regulated. This may not be typical of your usual way of living. Most of us slide off our regimens occasionally, and some do so fairly frequently. Reflect carefully on your willingness to maintain tight control in order to have a responsible pregnancy. Although it does require effort on the part of the diabetic woman, many women have reported that it actually turned out to be less of a challenge than they had anticipated. A common comment from pregnant women with diabetes is that their growing abdomen serves as a constant reminder of why they're working so hard.

"I made a commitment to follow my diabetic regimen to a point of perfection. Neither birthday nor any other holiday succeeded in tempting me to deviate from my meal plan. I related to a cartoon I saw just before Christmas. Two little boys in a department store were standing before a Christmas display. One boy said to the other, 'I'm so good at this time of year I can hardly stand myself.' While I understood that feeling, I also made the surprising discovery that it actually became easier and easier simply to make no exceptions. And I had a tremendous amount of support from the medical team.

"The team of mother, father, obstetrician, diabetologist, dietitian, and nurse worked hard to make my pregnancy successful. I was extremely thankful to have an upbeat, 'human' medical team whose humor and warmth reinforced the excitement of a pregnancy instead of treating it like a high-risk, complicated medical problem. Whenever the seriousness of the situation did arise, I felt supported rather than fearful. For example, my diabetes doctor told me that any sign of infection, high sugars, or ketones should be reported immediately and not be left until tomorrow. It wasn't frightening to hear him say that, just reassuring to know that he would be there to help.

"Besides wonderful medical support, I was blessed with a supportive husband who gave me a steady diet of love and humor. As my abdomen increased, I began to wonder how much longer I should inject my insulin abdominally. Although my obstetrician gave me the answer 'as long as it is both physically and psychologically comfortable,' it was my husband's response that took the prize. He told me, 'Just keep injecting in your abdomen until you hear someone say "ouch."' Humor gives wonderful perspective."

Laboratory tests are an important part of support in a diabetic pregnancy. Each test and each visit to your medical team is an excellent reminder that you are not alone. Skilled people are doing everything they can to help you.

The baby's birth does not signify the end of the close working relationship between the mother and medical team. If you choose to nurse your baby, you must be well informed about your caloric needs for milk production as well as the ongoing balancing act with insulin. Throughout pregnancy, insulin requirements increase. Toward the end of a pregnancy, a woman may be taking two to three times as much insulin as in her prepregnancy days. At the time of birth, insulin requirements drop dramatically and a woman becomes extremely sensitive to insulin. Some women require no insulin immediately following delivery. The nursing mother may drop bedtime insulin entirely as her body burns many calories overnight for the production of milk. The teamwork continues. The baby is its newest member.

Because information on diabetic pregnancies is continually changing and growing, we encourage you to rely more on your medical advisors than on any printed information. Reflect on the issues. Make informed, responsible choices.

To Pregnant Women Whose Diabetes Is Not In Good Control... The advice given so far on preparing for a diabetic pregnancy may raise fears in anyone who is already pregnant and maintaining less-than-excellent blood glucose control. Have you endangered either your baby's health or your own? There is no simple answer. You must discuss your situation with an obstetrician experienced in diabetic pregnancies.

In the past, when tight control was not yet possible, many women had successful pregnancies with only minor difficulties. Statistically, these women and their babies were in greater risk, but each individual pregnancy had its own outcome. Even if your control has been moderate to poor, you may still have few problems if you regulate your blood glucose levels now. Discuss this fully with your medical team.

Beyond this, you may want to explore the techniques for working through possible resistance to maintaining good control in Chapters 3 and 15.

Vaginitis

Some women report that their diabetes was diagnosed when they went to see their doctor about severe vaginal itching. This problem is usually due to yeast infection. Diabetic women have an increased incidence of yeast infections because yeast grows more rapidly in glucose. The infections occur more frequently when blood sugars are high enough that glucose is present in the urine. Your doctor can prescribe treatments for yeast infections, but prevention is better. Generally these infections can be prevented by keeping the urine free of sugar.

Recently, a well-controlled study showed that eating 8 ounces of yogurt each day decreased the number of yeast present in the vagina as well as the number of yeast infections. It is important to make sure that the yogurt you buy in the market contains live (not pasteurized) lactobacilli acidophilus. The L. acidophilus presumably directly inhibits yeast growth and survival. (Clearly, this treatment is great if you like yogurt. Of course, you must count the yogurt in your diet.)

If you choose to keep blood sugars in a normal range, refer to Chapter 5, "The Intensive Regimen." Using this chapter as a guide, discuss improving your regimen with your physician.

Menopause

At some point in middle age, women cease having periods. Because certain hormones are no longer present, the need for insulin usually drops. However, if the hormones are replaced, then insulin requirements will be affected by the estrogen and progesterone. According to Dr. Lois Jovanovic, a noted authority in diabetic women's issues and herself a diabetic, the insulin requirements with hormone replacement are determined by how closely the hormone doses match the woman's needs. Higher doses of hormones require higher doses of insulin.

Day-to-day variations during menopause are far easier to handle with blood glucose monitoring. Some women experience profuse sweating during menopause and wonder if it is caused by hypoglycemia or by their "change." With blood testing, a woman can generally figure out what's happening and get in control of her life.

Hormones do affect blood sugar levels. You can choose whether or not to take hormones. Because a history of cancer is another factor to consider in making this decision, it is best to discuss all the factors with your carefully selected medical advisors. Remember that you are a unique person, and the effect your hormones have on your blood sugar levels may be different from what you hear from other women or read about. When books describe what is normal, they are more accurately describing what is average. Since few of us are "average," you should work with your medical team to understand your unique reactions. Doing this is another leg of the journey toward personal growth and fulfillment.

It is comforting to have support for the physical needs of diabetes. But there is another type of support that is equally important, if not more so. That is emotional support.

Emotional Issues

I believe that women who have diabetes have a distinct advantage over men who have diabetes. Traditionally, women have found it easier to connect with friends on an emotional level. To receive emotional support, one needs to understand the language and be willing to engage in the process of both seeking and receiving it. The language of emotional support includes "I feel... I need... I am angry, fearful, lonely because..." "It makes me feel so good when..." Getting emotional support includes a willingness to begin conversations with phrases like these. The process also requires time and an appropriate setting. A fifteen-minute commute on the way to work won't do it. A meeting in a relaxed atmosphere like a restaurant or your home, with an hour's worth of time, is more likely to allow the process to work.

People who feel reticent to begin talking with their friends about the feelings they have about diabetes may find it very helpful to attend a meeting of the local American Diabetes Association. Meeting others who have diabetes often creates an instantaneous bond that connects people on an emotional level.

A variety of support groups are available to people who are interested in group interaction. These allow people who have diabetes and are feeling "stuck" to meet one-to-one with others who have diabetes. This effective program provides two-way benefit, as both the giver and the recipient find support. If this type of program appeals to you, check with your local ADA chapter or call 1-800-DIABETES for a local referral. Whether it's through a formalized program of social support or the casual warmth of two friends having coffee, take the step toward connecting on a feeling level. It may seem awkward at first, but keep at it. The rewards are great.

Dating and Marriage

Some women are reluctant to tell their dates that they have diabetes. If you are dating, consider the following scenarios.

  1. Which situation would be better?

Living Well As A Diabetic Woman

a. You have an insulin reaction when you are with a man who knows you have diabetes.

b. You have a reaction when you are with someone who hasn't a clue as to why your behavior is changed.

2. You are dating someone who needs to eat at a particular time. Would you prefer to have your date tell you that? Or, would you prefer to have him jeopardize his health to eat a fashionably late dinner?

3. Do you really believe that diabetes is such an awful disease that someone would not want to date you because of it?

a. If your answer is yes, you should talk to a diabetes educator who can help you to adapt to diabetes and have a fun and full social life.

b. If your answer is no, remember that you can influence the way your date thinks about diabetes. Present it positively, as a disease that can be controlled through a healthy lifestyle.

"A touching and reinforcing moment for me came at a party, one evening when I overhead my husband say to the group of people with whom he was visiting: 'The best thing that ever happened to me was marrying someone with diabetes. We live such a healthy life.'

"Dating was not particularly problematic for me in terms of my diabetes until marriage became an issue. It is at major decision points in life—such as marriage, career, children—that one is confronted again with accepting the fact that diabetes, like any chronic disease, is unavoidably a part of life and of that decision.

"While my husband and I were dating, I wondered about what diabetes would mean for him if were married. But I did like his attitude. He was at ease—never treating me like a 'diabetic,' but rather as an attractive (to him) young woman. And he had just the right measure of concern; that is, he asked questions about appropriate restaurant choice, timing of meals, and what, if any, dessert I would eat when we ate at his parents' house for the first time. Humor helped us through the rough spots (and it still does!).

"But somewhere in my subconscious a shadow was lurking, and I couldn't quite make out what it meant. A wonderfully sensitive physician helped me bring it into the light so that I could see it and deal with it. It was this: Just before I became engaged, I visited my doctor. In the waiting room, I met a young woman exactly my age who was losing her sight as a result of diabetes.

"Suddenly I had an urgent need to know the future. I wanted my doctor to look into a crystal ball and tell me what course my diabetes would take, so that I would have some idea of what 'for better or worse' might mean to my husband.

My doctor gently explained to me that no one knows what the future will bring. Perhaps the most profound lesson that diabetes has taught me is this: Diabetes does not make life any more uncertain. It simply makes us more aware of the uncertainty of life."

People blessed with the awareness that life is uncertain are in a unique position to enjoy life more fully. Time is more likely to be savored than wasted. All of life's experiences become a potential source of wonder. The embarrassment of saying "I love you" gives way to appreciation for having the courage to say it.

It is helpful to be able to identify what makes your life fulfilling, because that's what will motivate you to handle any challenge that threatens your enjoyment of life. Your desire to live fully will mobilize the great inner strengths that you have.

"My husband and I wed and have enjoyed healthy, happy times. Four years after we married, we had a child. I knew that our son would never see his mother coping with stress by taking alcohol or drugs. My early experiences had already set healthy stress-management habits of diet and activity.

"Our family life has been full. I have felt great and participated actively and fully in my teaching career as well as having a social life of partying, cross-country skiing, and bicycling."

Most women fully expect to enjoy retirement with their husbands. They also expect to watch every hockey game of their children as they grow up. They look forward to graduation, weddings and grandchildren. Without the challenge of a chronic disease, it is easier to deny that untimely death could ever rob them of their lifelong plans. Besides a mighty important lesson about the uncertainty of life, diabetes can give one the gift of appreciating how precious life is. It's an odd and profound gift that is difficult to explain. It's like appreciating the fragile, exquisite beauty of a snowflake with the understanding that it may be the last one you'll ever see along with the faith that it isn't. Perhaps the oddest part of the gift is the realization that we receive this gift through suffering. The painful awareness of our mortality actually gives us the gift of appreciating life.

Although there surely are times when diabetes causes us to grapple with life's most profound issues, there are plenty of times when having diabetes is little more than a minor inconvenience. Balancing the emotions of those very different viewpoints is important to one's overall well-being.

"At about the six-week point in my pregnancy (before it had been confirmed), I attended a diabetes and pregnancy conference. It was directed to health professionals and contained (to me, because I suspected I was pregnant) a ton of horror. I heard someone talk about the possibility of brain damage to the baby if ketones were present in the early weeks of development. That horrified me because I had been experiencing fasting ketosis recently. I went to my doctor immediately following the conference. He explained that in the early weeks of fetal development the body's need for calories is greatly increases, and that's why I had ketones in my urine. An increase in calories and insulin took care of the physical problems.

"I resolved to avoid similar conferences during my pregnancy to alleviate my emotional discomfort. But this is not to recommend ignorance as bliss. Education is a most important ally. I sincerely believe that one must strive for the balance of knowing what you need to know and then avoiding a mental diet of facts that only frighten and immobilize the spirit. I knew that my carefully selected physicians knew the facts, dangers, and cautions of a diabetic pregnancy. I allowed them to do the worrying. I concentrated my efforts on doing all that they recommended and then did everything possible to keep mind and spirit positive and hopeful."

To follow a self-care regimen, we need to accept the seriousness of diabetes as well as our personal vulnerability. Then, we also need hope. We need to understand all of our options for health and act on them. Reflect on the issues that cause you emotional discomfort. Talk them over with a trusted advisor. Act to prevent problems, and promote health and well-being. By taking positive action, you will gain an overall sense of control over your life.

Career Concerns

Until the mid-eighties, women were bombarded with advice about what to do with their lives. We were urged to seek nontraditional careers. We were told to rebel against being "just homemakers." But now the pendulum seems to be swinging toward more reasonable advice: Women should be able to choose whatever they want to do—have a career, go to school, stay at home, do volunteer work, or combine any of these choices. If the choices they make are manageable and fulfilling, women can find satisfaction and harmony in their lives. If they undertake either too little or too much, the effects are negative and stressful. Balance is essential to anyone who wants a happy, healthy life. We need enough meaningful activity to give life excitement and a sense of purpose, but not so much activity that we are overwhelmed by demands on us. All men and women struggle with this balancing of life. When diabetes is present, it is simply another ball to juggle.

Reflect on your own life challenges as I share a few of mine.

Diabetes goes with me:

▷ Into the hospital where I do volunteer work. I attend monthly meetings from 4:00 until 6:00 p.m. To keep balance, I do a blood test just before the meeting and then help myself to the fruit and crackers offered if I need them. My own supply of dried fruit is ever at hand should I need more.

▷ On national and international airplane flights. I juggle time-zone changes and insulin requirements according to my doctor's good advice. With snacks like dried fruit and granola bars in my purse or briefcase, I can cope when a meal flight ends up serving no food. I always carry my blood glucose meter with me on the plane. Extra tests reassure me that I am remaining in balance.

▷ Up to the podium as I make presentations. A blood test before speaking tells me if my jitters are simply from nervousness or if I am hypoglycemic.

▷ Into those "one-hour" meetings that begin at 11:00 a.m. and end at 1:00 p.m. Inconspicuous snacks like LifeSavers keep me going without interrupting the meeting.

Diabetes is ever present when I'm working too many hours and forgetting to balance my work with exercise (for the body). I have seen tests of 400 as a result of the distress of imbalance. It is tempting to curse my diabetes, saying "If it weren't for that darned diabetes, I could keep up the same pace as my friends do!" But then I look at the picture more carefully. What is really happening is this: Diabetes tells me when life is out of balance and my body is asking me not to abuse it. Diabetes, in this case, is a blessing in disguise. In fact, I often find myself cautioning my nondiabetic friends to take better care of themselves. Although they know the harmful effects of stress, they don't have a tool (like my blood glucose meter) to tell them that their stress is harming them.

Living Well As A Diabetic Woman

The heart of life is neither male or female, for it beats for all. The skills we need to live well with diabetes are the very same skills that anyone needs to meet the inevitable pain and challenges of life. To experience joy and soul-satisfying growth, we need to believe that diabetes has that gift to give. Great philosophers teach us that pain hollows us out, allowing us to hold more joy. They even suggest that pain holds as much wonder as joy. Indeed, joy and sorrow are inseparable in the same way that pain and growth often come together.

With maturity, we all become philosophers to some degree. If we can accept the philosophy that pain brings growth, then we have the foundation upon which to build a healthy life. Nietzsche said that people who have a *why* to life can bear almost any *how*. With this belief, we accept diabetes as one more building block of life.

Chapter Twenty

Living Young
With Diabetes

Believe it or not, every grown-up has a child inside that remembers what it's like to be a kid. The authors of this book asked the kids inside them to write about having diabetes when they were young. Cathy was 10, Gary was 12, and Ernie was 14 when their diabetes started.

You're really lucky to be a kid now. The doctors and nurses today know so much more about diabetes than when we were kids. They're good at helping you learn all the things you need to know about taking care of yourself. They've finally figured out that kids can do all kinds of complex things, like testing their own blood sugar. Children are a lot smarter than most grown-ups probably realize.

Having diabetes keeps us on our toes—more than most people. Some great entertainers, public figures, and athletes have diabetes. Wade Wilson, Mary Tyler Moore, Halle Barry, Sylvia Chase, and Catfish Hunter—have diabetes, and it hasn't stopped them. It doesn't have to stop you. With diabetes or without, there is a world of things we can accomplish if we really want to.

The kid inside Ernie says:

One dumb thing I had to get over when I was a kid was pretending not to have diabetes. For a long time, I ate whatever I wanted (usually when no one was looking). I even forgot shots and ended up in the hospital in a coma one time. I thought if I acted like I didn't have diabetes, it would just go away. But it didn't.

I think I would have been a lot happier if I had taken better care of myself. I don't mean being perfect! But I wish I had remembered my shots, done my tests regularly, and not eaten sweets so often. I guess I thought the doctor and my mom and dad were the ones I did these things for, and I resented them for that. Now I know you do those things for yourself, not for anybody else.

Sometimes having diabetes makes me feel sad or angry or afraid. Don't ever think you shouldn't have these feelings. They are a natural part of you, and there's no reason to pretend you don't have them. When I kept my feelings inside, I ended up doing things that were worse than saying "I'm angry."

The kid inside Gary says:

My doctor wanted me to meet another young person with diabetes while I was still in the hospital. (When I was a kid, you had to stay in the hospital for several days just to get regulated). I was embarrassed to meet this person. It was even worse because he was coming to the hospital just to see me. I don't remember his name, but he was just a little older than me and he seemed nice. I remember him telling me that taking insulin gets to be a habit, like brushing our teeth. It helped me to talk to someone else who had diabetes. It took away some of my fear. At the time, I didn't think it was that important to me. But it was. I still remember it! It made me realize that even the most difficult things can be learned and become part of our routine. As humans, we are much more adaptable than we can imagine.

In a way, diabetes really helped me grow up. I learned about taking responsibility. I learned how to talk about diabetes and even other things without being ashamed. I learned how to talk to the coaches at school and the dietitian in the school kitchen. I learned how to arrange my life so that diabetes didn't interfere too much. I learned how to go out with my friends and do what they did and still keep my diabetes under pretty good control.

The kid inside Cathy says:

When I was little, they didn't even have blood sugar testing you could do at home. Blood tests are a lot better than testing your urine. They help you know if you have enough energy for playing hard without having reactions. But remember, those test numbers are just facts to help you. They don't say whether you're a good person or a bad person. They just tell what your blood sugar is, so you can figure out how to change your insulin, food, or exercise.

It's a little like being a scientist. If your blood sugar is higher or lower than you want it to be, you can usually figure out why. Maybe you ran extra hard today. Maybe your snack was bigger than usual. Maybe you've got a bad cold. Maybe you got angry at your brother. When you figure out the reason your blood sugars are off, you're not only a scientist, you're a detective, too!

My doctor first told me I had diabetes when I was in the hospital for a broken arm. A clown came to my room to cheer me up and give me a balloon. I said, "I just have a broken arm and diabetes. I'm not sick!" I went on feeling that way and never saw diabetes as a reason not to do anything. I did everything my friends did, except for eating a lot of sweet things.

I asked my mom if having diabetes would make me different from the other kids. She told me, "You'll be stronger and more in charge of your life. You'll learn how to take care of yourself and eat the right things. That will mean our whole family will benefit because we'll learn to take care of ourselves from you."

All three of us say:

We know having diabetes is a problem sometimes, but we want you to remember that having diabetes doesn't mean you're sick. You just have to watch some things other kids don't ever have to think about. (Some people think that makes

Diabetes: A Guide to Living Well

us smarter than other people.) But most of the things we are supposed to do are healthy for everybody.

You'll be learning about diabetes for a long time, probably the rest of your life. We hope there will be a cure for you to learn about someday. Scientists are working on it now, but nobody's sure when they'll find it. Until they do, take good care of yourself so the cure will work for you.

To The Parents Of A Youth Who Has Diabetes...

Credo for the parent of a child with diabetes

My child is an essentially healthy person who happens to have some qualities that need special attention, not a sick child who must be protected.

My child is capable of learning to handle all aspects of diabetes care over time, not someone who must remain dependent on me.

My child will learn to take good care of diabetes by following my model of healthful behavior and by receiving positive rewards, not from threats of the consequences of diabetes.

I will find the right balance between my responsibility as a parent and my child's growing responsibility for his or her own life, including the care of diabetes.

When I feel I can't cope, I will get the help I need to go on living well and aiding my child to live well. I do not need to sacrifice my life to diabetes.

To live well with childhood diabetes calls for a unique partnership between you and your child, one that can enrich and deepen your relationship. You can learn together, adapt together, and feel together as you meet the demands of this condition. With a preteen, especially, you become an authoritative source of information and guidance as you learn about diabetes. At the same time, you respect and support your child's growing capacity for self-management and participation in decision making.

Having a child with diabetes presents enough special challenges that you deserve a book specifically addressing your child's and your unique needs. Fortunately, there are several excellent ones that we suggest you read if you are the parent of a youth with diabetes. These books are listed at the end of this chapter, together with several other resources specific to parents and youth.

We begin with an often-neglected subject: your own needs as the parent of a youth with diabetes.

Take Care of Yourself!

Many of the techniques for living well described in this book apply to your life as well as your child's. Your maintenance of psychological health, good diet, and exercise programs become a model for your child. This is the very best way of teaching—to be what you want your child to become. With this understanding, taking care of yourself helps both you and your child. And you avoid the useless martyr role—sacrificing yourself for someone else's well-being.

Use the tips for stress management and coping included in Chapters 3, 12, and 15, and find a support group for parents through your local chapter of the American Diabetes Association. Parents with experience can help you cope with your problems and guide you in handling the problems that come up with your child. (See Chapter 14 for more on support groups and networks for both you and your child.)

Adapting the Living Well Approach to Your Child's Situation

The underlying approach of this book is respect for the capacity of the individual person with diabetes to make wise self-care choices. We believe the diabetes regimen must be individualized; that the desire to follow it grows when parental attention is positive rather than threatening; and that living well is a matter of one's whole life, not just blood sugar levels.

As the parent of a child or teenager, you may wonder if these beliefs are fully applicable without risk to your child. Can a child of 5 or 6 make wise choices to handle precise techniques like insulin injections or home blood glucose testing? What will control the rebelliousness of your teen other than threats of future catastrophes if he or she doesn't shape up?

Many parents and youths have demonstrated this approach by sharing responsibility fully, discussing decisions together, and gradually passing responsibility on to the growing child. Children as young as 5 have learned to use meters accurately to test blood sugar levels and to give their own insulin. Children in the pre-teen age range (we've heard about a few even younger) are using insulin pumps successfully. Rebelliousness may be an inevitable part of the teen years, but there is little evidence that coercion and threats are an effective way of handling it. The Living Well approach gives a teenager positive reinforcement and opportunities to learn to make more responsible choices.

Balance and Individualization

We have emphasized the need to design a diabetes treatment program specific to the needs and character of the individual throughout this book. Now we must consider two or three individuals—the child and the parents—as well as the rest of the family. Living well with youthful diabetes demands a balance between lives of all the family members and an adaptation to the unique pattern of the individual family.

Different families have very different patterns concerning responsibility, decision making, participation, emotional support, health practices, and other areas important to diabetes care. You must find a way of dealing with the demands of diabetes that fits your family's patterns. But you may need to change patterns that unintentionally undermine your child's ability to live well. He or she may find it difficult to follow a healthful lifestyle if the rest of the family eats an unhealthy diet, doesn't exercise, and handles stress poorly. Becoming responsible for his or her own care will be hard if the parents are either too protective or too dominating.

My Family Profile

To identify your family's patterns, explore your answers to this questionnaire. You can gain insight into your own family's patterns and how they may affect your youth with diabetes.

1. How are decisions made in your family?

_____

_____

Do you discuss issues together?

_____

_____

Do you explore alternative options to choose from?

_____

_____

Who participates in the actual decision making?

_____

_____

What matters do the children decide on their own?

_____

_____

In what areas are the children simply given orders?

_____

_____

2. How well do the children follow either their own decisions or suggestions, and orders given by parents?

_____

_____

Parent's opinions

_____

_____

Children's opinions

_____

_____

How well do the parents follow either their own decisions or directions given by external authority?

_____

_____

3. When a child disobeys or acts irresponsibly, how do the parents respond?

_____

_____

What is done to help the child act differently?

_____

_____

Do these things work?

_____

_____

4. In your family who has taken the responsibility to learn about diabetes?

_____

_____

_____ Mother   _____ Grandparent

_____ Father   _____ Other

_____ Child

5. Does the family as a whole follow a healthful lifestyle? _____

A moderate and balanced diet? _____

Regular exercise and activity? _____

Effective stress management? _____

Emotional stability? _____

6. What major challenges other than diabetes face you and your family?

_____

_____

Your answers may suggest areas where your family could strengthen its ability to cope with diabetes and other life challenges. Parents can use the results of this exercise to discuss possible changes, first between themselves and then with the whole family.

Ages And Phases Of Youthful Diabetes

The age of your child will determine how you adapt this book to your situation. In this section, we will make a few suggestions for different ages. Whatever the age of the child, we recommend you seek health care professionals who are knowledgeable and experienced in working with youthful diabetes. Diabetes care, particularly for children and teenagers, is best managed by an experienced team, including a physician, diabetes nurse educator, dietitian/nutritionist, and others as needed. This is even more vital now that we know from the DCCT that blood sugar control matters. It is logical that starting good blood sugar management early on increases the odds of avoiding serious complications.

Infancy to Age 4 or 5

If you have a young child with diabetes, this book will be a major educational source for you, but you will need further guidance in many aspects of caring for and educating your child. Your health care team and diabetes support network will play an important role, even more than with older children. The Introduction and Chapter 1 offer basic attitudes and practices that you can draw on in your parenting. Chapters 3, 12, and 15 will help you help yourself as well as your child with the emotional challenges of diabetes. When your child approaches school age, you can cautiously begin sharing responsibility for day-to-day diabetes tasks. As the young one demonstrates expertise under your supervision, you will gain confidence and a sense of what he or she can handle.

Age 5 to Puberty

As your child matures, you will be able to start passing on more and more responsibility for details of self-care. From this time, you will be able to use diabetes classes, support groups, and camps to supplement your roles in education and emotional support. Use *Diabetes: A Guide to Living Well* as a source book for answering questions and offering guidance. You and your doctor and other health care team members will help determine regimen choices for the child to consider. You will work together to build the positive motivation needed for following the resulting team program.

Teenage years

At this time, the basic approach presented throughout this book may be the most effective way of bypassing or quieting rebellion against diabetic regimen. See your child as capable of making responsible choices, as needing to participate fully in decisions about his or her health and lifestyle, and as the final authority over what he or she actually does with his or her life. With this point of view, there is a basis for negotiation that cannot exist if you hold onto this responsibility and authority. You are also more likely to keep communication open about what is going on with diabetes in your teen's life. Children who learn well from written material may be able to start working directly with *Diabetes: A Guide to Living Well*, although you may need to help. (This book is written at the high school level.)

Choosing The Level Of Regimen

For all but the very young, your doctor/health care team, your child, and you must work together to find a level of diabetic regimen and control that will work for all parties. Often the physician advises moderating or adapting the intensive regimen because of the greater dangers of insulin reactions in childhood. Children are usually much more active and engage in their activities with such intensity that the onset of reactions may be difficult to notice. Often they wish not to appear different because of their diabetes, and they may want to hide their vulnerability. The level of awareness demanded by the intensive regimen might cause some children to become preoccupied with their illness and some parents to become obsessive about it.

On the other hand, with the right combination of child, parents, and doctor, many children have learned to manage diabetes very carefully and live full, exuberant lives. Today, there are many variations of insulin regimens that provide great flexibility and can minimize the risk of reactions. The decision about the level of regimen a child is to learn to follow must be reached through thoughtful discussion between the whole family and the physician/health care team. The factors you will need to balance include

1. The long-term value of avoiding chronic high blood sugar levels.
2. The need to avoid frequent insulin reactions.
3. The feelings of your child and yourself.
4. Your child's age and learning skills.
5. Your child's growth pattern and overall health (chronically high blood sugar can slow growth and the onset of puberty).
6. Your child's activity patterns, sports schedules, lifestyle, and other personal preferences.

Diabetic Complications

Diabetes carries with it the risk of secondary disorders that may develop later in life. No subject in parenting requires more sensitivity than these possible complications. Along with insulin reactions and diabetic coma, they constitute a major threat and source of fear for parents and children alike. When your child begins to be aware of diabetic complications, you will need to convey carefully the nature of the threat and tell your child what to do to reduce the risk. (Your child may come to you in distress after hearing of a relative or friend of the family who has diabetes and has developed serious complications.) There are several important points to make:

> Some people with diabetes develop a complication, but many do not. The authors of this book, after well over 120 years of diabetes altogether, all see clearly, have no kidney disease, and have only minor complications.

> People with diabetes can do many things to lessen their risk of developing complications.

> Treatment for diabetic complications is improving; in many cases, treatment enables the person with diabetes to avoid disabilities altogether.

> If your child is old enough, discuss the concept of risk, and how everyone is at risk and has to learn to deal with the fears this produces. Life has threats, but we live well by remembering life's promises more than the threats.

> In general, answer the questions your child brings up, but don't flood him or her with too much information. Keep a balance between the facts and the emotional reassurance you offer.

You should not force information about complications on your child, and, above all, you should never use threats of dire consequences to encourage your child to follow regimen. Either practice is likely to build more anxiety than adherence. Carefully inspect any booklets or audiovisual presentations on complications before using them. Old educational materials often use frightening, worst-case photos and threatening language. Even current publications on complications are seldom written with sensitivity to the emotional needs of the reader.

Before discussing complications with your child, read Chapter 16 and the sections on preventive measures in Chapter 18. Deal with your own feelings about these threats first, so you can be calm in helping your child.

Diabetes Power Struggles

Any parents and children may develop power struggles over the children's behavior. With diabetes, however, these conflicts can take on an extreme level of emotion when "not doing the right thing" appears to threaten the child's very survival. As the parent, you may feel anxious, frantic, and possibly angry when your child "forgets" insulin repeatedly or eats excessive amounts of sweets. If your anxiety causes you to try to force your child to follow a regimen, you may simply incite your child to rebel even more.

You can do several things to avoid turning a matter of such genuine concern into a full power struggle:

▷ Deal with your own feelings apart from the situation. Don't dump them on your child.

▷ Ask your child to help you understand what is happening and what changes are needed to handle the problem. Work with your child rather than giving commands.

▷ Look at your child's behavior in terms of what is happening in his or her life. How does having diabetes function to reward the child with attention; to allow him or her to escape obligations or responsibilities; or to express feelings he or she can't express directly? How can you help satisfy these needs directly?

▷ Are there barriers—knowledge or skill related, social, attitudinal, or environmental—that are impeding the desirable behaviors?

▷ Set goals together, with a clear understanding of how you will both know when they are met. If it fits your parenting style, set appropriate rewards and penalties.

▷ Work with the basic understanding that you have a problem to solve together, not that your child is the problem.

Finally, understand that in some matters of regimen there is room for a few little vacations. Sweets, for instance, are not poison to a person with diabetes; they are simply something to be eaten with moderation. Don't let your child think that the only time he or she can eat a dessert or piece of candy is during an insulin reaction. Dietitians have found that regular nondietetic ice cream at mealtime does not increase blood sugar level seriously, so long as it is not covered with lots of gooey toppings.

Diabetic For A Day

Parents and diabetes professionals have gained remarkable empathy by living as someone with diabetes for a day or more. They test their blood several times a day, take injections of sterile water, watch their food plan, and follow an activity or exercise program. If you care to enter into your child's reality in this way, you will discover a new level of respect for what he or she must do each day. And your youngster will be delighted that you have taken this dramatic step to see the world in this new way.

The empathy this simulation teaches is the foundation for good parenting. When your love for your child is supported by this sort of respect and understanding, you both find that you can live well with diabetes.

Books For Parents Of A Youth With Diabetes

Kid's Corner. For children with diabetes. Children aged 8 to 12 have fun as they learn about diabetes through this booklet of puzzles and games. Order from the American Diabetes Association, 1-800-232-6733.

A Book on Diabetes for Brothers and Sisters. Linda Siminerio. Children's Hospital of Pittsburgh, Pennsylvania.

Sweet Kids: How to Balance Diabetes Control and Good Nutrition with Family Peace. Betty Page Brackenridge and Richard Rubin. This is a terrific new book for parents and other caregivers. Order from the ADA also.

In Control: A Guide for Teens with Diabetes. Jean Betschart and Susan Thom. A readable, straight-talking book directed specifically at teenagers, but parents will certainly benefit as well. Deals with all the tough teenage problems and decisions. Available from Chronimed Publishing, 1-800-848-2793.

A Magic Ride in Foozbah-Land. Jean Betschart. With full-color illustrations, this book guides 3- to 7-year-olds and their parents through an amusing tale that leads to a better understanding of diabetes and how to manage it. Available from Chronimed Publishing, 1-800-848-2793.

Chapter Twenty-One

Living Well
In The Future

Introduction

The pace of diabetes research continues to accelerate. As researchers march toward a "cure," what will this mean for those of us with diabetes? First, it will become easier and easier to control our blood sugar, either through new technological devices or advances in pancreas and islet cell transplants. Second, new ways to prevent or treat complications will be discovered. Third, researchers are investigating the feasibility of actually preventing the development of diabetes in those at risk. Intimately tied to each of these areas will be a better understanding of the immune reactions that cause diabetes, as well as the genes that predispose or prevent the development of diabetes and its complications.

Easier Blood Sugar Control

External insulin pumps worn outside the body have been available for several years. However, implantable pumps (about the size of a hockey puck but likely to become smaller) surgically inserted under the skin are in the final phases of experimental trials. The pump is filled approximately monthly by injecting very concentrated insulin into a reservoir in the pump, which then releases insulin as programmed by a hand-held remote control device. Instead of under the skin (subcutaneously), the insulin is released directly into the peritoneal cavity (the space between the abdominal wall and the organs in the abdomen) close to the liver. This is a more normal, physiologic way to absorb the insulin, and this tends to improve and smooth out blood sugars compared to subcutaneous delivery. However, the user must still test blood sugars frequently—and this means pricking the finger each time. On the horizon are two advances that will alleviate this concern: the noninvasive glucose meter and the implantable glucose sensor.

Several companies and researchers are developing meters that can read sugar levels within the body without drawing even a drop of blood! One device measures the absorbance of laser or near infrared (NIR) light beams directed through the skin in blood vessels of the finger or wrist. Another directs the laser beam into the watery fluid near the front of the eye (the aqueous humor) and calculates the sugar based on the deflection of the beam caused by the sugar concentration. A third is worn like a wrist watch and uses a tiny electrical current to draw body fluid into a disposable pad attached to the watch. It then makes the necessary calculations. Another samples the glucose level in the fluid between the cells of the body (interstitial fluid), sampled from the forearm area where there are fewer pain receptors. Over 20 companies are in various stages of product development, using these technologies or some variation. They will proceed through their trial periods, fail or become approved by the FDA, and will be marketed to health professionals and the public—but at a cost (at least initially); probably 10 to 50 times the cost of invasive meters! And the field so far has had many false starts and failures.

Work is also proceeding to develop an implantable glucose sensor. In the past, development has been plagued by technical problems: The sensor clogs or accuracy fails in a few months. Work in progress includes a very fine disposable sensor, that would be inserted under the skin and left in place for 5 to 10 days. An external device would take readings transmitted by telemetry. It is likely that the technical problems will be solved in the next few years, and the implantable sensor, in conjunction with the implantable pump, will create a true artificial pancreas.

Manufacturers are making more and more comfortable lancets (thinner and sharper), lancet devices (adjustable penetration, smoother action), needles (thinner and sharper), and insulin delivery devices (easy-to-use-and-carry pens, and improved needle-free jet injectors).

In the meantime, progress is being made in the development of aerosolized insulin, either through a nasal spray or inhaled through the mouth, similar to the familiar inhalers for asthma. The oral inhalers appear to be less irritating than the nasal spray, and are absorbed more efficiently into the lungs and bloodstream. Long term effects of this method of delivery are still not known.

As for the traditional insulin preparations, we expect that in the next few years, all the animal-source insulins will be replaced by synthetic genetically engineered insulin. Animal ultralente already is no longer available in the United States. The engineered insulins are pure and not dependent on an external supply of animal pancreases. However, we hope manufacturers keep working to genetically engineer insulin with a variety of activity profiles (onset, peak, and duration) to add flexibility to the user's armamentarium. Insulin lispro (see Chapter 5), the very rapid acting regular insulin, is an example of these insulin analogs. In particular, we would like to see some tinkering to develop an Ultralente insulin that matches the longer duration and peak-free action of the old beef/pork Ultralente (see Ultralente anecdote in Chapter 5). One such analog insulin is already in clinical trials. It is intended to provide a relatively constant, "basal" level of activity, mimicking the body's own.

Amylin (Pramintide) is a recently discovered hormone that is also secreted by the pancreas and must be injected the same as insulin. It is now in clinical trials, and it is hoped that it will be useful for insulin users in smoothing out wide swings in blood sugars, avoiding hypoglycemia, and decreasing the rate of absorption of carbohydrates in the stomach.

Some substances from the worlds of alternative, complementary or "integrative" medicine may prove helpful in blood sugar regulation, particularly in Type 2 (noninsulin dependent) diabetes.

First, a chromium supplement (in the form of a pill—chromium picolinate) has been shown not only to decrease blood lipids (total cholesterol and LDL) by about 10 percent but also blood glucose by about 25 percent. It was particularly effective in American Indians, who have a high incidence of noninsulin-dependent diabetes. A more recent well-controlled study showed that 4 months of high doses of chromium picolinate (500 micrograms twice a day) reduced blood sugar levels and cholesterol significantly in people with Type 2 diabetes. The drug appears to have few toxic or side effects, but these results are still preliminary. Furthermore, the study participants lived in China, and may have had a chromium deficient diet.

Another nutritional supplement, lipoic acid, a naturally occurring antioxidant in our body, may have some benefit in those with diabetes. It may improve regeneration of damaged nerves in diabetic neuropathy, and decrease the glycation that we discussed in Chapter 18. It may also lower blood sugar levels. A typical dose is 50 to 200 mg per day, but much more study needs to be done before this can be a general recommendation. Another small but controlled study in Finland showed that ginseng (200 mg once daily) lowered fasting blood sugars and improved mood, vigor, and sense of well-being in people with Type 2 diabetes.

Progress has also been significant on the transplant front. First, survival of pancreas transplant recipients has continued to improve, and their new pancreases are producing insulin for longer periods of time. Second, islet cell transplantation researchers are exploring ways to prevent the recipient's rejection of the foreign tissue. Various materials are being tested to coat or encapsulate the islet cells, preventing the cells from being attacked but allowing insulin and glucose to pass through.

An alternative approach uses targeted antibodies (genetically engineered monoclonal antibodies) to prevent the patient's own immune mechanisms from destroying the transplanted cells. Another method has been used in rats to fool the body into believing that the transplanted cells were its own. The islet cells were transplanted into a gland in the neck called the thymus.

A limitation of some of the above methods has been the availability of sufficient tissue, either pancreas or islet cells, to treat all those who may benefit. A new method, using genetic engineering and a line of cells that can be grown in a test tube (hence suitable for large-scale production), may produce an artificial beta-cell. It uses mouse pituitary cells that have been engineered to produce insulin and respond to glucose. However, additional work needs to be done to remove some of the "bugs" (for instance, cells start releasing insulin before blood sugar is high enough and also secrete a mouse hormone that may affect humans). Another innovative procedure, using a highly modified virus that was coded to produce insulin, "infected" animal livers so that insulin could be manufactured in the liver rather than in the pancreas. The prospects are good that one or more of these transplant approaches will soon be successful.

Prevention And Treatment Of Complications

We believe the next decade will see considerable research in the genetics of both Type 1 and Type 2 diabetes. One particularly exciting area will be the detection and study of those genes that either predispose someone to the development of complications, or protect them against complications. As we discussed in earlier chapters, some of us in optimal control of our diabetes will develop complications, and others in poor control will manage to avoid most if not all complications. Our own genetic makeups will likely explain some of this variability. For example, a study suggested that a particular kind of diabetic neuropathy (cardiovascular autonomic neuropathy) was strongly associated with a particular genetic marker. The Diabetes Control and Complications Trial (see Chapters 4 and 18) can provide an excellent pool of people to study genetically for this purpose, since data on their level of control and their development of complications will already have been collected.

Several drugs are being developed and tested that hold the promise of preventing or treating complications. Some of these were mentioned in Chapter 18, like ACE inhibitors for preventing nephropathy, and sorbinil or tolrestat for treating neuropathy. Much more study needs to be done. Pimagedine (aminoguanadine) is a drug that inhibits glycosylation, and is currently in clinical trials. If successful, this would be a very promising new medication to prevent complications. Since many diabetic complications involve abnormalities of the blood vessels, particularly the new growth of abnormal vessels as in retinopathy, trials of drugs that retard vessel growth (angiogenesis inhibitors) are being considered for people with diabetes. One example is alpha-interferon, which has been used in the treatment of leukemia and AIDS. However, the potential benefits must be weighed against cost and side effects, particularly where a generally satisfactory therapy (laser photocoagulation) already exists.

Preventing The Development Of Diabetes

Researchers know that Type 1 diabetes is an autoimmune disease—in which the person's own antibodies attack insulin-producing beta cells of the pancreas. Only recently have researchers been able to determine those who are the most likely to develop diabetes before most of their beta cells have been destroyed (a slow process) and before they have developed typical clinical symptoms. The National Institutes of Health, together with the American Diabetes Association and the Juvenile Diabetes Foundation, began a nationwide study to identify those relatives of people with diabetes who might be at risk for developing diabetes themselves, and then see if they would prevent or delay its occurrence. Small doses of injected insulin will be used to "rest" the pancreas or foil the immune system (oral insulin crystals). The study, called the Diabetes Prevention Trial (DPT-1) is now slated to end in the year 2002. For more information, call 1-800-HALT-DM1.

The NIH has also launched a nationwide study for the prevention or delay of Type 2 diabetes in those at risk, called the Diabetes Prevention Program (DPP or DPT-2). The study will identify those with impaired glucose tolerance (IGT), which precedes full diabetes. Volunteers will be divided into four groups: one will receive intensive guidance to change lifestyle behaviors (primarily eating habits and physical activity) designed to decrease weight by 7 percent; a second will receive metformin, and the third group will receive troglitazone, both new drugs that lower blood sugar (see Chapter 6); the fourth group is the control group, and will receive placebos instead of the drugs and simply information on diet and physical activity. Call 1-888-377-5646 or 1-888-DPP-JOIN toll-free for more information and a list of participating centers.

Research is also beginning on a large scale to identify the genes responsible for both Type 1 and Type 2 diabetes. Just as the cloning and sequencing of the gene responsible for cystic fibrosis have stimulated further research into the cause and cure for cystic fibrosis, so too will genetic research into diabetes help advance treatment for people with diabetes. The National Institutes of Health and the American Diabetes Association (assisted by grants from private industry) have begun major projects to develop family trees and establish banks of cells from family members that can be studied by a wide range of collaborating researchers, all hoping to identify the many different genes involved and their complex interplay.

To conclude, we believe that there is a very good chance that some form of "cure" will be a reality in the new millennium. The future prospects are truly exciting for those of us with diabetes.

A Diabetes Survival Kit

Living well with diabetes begins with staying alive. And one of your highest priorities should be to learn how to prevent and treat the three most immediate potential health threats to you and your diabetes management.

1. Insulin reactions or low blood sugar (hypoglycemia) can lead to confusion and unconsciousness. You need to know what causes very low blood sugar, the symptoms that you experience, and the treatment. Chapter 9 provides the details of low blood sugar and how to deal with it.

2. Diabetic coma. If you have Type 1 diabetes, you also need to learn the causes and symptoms of diabetic ketoacidosis and coma, which can result from very high blood sugar (hyperglycemia), omitted insulin shots, poorly managed illness or infections, or extreme stress. The Diabetic Ketoacidosis and Sick Day Management section that follows discusses diabetic coma. Diabetic coma is rare in Type 2 diabetes.

3. Handling infections. Small infections can become severe, and severe ones can lead to diabetic coma. The following section, on Keto-acidosis and Sick Day Management, and the foot-care section of Chapter 18 are good sources of information on handling infections.

These three threats require that you

▷ Never omit an insulin injection unless your doctor okays it.

▷ Always carry candy, sugar, or glucose tablets with you to treat reactions.

▷ Always wear a diabetes identification bracelet or necklace.

▷ Treat all wounds, scratches, and punctures to prevent infections.

▷ Report illness or infections to your doctor, especially when they increase blood sugar levels or when you have ketones in your urine. See your doctor without delay if you need treatment.

Diabetic Ketoacidosis and Sick Day Management

Diabetic ketoacidosis—or ketosis—is a condition of Type 1 diabetes in which blood glucose and ketones rise to high levels. This state can be dangerous for a person with diabetes, leading to diabetic coma if not treated. It usually responds to prompt treatment, however, so you should know the symptoms and steps you can take when the symptoms occur.

Causes

▷ The physical stress of illness or infected wounds

▷ Great emotional stress

▷ Chronically high blood sugar levels combined with stress

▷ Omitted insulin

▷ Any combination of the above

Initial Signs and Symptoms

▷ Positive urine ketone and glucose tests

▷ High blood sugar tests (above 240 mg/dl [13.3 mmol/L])

▷ Dehydration, thirst, dry mouth

▷ Excessive, frequent urination

▷ Nausea, vomiting, abdominal pain

▷ Fatigue or weakness

▷ Fever

▷ Blurred vision

Signs and Symptoms as Condition Advances Toward Diabetic Coma

▷ Flushed, dry skin

▷ Fruity odor on breath

▷ Sunken eyes

▷ Deep, labored breathing

▷ Pulse usually rapid

▷ Unconsciousness

You may need to be treated in the hospital if your condition advances toward diabetic coma or does not respond to home treatment. Stay in touch with your doctor from the very first signs of ketosis. (Note that insulin reactions, which can also lead to unconsciousness, are marked by much more rapid onset than ketosis, shallow breathing, normal-smelling breath, and low blood sugar.)

Any level of ketosis marked by a positive test for ketones in your urine needs your immediate attention. (People with kidney disease, especially, should be aware of the symptoms and begin treatment immediately when urine tests show ketones.)

Test urine and blood frequently: When you are ill—especially when you are vomiting, have diarrhea, or are feverish—you should test your urine for ketones and test your blood glucose. Infected wounds also can produce ketosis. Test every two or three hours until the results are normal.

Confer with your doctor: When you are ill and have ketones in your urine, ask your doctor for guidance in handling the situation. Your doctor will usually suggest extra shots of regular insulin to bring blood glucose and ketone levels down. The amount of insulin needed will be determined according to your body weight, blood sugar level, and severity of illness.

(After you have dealt with this level of illness a few times, your doctor may tell you that you know enough to handle it with minimal medical guidance. But any time you do not see improvement within six or eight hours, ask for your doctor's help.)

Continue taking insulin: You should never omit insulin, even when you are ill and unable to eat solid food. The stress of illness itself raises blood sugar levels.

Continue eating: You need to continue eating and drinking foods and fluids with caloric value, even if your blood sugar is high and you are vomiting or have diarrhea.

Take in at least 10 to 20 grams of carbohydrate every one to two hours. Possible sources include: 1/3 cup flavored gelatin, 1/2 cup vanilla ice cream, 1/2 cup custard, 1/2 cup orange juice, 3/4 cup gingerale (not diet), 1/2 cup regular cola, or 1 cup Gatorade.

If you have trouble keeping food down, take smaller quantities every fifteen to thirty minutes.

Limit activity: When you have high blood sugar and ketones in your urine, don't exercise, even if you feel able. Exercising at this time can actually raise blood sugar.

Resources For
Living Well

As you've learned, living well with diabetes is a process; a process that relies on how you respond to information from a number of sources, such as blood glucose tests, your physician, or others with diabetes. Here, we list a variety of resources that may be helpful to you or a family member. We have done our best to provide the most current information; however, as you might imagine, addresses, publications, and even organizations themselves change quite frequently.

Diabetes Identification

You should wear, at all times, a bracelet or necklace identifying you as having diabetes and giving a number to call for information in case of emergency. The following service provides attractive I.D. bracelets and necklaces and maintains 24-hour hotlines, where details of your diabetes care are available to medical personnel from anywhere in the world.

Medic Alert Foundation International
P.O. Box 1009
Turlock, CA 95381
(800) 432-5378

Organizations and Sources of Information

American Diabetes Association
1660 Duke Street
Alexandria, VA 22314
Or call 800-806-7801 for membership inquiries; 800-DIABETES to reach the Diabetes Information and Action Line and customer service

The American Diabetes Association (ADA) supports research, education, and public awareness programs relating to both Type 1 and Type 2 diabetes. A membership fee of $24 a year provides monthly issues of *Diabetes Forecast* and automatic membership in a local chapter.

Juvenile Diabetes Foundation International
120 Wall Street, 19th Floor
New York, NY 10005
800-223-1138

The Juvenile Diabetes Foundation (JDF) is a volunteer organization specializing in insulin-dependent diabetes. It has a network of chapters worldwide and raises funds for diabetes research. Chapters provide helpful brochures as well as personal contact. A quarterly newsletter is published for JDF members.

National Diabetes Information Clearinghouse
1 Information Way
Bethesda, MD 20892-3560
301-654-3327

The National Diabetes Information Clearinghouse (NDIC) works to increase knowledge and understanding about diabetes among patients, health professionals, and the public. It provides responses to inquiries, and resources for patient education, including publications, professional and patient education programs, and an online data base. Call or write to request NDIC's publications list. *Diabetes Dateline* is the organization's newsletter.

American Association of Diabetes Educators
444 North Michigan Ave., Ste. 1240
Chicago, IL 60611

For the names of diabetes educators in your area, call 800-TEAM-UP-4, or write to them for more information.

The American Dietetic Association
National Center for Nutrition and Diabetes
216 West Jackson Blvd.
Chicago, IL 60606-6995

To listen to recorded messages or to obtain a referral to an registered dietitian in your area, call 800-366-1655.

Joslin Diabetes Foundation, Inc., Publications Department
One Joslin Plaza
Boston, MA 02215

Joslin Clinic was the pioneer treatment center for diabetes care. The Foundation provides information and literature concerning diabetes.

HCF Diabetes Foundation
P.O. Box 22124
Lexington, KY 40522

The HCF Diabetes Foundation publishes *Diabetes and Nutrition* ($6 per year), a newsletter based on the work of James W. Anderson, M.D., concerning the healthful benefits of high-carbohydrate, high-fiber diets. Other publications are available.

International Diabetes Center (IDC)
Park Nicollet HealthSource
3800 Park Nicollet Boulevard
Minneapolis, MN 55416
612-927-3393

The goal of this organization is to help persons with diabetes have fulfilling and active lifestyles. IDC publishes books and pamphlets. For a catalog call, 800-372-7776.

Diabetes Health Care
P.O. Box 114
Van Nuys, CA 91408
800-972-2323

Provides general diabetes information. (Also see listing under Diabetic Supplies.)

Other sources of information include companies that produce diabetic supplies. You may request specific booklets and catalogs of publications from the following:

Bayer Corporation, Diagnostics Division
511 Benedict Ave.
Tarrytown, NY 10591

Boehringer Mannheim Corporation
P.O.Box 50100
Indianapolis, IN 46250-0100

Eli Lilly & Co.
Lilly Corporate Center
Indianapolis, IN 46285
Monoject Division
Sherwood Medical
St. Louis, MO 63166

Miles Laboratories, Inc., Ames Division
One Becton Drive
Franklin Lakes, NJ 07417-1883

Pfizer Laboratories
New York, NY
Novo Nordisk Pharmaceuticals
120 Alexander St.
Princeton, NJ 08540

Diabetes Magazines and Newspapers

American Diabetes Association
Membership Services Division
P.O. Box 61054-0363
Mt. Morris, IL 61054
1-800-806-7801

Diabetes Forecast is the most complete magazine for people with diabetes. Published by the American Diabetes Association, it includes reports on new research, personal stories, practical tips on diabetes care, and articles for children. Membership is $24 per year. Reprints and special topic packages are available.

Diabetes Interview
3715 Balboa Street
San Francisco, CA 94121
1-800-488-8468

Diabetes Interview is a monthly newspaper from publisher and editor-in-chief, Scott M. King, who has had Type 1 diabetes for more than 20 years. The newspaper features a variety of articles, all reviewed by a medical advisory board.

Diabetes Self-Management
P.O. Box 52890
Boulder, CO 80322-2890
1-800-234-0923

Diabetes Self-Management is a bimonthly magazine containing practical self-care articles. Subscription is $18 per year.

Two Types
Patients Publishing Co. Inc.
454 E. Paces Ferry Rd.
Atlanta, GA 30305

Calling itself the "official diabetes lifestyle magazine," *Two Types* is a monthly magazine that features articles on topics such as travel, cooking, family support, and new products. Subscription is $29.95 per year.

On-Line Diabetes Information

The following is a selection of diabetes-related internet sites.

American Diabetes Association
http://www.diabetes.org

American Dietetic Association
http://www.eatright.org

National Institutes of Health, National Institute of Diabetes and Digestive and Kidney Diseases
http://www.niddk.nih.gov/

Diabetes Interview on-line newsletter
To get on mailing list, send the message "subscribe diabetes-news" to listserve@netcom.com

Diabetes Self-Management
http://www.diabetes-self-mgmt.com

Some Books On Diabetes

The following books are available from Chronimed Publishing:

Weight Management for Type II Diabetes, by Jackie Labat, MS, RD, CDE, and Annette Maggi, MS, RD. (1997) This guide combines nutrition and exercise information, helping readers to set reasonable goals, develop lifestyle habits that last, and manage stress.

A Touch of Diabetes, revised and expanded edition, by Lois Jovanovic-Peterson, MD, Charles M. Peterson, MD, and Morton B. Stone. (1995) Everything people with newly diagnosed Type 2 diabetes need to know, from curbing potential complications to counting calories, is in this book.

In Control: A Guide for Teens with Diabetes, by Jean Betschart, MN, RN, CDE, and Susan Thom, RD, LD, CDE. (1995) For 12 to 18 year olds, this book answers the questions teens with diabetes are faced with.

Diabetic Low-Fat & No-Fat Meals in Minutes, by M.J. Smith, RD. (1996) Contains more the 250 recipe favorites and diabetic menus for 60 days.

Learning to Live Well With Diabetes, by Donnell D. Etzwiler, MD, and others from the International Diabetes Center. (1991) This comprehensive and easy-to-understand manual helps people with diabetes work with their diabetes team to improve control and quality of life.

Exchanges for All Occasions: Your Guide to Choosing Healthy Foods Anytime Anywhere, fourth edition, by Marion J. Franz, MS, RD, CDE. (1997) This book helps everyone use the exchange system for meal planning in almost any situation.

Other books available in bookstores or libraries:

The Physician Within: Taking Charge of Your Well-Being, by Cathy Feste. (1995) Published by Henry Holt & Company, this book is about self-motivation for people who are trying to follow either a pattern of healthy living or a specific medical regimen.

Psyching Out Diabetes, by Richard R. Rubin, PhD, June Biermann, and Barbara Toohey. (1992) This book helps readers overcome the fear, denial, depression, grief, frustration, embarrassment, and guilt that get in the way of good diabetes control.

Diabetes: A Practical New Guide To Healthy Living, by James W. Anderson, MD. (1991) Warner Books publishes this guide for general diabetes management written by Dr. Anderson, with a special section on the HCF diet plan. Order from HCF Diabetes Foundation, P.O. Box 22124, Lexington, KY 40522.

Stop the Rollercoaster: How to Take Charge of Your Blood Sugars in Diabetes, by John Walsh, PA, CDE, Ruth Roberts, and Lois Jovanovic-Peterson, MD. (1995) This book provides help for those who use insulin and experience inexplicable blood sugar highs and lows.

The NutriBase Guide to Carbohydrates, Calories & Fat in Your Food, by Art Ulene, MD. (1995). From Avery Publishing Group comes this comprehensive listing of nutrient information for over 30,000 foods.

Everyday Cooking with Dr. Dean Ornish, by Dean Ornish, MD. (1996) This book features 150 healthy recipes that are easy and inexpensive to prepare.

Diabetes: Caring for Your Emotions as Well as Your Health, by Jerry Edelwich, MSW, and Archie Brodsky (1986).

The Diabetic's Book: All Your Questions Answered, third edition, by June Biermann and Barbara Toohey. (1994)

The Diabetic's Total Health Book, third edition, by June Biermann and Barbara Toohey. (1992)

The Peripatetic Diabetic, by June Biermann and Barbara Toohey. (1984)

The Diabetic Woman, revised edition, by Lois Jovanovic-Peterson, MD, June Biermann, and Barbara Toohey. (1996)

The American Diabetes Association publishes a large number of books and pamphlets. They can be ordered from: American Diabetes Association, Order Fulfillment Department, P.O. Box 930850, Atlanta, GA 31193-0850; or call 1-800-232-6733.

The American Diabetes Association Complete Guide to Diabetes (1996)

Family Cookbooks—Volumes I, II, III, and IV, from the American Diabetes Association and The American Dietetic Association

Sweet Kids: How to Balance Diabetes Control & Good Nutrition With Family Peace (1996).

Diabetes A to Z: What You Need to Know About Diabetes—Simply Put (1996)

Managing Diabetes on a Budget: How to Get the Most Out of Every Dollar You Spend (1996)

How to Get Great Diabetes Care: What You and Your Doctor Can Do to Improve Your Medical Care & Your Life (1996)

Films and Audiovisuals

Films, videos, and audiotapes are available on different aspects of diabetes care. Your library, local chapter of ADA, or your diabetes educator or doctor may have these resources. Some of the titles available are:

▷ Diabetes: Focus on Feelings

▷ The Sugar Film

▷ Gestational Diabetes—Great Expectations

▷ Know Your Diabetes: Know Yourself

Discount Diabetes Supplies

The following list is a sampling of companies that offer diabetes supplies. They all have toll-free numbers, so calling to check on prices is free to the caller. Also inquire about any specials they may be offering.

Diabetes Health Care
P.O. Box 114
Van Nuys, CA 91408
1-800-972-2323

The Diabetes Mall
1030 West Upas St.
San Diego, CA 92103
1-800-988-4772

Diabetes Self Care
P.O. Box 12568
Roanoke, VA 24026
1-800-258-9559

Diabetic Express
P.O. Box 80037
Canton, OH 44708
1-800-338-4656

Diabetic Care Center
31122 Vine Street
Cleveland, OH 44095
1-800-633-7167

Diabetic Promotions
P.O. Box 5400
Willowick, OH 44095-0400
1-800-433-1477
(216) 934-6185

Diabetes Supplies
275 Curry Hollow Road
Pittsburgh, PA 15236
1-800-622-5587

Home Service Medical
P.O. Box 59024
Minneapolis, MN 55459
1-800-888-5651

H-S Medical Supplies
P.O. Box 42
Whitehall, PA 18052
1-800-344-7633

Hospital Center Pharmacy
433 Brookline Ave.
Boston MA 02215
1-800-824-2401

Jocelyn Bischoff's Diabetic
2200 Airport Blvd.
Freedom, CA 95019
1-800-537-0404

National Diabetic Pharmacies
2157 Apperson Drive
Salem, VA 24153
1-800-467-8546

Self Care, Inc.
4827 Geary Boulevard
San Francisco, CA 94118
1-800-252-5885

415-664-1100

Sugar Happy Diabetes Supplies
824 Miranda Creek Court
Alamo, CA 94507
1-800-347-4848

Index

acarbose, 127, 128
acetohexamide, 126
activity guidelines, 211-212
activity, 199-212
  benefits of, 199-201
  blood glucose levels and,
    82-83, 111-112, 206-208
  hyperglycemia and, 148, 207
  insulin injections and, 78, 110,
    206-207
  level of intensity, 208-210
  personal profile, 202-203
  precautions, 206
  reducing risks of complications,
    283
  starting a program, 203-205
  strenuous, 207
    blood glucose and, 84, 169
    insulin reactions and, 166
  stress and, 222
  stretching, 210-211
  timing of, 206-207, 210
  Type 2 diabetes and, 120
  types of, 204-205
acupuncture, 222
adolescence, 43, 89, 328
adult-onset diabetes (see Type 2
  diabetes)
albumin, 291
alcohol, 190-191
  blood glucose levels and, 78-79
  insulin reactions and, 162
alpha-glucosidase inhibitors, 127

alpha-interferon, 337
alprostadil, 297
Amaryl, 126
American Association of Diabetes Educators, 23, 115, 227,
  334
American Diabetes Association
  California Affiliate, 230
American Diabetes Association,
  20, 22, 115, 343
  nutrition guidelines, 177
American Dietetic Association,
  344
aminoguanadine, 337
amylin, 335
animal insulin, human insulin vs.,
  76
antihistamines, 79
autogenics, 221-222

basal rates, insulin, 86-87, 103
behavior, stages in changing, 2-3
beliefs, personal, diabetes care
  and, 253-261
beta blockers, 79
  insulin reactions and, 162, 170
biguanides, 126-127
birth control, 309
blood glucose levels
  activity and, 82-83, 111-112,
    206-208
  effects of insulin injections, 75-
    79
  emotions and, 84-86

control, diabetes, benefits of, 42-44

determining present level of, 36-41

conventional insulin regimen, 96

coping, 8-9, 21, 27-31

Coumadin, 79

counselor, role of, 228-229

crises, handling, 27-31

dating, women and, 315-316

dawn phenomenon, 77

DCCT (Diabetes Control and Complications Trial), 2, 19, 42

insulin reactions and, 164

decongestants, 79

dehydration, blood glucose levels and, 84

dentist, role of, 228

depression, 85, 236

dexfenfluramine, 125

DiaBeta, 126

Diabetes Care, 118

Diabetes Coalition of California, 230

Diabetes Control and Complications Trial (DCCT), 2, 19, 42

Diabetes Forecast, 118

Diabetes Interview, 118

Diabetes Self-Management, 118

Diabetes Spectrum, 118

diabetes care guidelines, 231-233

diabetes care

a contract with yourself, 13

balancing other concerns, 8-9

breakthroughs, 1-2, 333-338

coping techniques, 8-9, 14, 21, 27-31, 235-249

"honeymoon" period, 93

past vs. present methods, 33-34

rewards, 10-11

setting goals, 11

diabetes educator, role of, 228

diabetes prevention, 337-338

diabetes supplies, 158

diabetes

initial tasks following diagnosis, 17-26

steps to managing, 3-15

diabetic coma, 43, 84, 167-168

Diabinese, 126

diagnosis of diabetes

initial tasks, 17-26

related questionnaire, 23-26

Type 2 diabetes, 120, 122

dialysis, 294

diuretics, 79

drugs

prescription, 78-80

recreational, 78-79

Dymelor, 126

emotional support, 58-59

complications and, 276, 279

stress and, 220

women and, 315, 317-318

emotions, 21, 22-26, 235-249

blood glucose levels and, 84-86

diabetes care and, 253-261

estrogen supplements, 79

exercise (see activity)

expenses, reducing, 44-45

eye disorders, 228, 286-290

DCCT and, 42

stress and, 214-215

vitamin supplements and, 285

family concerns, diabetes and, 321-332

fast food, 185

fat, dietary, 177-178

absorption rates of, 81

insulin and, 77

percentage in diet, 178

fatigue, blood glucose levels and, 84

females
  blood glucose levels and, 86-89
  diabetes and, 43, 307-320
  intensive regimen and, 48
Fen-Phen, 125
fenfluramine, 125
Feste, Cathy, 307
fiber, dietary, 180
  absorption rates of, 81
  content in foods, 194
food, 175-198
  blood glucose levels and, 81-82
  complications and, 275
  fast, 185
  glycemic effect, 176, 193
  healthy tips, 185-191
  information resources, 183,
    196-198
  insulin injections and, 78
  reducing risks of complications,
    283
foot care, 228, 296, 297-299,
  304
frozen shoulder, 300
fructosamine test, 70

Gantrisin, 79
glimepiride, 126
glipizide, 126
glucagon, 167
Glucophage, 126-127, 159
glucose test, urine (see urine glucose tests)
glucose, blood (see blood glucose)
Glucotrol, 126
Glutose, 167
glyburide, 126
glycated hemoglobin (see hemoglobin A1c)
glycemic effect, food and, 81,
  176, 180-182, 193
glycosylated hemoglobin (see
  hemoglobin A1c)

Glynase, 126

HbA1c (see hemoglobin A1c)
health care team
  choosing of, 122-123
  working with, 227-234
heart disease, 300-304
  activity and, 200
  dietary cholesterol and, 178,
    179
  resources, 305
hemoglobin A1c
  complications and, 42, 131
  definition of, 69
  kidney disease and, 292
  moderate regimen and, 136
  target levels, 42, 65
"honeymoon" period, diabetes
  care and, 22, 93
hormone supplements, 314
hormones
  blood glucose levels and, 86-89
  hypoglycemia and, 49
hospitalization, diabetes diagnosis and, 18
Humalog (see lispro)
human insulin, animal insulin vs.,
  76
hyperglycemia
  activity and, 148, 207
  complications of, 43
hypertension, 301-303
  complications and, 282
  kidney disease and, 293
  reducing risks of complications,
    284
  salt and, 191
hypoglycemia, 159-174
  alcohol and, 162
  causes, 160
  children and, 173, 329
  intensive regimen and, 35, 45,
    163-164
  preventing, 168-172

drawbacks, 35, 44-46
economic costs of, 44-45, 63-64
establishing a routine, 90-91
insulin injection plans, 95-101
insulin pump and, 100-103
insulin reactions, 164-165
insulin regimen, choosing, 92-93
laboratory tests, 112-113
maintaining motivation, 115-117
pregnancy, 48
related tasks, 47, 55-56
urine testing, 66
intermediate insulin, 76
International Diabetes Center, 345
internet resources, 347
Isoniazide, 79

jet injection insulin devices, 95
joint disorders, 299-300
Joslin Diabetes Foundation, 345
Juvenile Diabetes Foundation International, 23, 230, 344
juvenile-onset diabetes (see Type 1 diabetes)

ketoacidosis, 43, 84
management guidelines, 340-341
ketones, 66, 138, 155, 341
activity and, 83
Somogyi reactions and, 77, 135, 160, 163-164
stress and, 216
kidney disease, 290-295, 337
DCCT and, 42
hypertension and, 303
intensive regimen and, 35
metformin and, 127
vitamin supplements and, 285

Kumamoto Study, Type 2 diabetes, 42, 119

laboratory tests, 69-71
intensive regimen and, 112-113
moderate regimen and, 133, 148
lancing devices, 63, 334
Lasix, 79
lente, 76
limbs, complications of, 297-299
lipids tests, blood, 70-71
lipoic acid, 335
lispro, 75-76, 87
injection sites, 78
insulin pumps and, 102
Type 2 diabetes and, 128
loose regimen, 153-158
blood glucose tests and, 154
insulin reactions and, 164
related tasks, 51, 153
urine glucose tests and, 154-155

managing diabetes, steps to, 3-15
MAO inhibitors, 79
marijuana, blood glucose and, 79
marriage, women and, 316-317
massage, 222
meal planning (see food)
meals (see food)
medications, Type 2 diabetes, 34, 126-129
weight loss, 125
meditation, 222, 224
menopause, 89, 314
menstruation, 86-89, 308
mental health, 228-229, 236
metabolic record keeping, 66-69
metabolism, diabetic, 72-74
meters, blood glucose (see monitors, blood glucose)
metformin, 126-127, 128, 159
Micronase, 126

moderate regimen, 131-151
  adjusting insulin dosages, 143-148
  blood glucose tests, 134-136
    target levels, 135
  insulin plans, 139-142
  insulin reactions, 164
  maintaining motivation, 149-150
  related tasks, 49-50, 131-132
  urine glucose target levels, 135
monitors, blood glucose, non-invasive, 63, 334
Monojel, 167
motivation
  intensive regimen and, 115-117
  moderate regimen and, 149-150
muscoskeletal disorders, 299-300
MUSE, 297

Nardil, 79
nephropathy, 290-295, 337
  DCCT and, 42
  vitamin supplements and, 285
nerve disorders, 295-299, 337
  DCCT and, 42
  insulin reactions and, 162, 170
neuropathy, 295-297, 337
  DCCT and, 42
  insulin reactions and, 162
nicotine
  reducing risks of complications, 284
  stress and, 222-223
non-insulin-dependent diabetes (see Type 2 diabetes)
NPH, 76
nutrition guidelines, American Diabetes Association, 177, 183

on-line resources, 347
oral medications (see medications and Type 2 diabetes)

organizations, diabetes, 343-346
Orinase, 126
orlistat, 125

pain, blood glucose levels and, 84
parenting a child with diabetes, 323-332
Parnate, 79
pharmacist, role of, 229
phentermine, 125
Physician Within, The, 307
physician
  role of, 227-228
  working with, 19-20
pimagedine, 337
podiatrist, role of, 228
postprandial blood glucose tests, 64
Pramintide, 335
prayer, 222
Precose, 127
pregnancy, 309-313
  blood glucose levels, 89
  intensive regimen, 48
  renal threshold, 136-138
preprandial blood glucose tests, 65
prescription drugs, 78-80
propranolol, 79
protein
  absorption rates, 81
  percentage in diet, 178
proteinuria, 291
psychiatrist, role of, 228-229
psychologist, role of, 228-229
puberty, 89, 328
publications, diabetes, 118, 346-349
pump (see insulin pump)

reactions, insulin, 45, 135, 159-174
  activity and, 82-83
  alcohol and, 78-79